KIDNEY PHYSIOLOGY AND TREATMENT OF KIDNEY DISEASES

Dr. Shipra Chandra

ALLIED
HEALTH
PRESS

Kidney Physiology and Treatment of Kidney Diseases

Author: **Dr. Shipra Chandra**

Allied Health Press
4164 Lakeshore Road
Burlington ON L7L 1A4
Canada
www.alliedhealthpress.com
Email: orders@arclereducation.com

ISBN: 978-1-77956-268-5

ABOUT THE AUTHOR

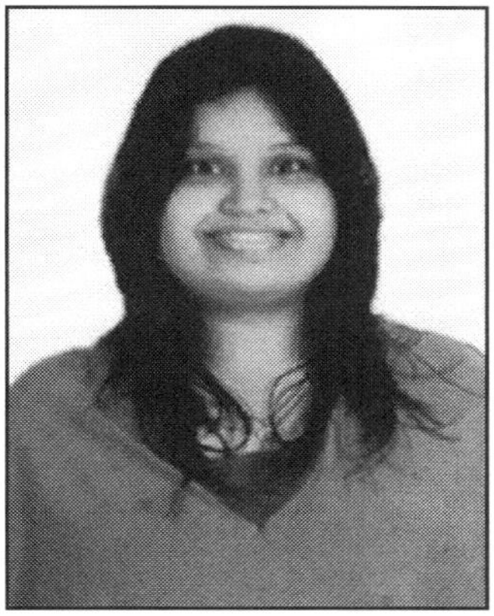

Dr. Shipra Chandra born in Delhi in 1983, completed school from a government school in Delhi in 2001 with First division. Being a science student , took admission in Chemistry Honors at Kirori Mal College, Delhi University. But the wonders of Human Body always fascinated me and I continued preparing for Pre Medical Test (PMT) despite being in a reputed college and course.

By the Grace of God and blessings of my family I secured 5th rank in CPMT 2002 along-with being waitlisted at DPMT and securing rank in AIEEE exam. Joined MBBS on 14/11/2002 at the most prestigious King George Medical College, Lucknow, U.P. Completed MBBS in First division in 2008 and joined AIIMS, New Delhi Department of Emergency Medicine for work experience in 2009 but continued the preparation for Post Graduation Entrance Test and cracked the UP-PGME in 2010 and was allotted MD Physiology from King George Medical University.

After completing the MD in 2013, I again cleared AIIMS, New Delhi entrance test for Senior Residency. Learned a lot during my 3 year tenure from 2013 to 2016 at AIIMS. Following which I joined Fortis Hospital Shalimar Bagh and continued search for a Government Job. Gave the interview at U.P. Public Service Commission in 2017, cracked it and joined as Assistant Professor at Sarojini Naidu Medical College, Agra in 2017. I have 7 research publications , one book chapter and guided 3 MD students during my tenure . Promoted to the post of Associate Professor in 2022 and currently working in the same capacity.

Word Roots, Prefixes, and Suffixes by Chapter

Chapter 1 Anatomy and Function of the Kidneys

albumin/o albumin

arteriol/o arteriole

azot/o urea, nitrogen

blast/o developing cell, germ cell

cyst/o bladder, sac

-emia in the blood

glomerul/o glomerulus

hydr/o water

Chapter 2 Renal Physiology: Acid-Base Balance and Blood Pressure Regulation

plasm/o plasma

angi- blood vessels angiotensin (hormone causing constriction of blood vessels)

hepat- the liver hepatocytes (main functional cells of the liver)

pneumon- the lungs pneumonia (an infection in the lungs)

nephr- kidney

-cele pouching, hernia

Chapter 3 Urine Formation and Concentration Mechanisms

ur-,urin-, of or pertaining to urine, the urinary system

-pathy, disease

-ule, small

ureter/o-, ureter

-uria, urine condition

-iasis, used to describe something abnormal

olig/o, refers to scanty or little

Chapter 4 Renal Endocrine Functions

hypo- below, under, deficient

para- around, beside, beyond, abnormal

syn- joined, together

adren/o adrenal glands

adrenal/o adrenal glands

calc/i calcium

glyc/o sugar

natr/o sodium

Chapter 5 Assessment of Kidney Function

Nephr- Kidney

Glomerul-Glomerulus

Pyel- Renal pelvis

-uria Urine condition

Cyst- Bladder

Chapter 6 Acute Kidney Injury (AKI)

-plasty Surgical repair

-pexy Surgical fixation

-itis Inflammation

-pathy Disease

Chapter 7 Chronic Kidney Disease (CKD)

Ren- kidney

opathy nephropathy

-emia uremia

Pyel- pyelonephritis

-ectomy nephrectomy

Chapter 8 Glomerular Diseases

Renal- Relating to the kidneys

Nephro- Referring to the kidneys

-Pathy Disease or disorder

Hyper- Excessive or above normal

Chapter 9 Cystic Diseases of the Kidney

cerebr- brain

chel- claw

corp- body

-emia blood

Chapter 10 Polycystic Kidney Disease (PKD)

ren/o (kidney)

pulmo/o Lung

pyel/o Renal collecting system

dys- (painful, abnormal, difficult, labored)

Table of Contents

LIST OF FIGURES

LIST OF TABLES

PREFACE

Chronic kidney disease (CKD) is a widespread health condition that affects a significant portion of the global population, with estimates suggesting a prevalence of between 8% and 16%. Despite its prevalence, CKD often goes unnoticed by both patients and healthcare providers. CKD is characterized by a reduced glomerular filtration rate (GFR) of less than 60 mL/min/1.73 m^2, albuminuria of at least 30 mg per 24 hours, or markers of kidney damage that persist for more than three months. These markers can include hematuria (blood in the urine) or structural abnormalities in the kidneys.

The burden of CKD is higher in low- and middle-income countries compared to high-income nations. While globally, the leading causes of CKD are diabetes and hypertension, other factors such as glomerulonephritis, infections, and environmental exposures like air pollution, herbal remedies, and pesticides are common in certain regions. Additionally, genetic factors can play a role in CKD risk, with traits like sickle cell trait and specific genetic variations (e.g., APOL1 risk alleles) increasing the risk, particularly in populations of African ancestry.

In the United States, the average rate of decline in GFR is approximately 1 mL/min/1.73 m^2 per year in the general population, and more than half of individuals have a lifetime risk of developing a GFR of less than 60 mL/min/1.73 m^2. Early detection and management of CKD by primary care providers are crucial, as progressive CKD can lead to serious complications, including end-stage kidney disease (ESKD), cardiovascular disease, and increased mortality.

The aim of the book "Kidney Physiology and treatment of kidney diseases" is to provide a comprehensive understanding of the physiological mechanisms underlying kidney function and the pathological processes that lead to kidney diseases. This book seeks to bridge the gap between fundamental physiological concepts and clinical practice, offering insights into the latest advancements in the diagnosis, management, and treatment of kidney diseases. Exploring the intricate workings of renal physiology, the book aims to equip healthcare professionals, researchers, and students with a deep knowledge of how the kidneys maintain homeostasis, regulate blood pressure, and manage waste excretion. It examines the various forms of kidney diseases, including acute kidney injury (AKI), CKD, glomerulonephritis, and polycystic kidney disease, discussing their etiology, pathophysiology, and progression. Furthermore, the book emphasizes evidence-based treatment strategies, highlighting both traditional approaches and cutting-edge therapies. It covers pharmacological interventions, lifestyle modifications, dialysis techniques, and kidney transplantation, providing a holistic view of patient management.

Integrating physiology with clinical application, this book aims to enhance the ability of clinicians to diagnose early, tailor treatments to individual patients, and ultimately improve outcomes for those suffering from kidney diseases.

Professional guidelines recommend a risk-based approach for the evaluation and management of CKD. Screening for CKD typically involves routine blood and urine tests. Symptoms of CKD can vary but may include hematuria, foamy urine (indicating albuminuria), nocturia (frequent urination at night), flank pain, or decreased urine output. In advanced stages, patients may experience fatigue, poor appetite, nausea, vomiting, metallic taste, unintentional weight loss, pruritus (itching), changes in mental status, dyspnea (shortness of breath), or peripheral edema (swelling).

The significant impact of CKD on health outcomes, early detection, and comprehensive management are essential to reduce the burden of this disease. The book is tailored for a diverse audience that includes medical students, healthcare professionals, and researchers specializing in nephrology. It serves as an invaluable resource for those seeking to deepen their understanding of kidney function and the complexities of renal pathophysiology. This book is also beneficial for practicing clinicians, such as nephrologists, internists, and primary care physicians, who are involved in diagnosing and managing kidney diseases. Additionally, it caters to advanced nursing practitioners, physician assistants, and other allied health professionals who provide care to patients with renal conditions. By offering a comprehensive overview of both the physiological mechanisms underlying kidney function and the latest therapeutic approaches, the book aims to enhance clinical practice and improve patient outcomes in the field of nephrology.

Chapter 1

ANATOMY AND FUNCTION OF THE KIDNEYS

Contents

Introduction

The excretion of extraneous water, electrolytes, metabolic products, and foreign materials such as toxins and medications is regulated by the kidneys. The body's fluid volume, pH, osmolality, and electrolyte composition are all maintained by the kidneys. The health of cells and organs depends on the stability of this environment. The kidneys perform this essential function with the assistance of many sensing systems that measure the volume of extracellular fluid and the osmolality of bodily fluids. The functions of the kidneys are significantly influenced by hormones such as atrial natriuretic peptide (ANP), angiotensin II, aldosterone, and antidiuretic hormone (ADH). Important endocrine organs, the kidneys also produce a range of hormones required for maintaining health, such as erythropoietin, renin, and 1,25-dihydroxyvitamin D3 (calcitriol).

Orientation and Directional Terms

Term	Definition	Illustration
Glomerulus	The glomerulus is a network of small blood vessels, or tuft, located at the beginning of a nephron in the kidney. It's the kidney's filtering unit, and each nephron contains a single glomerulus.	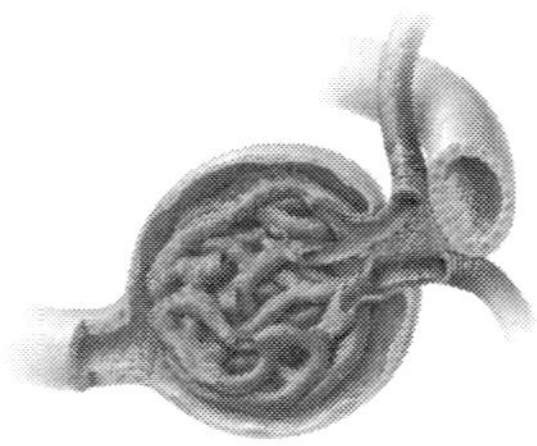
Nephron	A nephron is the basic structural and functional unit of the kidney. They are the microscopic structure composed of a renal corpuscle and a renal tubule.	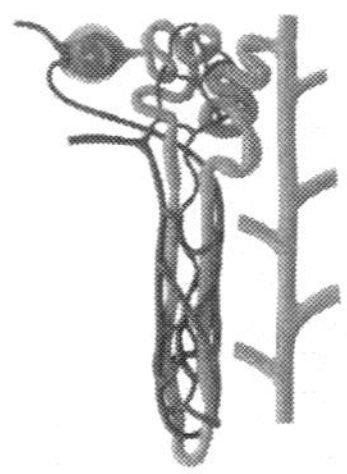
Renal artery	The renal artery is a major blood vessel that supplies oxygenated blood to the kidneys. The kidneys filter waste products from the blood and maintain electrolyte balance.	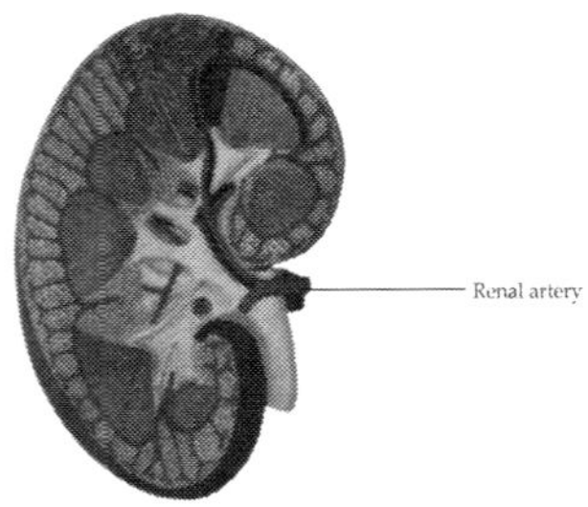
Renal corpuscle	The renal corpuscle is a structural and functional unit of the kidney that filters blood and produces urine. It's located in the kidney's outer layer, or cortex, and is made up of three main components: glomerulus, bowman's capsule, and mesangium.	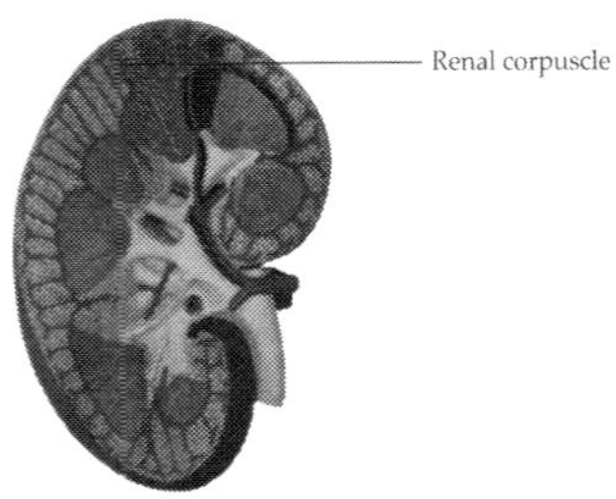
Vascular System	The vascular system is a network of blood and lymph vessels that move blood and lymph throughout the body.	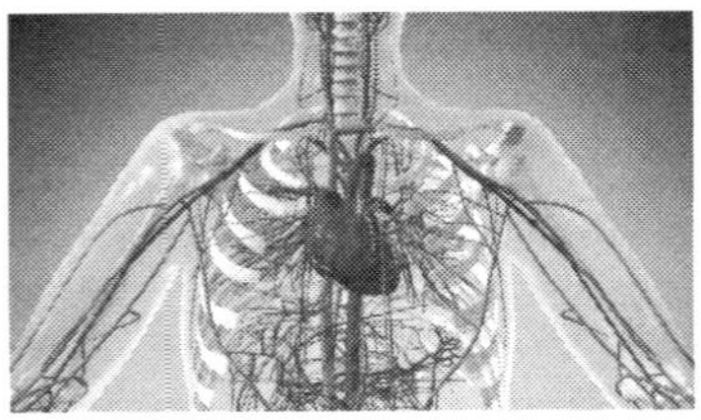

1.1. Anatomy of the Kidney

On either side of the midline in the abdomen, the kidneys are situated retroperitoneally, behind the peritoneal cavity. Each kidney is between 10 and 12 cm long and weighs about 150 g. The renal arteries, which branch off of the abdominal aorta, supply the kidneys with 20% of the cardiac output, or the maximum amount of blood per 100 grams of body tissue. The kidneys are extremely vascular organs. Nephrons are the 400,000–1,200,000 functional units found in each kidney. The renal veins subsequently empty the arterial blood supplying the kidney into the inferior vena cava (Hughson, Farris, Douglas-Denton, et al., 2003); (Figure 1.1).

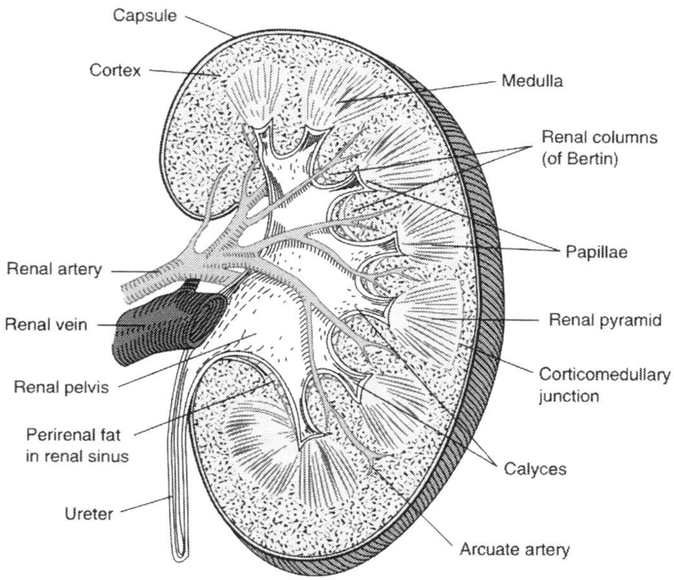

Figure 1.1. *Anatomy of the kidney. A coronal section through the kidney showing the renal cortex and medulla. The capsule surrounds the kidney. The cortex contains the glomeruli and the medulla, which are mostly tubules that drain into the renal calyces and then into the pelvis and connect to the ureter. The renal blood vessels (the artery and the vein) are shown in the hilum of the kidney. (Modified from Brenner B: Brenner and Rector's The Kidney, 7th ed. Philadelphia, Saunders, 2004.).*

Source: *A. Vishnu Moorthy, Bryan N. Becker, Frederick J. Boehm III, and Arjang Djamali. Pathophysiology of Kidney disease And Hypertension. Saunders, Elsevier. ISBN: 978-1-4160-4391-1.*

1.1.1. The Nephron

The glomerulus and tubule make up the nephron, which is the kidney's functional unit. Glomeruli are collections of specialized capillaries found in the kidney cortex's Bowman's capsule. The afferent arterioles allow blood to enter glomeruli, while the efferent arterioles allow blood to exit. Urine starts off as a glomerular ultrafiltrate, which is the blood minus plasma proteins, and it flows from the tubule to the glomerulus. The glomerulus is connected to the collecting duct, which eventually empties into the renal pelvis, by means of the kidney tubule's three distinct segments: the proximal tubule, the distal tubule, and the hairpin-shaped loop of Henle. Tubular reabsorption and secretion cause the glomerular ultrafiltrate's volume to decrease and its composition to alter as it passes through the tubules. Eventually, the urine empties into the bladder, where it is held until it is eliminated, via the renal pelvis, the ureter, and the bladder.

1.1.2. The Vascular System

The aorta gives rise to a single or occasionally double renal artery, which supplies each kidney. The afferent arteriole, which emerges from branches of the renal artery and supplies blood to the glomerular capillaries, and the efferent arteriole, which empties the glomerular capillaries, are what distinguish the glomerular capillaries from other types of arterioles. The efferent arteriole branches into a group of peritubular capillaries that closely encircle the tubules after the glomerulus. The kidney parenchyma thus contains two capillary beds arranged in series. This configuration is essential for tubular reabsorption and secretion as well as glomerular filtration (Figure 1.2).

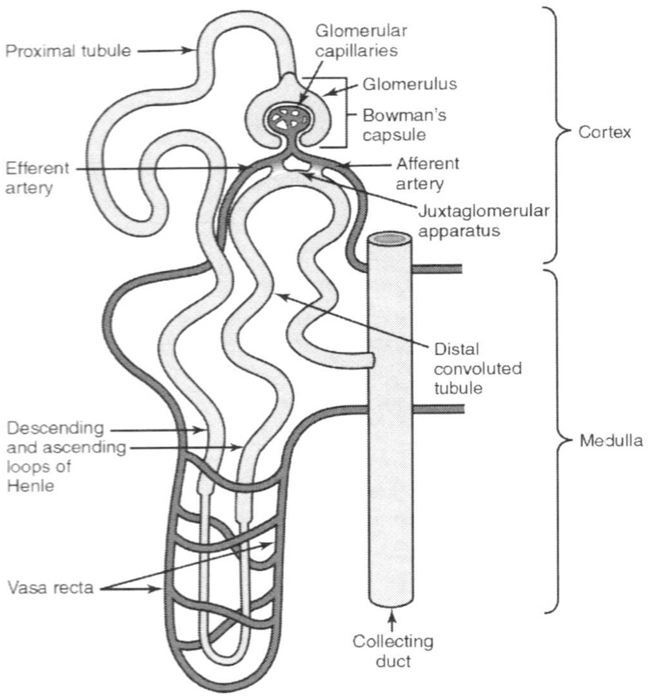

Figure 1.2. *The structure of the kidney showing the nephron and its vascular supply. The nephron with its various components: the glomerulus and the proximal tubule in the cortex, the descending and ascending loops of Henle in the medulla, and the distal tubule that returns to the glomerulus of its origin in the cortex and ultimately connects to the collecting duct. The afferent artery supplies the glomerulus. The efferent artery arises from the glomerular capillaries, branches one more time into the peritubular capillaries, and descends into the renal medulla as the vasa recta before connecting into the venous system.*

(Modified from Andreoli T, Loscalzo J, Carpenter C, Griggs R: Cecil Essentials of Medicine, 6th ed. Philadelphia, Saunders, 2004.)

Source: *A. Vishnu Moorthy, Bryan N. Becker, Frederick J. Boehm III, and Arjang Djamali. Pathophysiology of Kidney Disease and Hypertension. Saunders, Elsevier. ISBN: 978-1-4160-4391-1.*

The renal medullary portion receives its supply from the segments of postglomerular capillaries, also referred to as the vasa recta. The blood vessels known as the vasa recta are hairpin-shaped vessels that start in the cortex, travel through the medulla, and then return to the cortex where they connect to the venous system. Solutes and fluid that the tubules have reabsorbed are eliminated by the medullary circulation. Solutes enter the vessels and water exits them during the vasa recta's descending loops. This process is reversed in the ascending loops of the vasa recta: solutes exit the vessel into the interstitium and water enters the vessel. The vasa recta maintains a high medullary tonicity and reduces the removal of excessive medullary interstitial solutes through this process of counter-current exchange. Urine production requires this high medullary interstitial tonicity to be concentrated.

1.1.3. The Glomerulus

Glomeruli are collections of capillaries lined with a single layer of parietal epithelium epithelial cells and encircled by Bowman's capsules. The proximal tubule removes filtrate from the Bowman's space, while the afferent arteriole supplies and the efferent arteriole drains the glomerulus. The arrangement of glomerular capillaries between two arterioles makes them distinct (Figure 1.3).

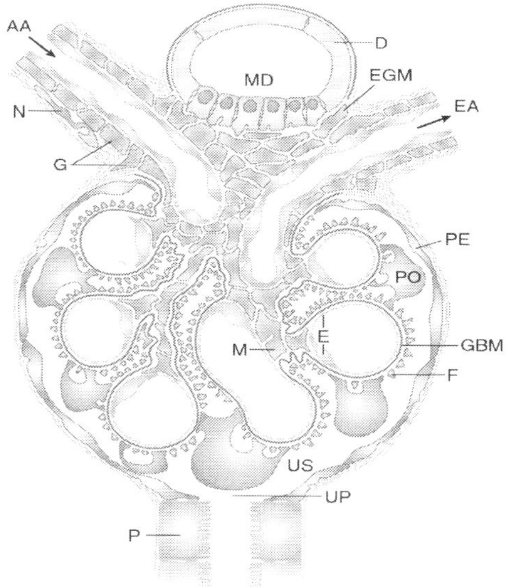

Figure 1.3. *The glomerulus with the capillary wall, the cellular constituents, and the Bowman's capsule. The mesangium with the matrix and the mesangial cell is noted. Also illustrated is the juxtaglomerular apparatus, which is comprised of the macula Densa and the renin-producing cells. AA, Afferent arteriole; D, distal tubule; E, endothelial cell; EA, efferent arteriole; EGM, extraglomerular mesangial cell; F, foot process; G, granules (renin); GBM, glomerular basement membrane; M, mesangial cell; MD, macula densa; N, nerve endings (sympathetic); P, proximal tubule; PE, parietal epithelial cell lining the Bowman's capsule; PO, podocyte; UP, urinary pole; US, urinary space.*

(Modified from Greenberg A: Primer on Kidney Diseases, 4th ed. Philadelphia, Saunders, 2005.)

Source: *A. Vishnu Moorthy, Bryan N. Becker, Frederick J. Boehm III, and Arjang Djamali. Pathophysiology of Kidney Disease and Hypertension. Saunders, Elsevier. ISBN: 978-1-4160-4391-1.*

Similar to capillaries found in other parts of the body, glomerular capillaries are lined by endothelial cells in the basement membrane. The individual fenestra, which is 70–100 nm long, fenestrates the glomerular endothelium. The glomerular basement membrane (GBM) is an acellular matrix that has two laminas: externa and interna on either side or a central lamina Densa. The GBM has a thickness of approximately 300 nm. It is made up of laminin and type IV collagen, two extracellular matrix proteins. Additionally, it contains glycoproteins that are negatively charged, like chondroitin sulfates and heparan. α-3, α-4, and α-5 collagen chains make up the triple helical collagen type IV molecule found in adult GBM. The GBM's tensile strength is derived from the cross-linked collagen chains (Maddox & Brenner, 2004; Briggs, Kriz, Schnermann, 2005; Alpern & Hebert, 2008).

The glomerular epithelial cell, also known as the podocyte, is a special type of cell found outside the glomerular bladder mass (GBM) in the glomerular capillaries. Podocytes were formerly more widely referred to as visceral epithelial cells. Large cells called podocytes give rise to numerous interdigitating foot processes that are attached to the GBM. The slit diaphragms, which are cytoplasmic connections, bind the neighboring foot processes, which originate from distinct podocytes. Between neighboring podocytes, the slit diaphragm creates a structure resembling a zipper. It functions as a size-selective barrier to keep molecules out of Bowman's urinary space. Its pores are roughly 40 nm across (Figure 1.4 (Nyengaard & Bendtsen, 1992) and; Figure 1.5).

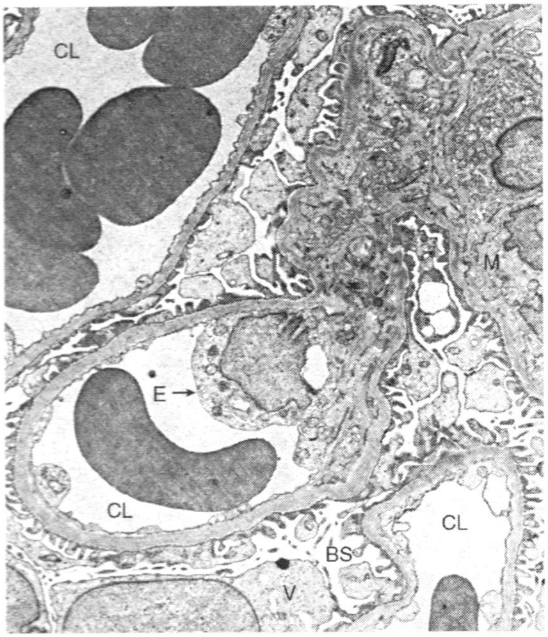

Figure 1.4, *Electron micrograph of a normal glomerulus showing the capillary loops (CL) with red blood cells. Bowman's urinary space (BS), endothelial cell (E), mesangial cell (M), and visceral epithelial cell (V) are also seen.*

(Modified from Brenner B: Brenner and Rector's The Kidney, 7th ed. Philadelphia, Saunders, 2004.)

Source: *A. Vishnu Moorthy, Bryan N. Becker, Frederick J. Boehm III, and Arjang Djamali. Pathophysiology of Kidney Disease and Hypertension. Saunders, Elsevier. ISBN: 978-1-4160-4391-1.*

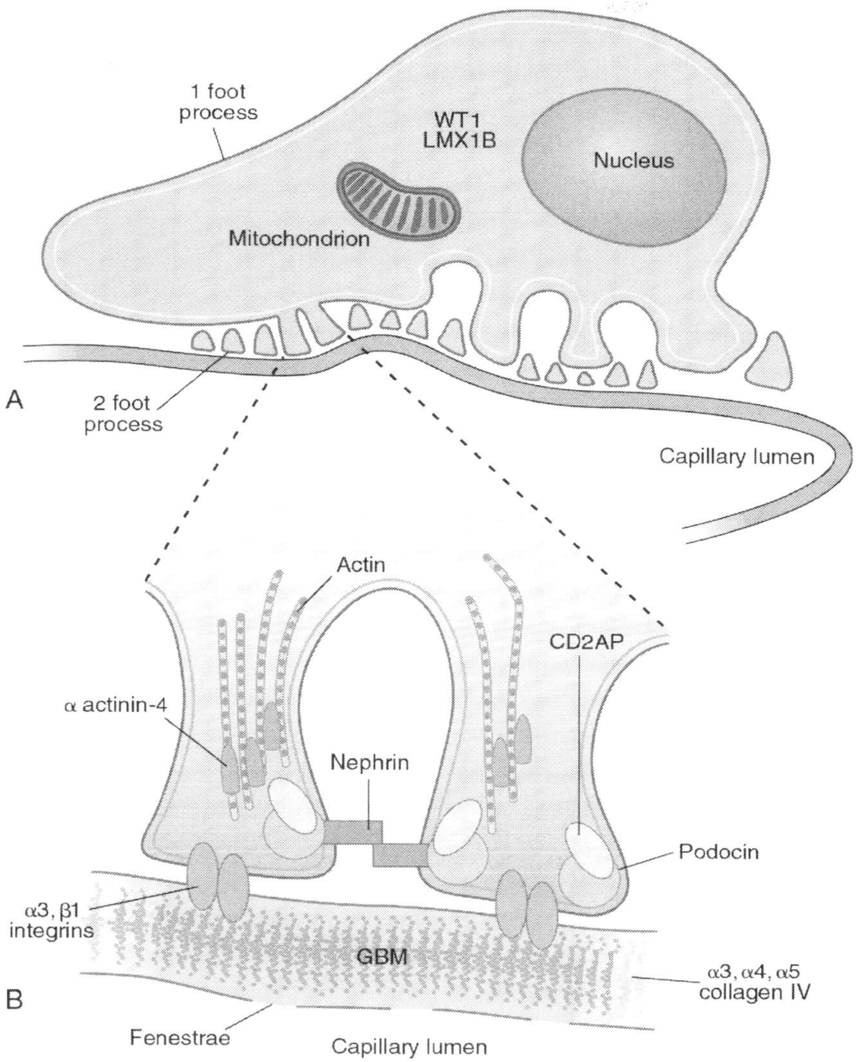

Figure 1.5. *A schematic view of the podocyte resting on a capillary loop. A, Primary foot processes give rise to secondary foot processes that are anchored to the basement membrane with integrins. B, Nephrin proteins extend from adjacent foot processes and interdigitate to form the zipperlike slit diaphragm. Nephrin is anchored onto the cell membrane by podocin and CD2AP. -Actinin-4 connects actin filaments to cellular structures. Inherited defects in proteins such as nephrin, podocin, CD2AP, and the transcription factors (WT1, LMX1B) have been found to cause focal glomerulosclerosis. Inherited defects in the α-3, α-4, and α-5 collagen type IV chains in the glomerular basement membrane (GBM) are seen in patients with Alport syndrome.*

(Modified from Greenberg A: Primer on Kidney Diseases, 4th ed. Philadelphia, Saunders, 2005.)

Source: *A. Vishnu Moorthy, Bryan N. Becker, Frederick J. Boehm III, and Arjang Djamali. Pathophysiology of Kidney Disease and Hypertension. Saunders, Elsevier. ISBN: 978-1-4160-4391-1.*

Nephrin, podocin, and α-actinin 4 are among the proteins that have been found in the podocyte and slit diaphragm. The glomerular capillary barrier's integrity depends on these proteins. Plasma proteins may leak into the urine and eventually cause renal failure due to inherited flaws in the genes that encode these proteins.

The glomerular capillary wall consists of the podocyte-formed filtration slits and the GBM. It acts as a barrier to keep protein and biological components out of the urine and to divide the blood in the glomerular capillaries from the ultrafiltrate in the Bowman's space. The filtration barrier is the term for this. The negatively charged proteins of the GBM exclude negatively charged molecules (e.g., albumin) from passing through the glomerular capillaries and into the ultrafiltrate. Research employing disparately charged (i.e., neutral, or cationic) dextran molecules has demonstrated the size- and charge-selective nature of glomerular capillaries. Larger, anionic molecules are held in the glomerular capillaries, while smaller, cationic molecules are readily filtered in the glomerulus.

The glomerulus contains mesangial cells, which are encircled by the mesangial matrix, in addition to endothelial cells and podocytes. Certain mesangial cells are attached to glomerular capillaries and can contract like smooth muscle cells. The reticuloendothelial system includes other mesangial cells. They release a range of cytokines and exhibit phagocytic activity. The mesangial matrix, which extends into the juxtaglomerular apparatus beyond the glomerulus's hilum, is less dense than the GBM.

1.1.4. The Kidney Tubule

The nephron's tubule is segmented into multiple sections. The various tubule segments differ in their architecture and functions in altering the volume and composition of the urine that is ultimately expelled. The glomerulus in the cortex gives rise to the proximal tubule. The proximal tubule descends into the medulla and becomes the loop of Henle after a tortuous path. Henle loops are shorter in the nephrons located in the outer zone of the renal cortex and longer in the deeper (juxtamedullary) nephrons, which extend nearly to the tip of the papillae. In close proximity to the glomerulus from which they originated, the distal convoluted tubules are formed by the sharp turn that the loops of Henle make and return to the cortex. At the glomerulus' hilum, a section of the distal convoluted tubule comes into contact with the afferent and efferent arterioles. The distal tubule's macula Densa cells are located here, and they can detect the amounts of sodium and chloride in the tubular urine. The wall of the afferent arterioles contains granular cells that contain renin; rich sympathetic nerve endings are also located in this region. The juxtaglomerular apparatus consists of the macula Densa and the renin-containing cells of the afferent arterioles. The collecting duct, which subsequently returns to the medulla and leads into the renal pelvis, is formed by the distal tubule (Maddox & Brenner, 2004; Briggs, Kriz, Schnermann, 2005; Alpern & Hebert, 2008).

1.2. Renal Blood Flow and Glomerular Filtration

Both glomerular filtration rate (GFR) and renal blood flow (RBF) are crucial for preserving healthy kidney function. GFR is the volume of plasma filtered in a given amount of time, whereas RBF is the volume of blood that flows through the kidney's glomeruli. Since RBF and GFR typically fluctuate simultaneously, an increase in RBF raises GFR.

1.2.1. Renal Blood Flow

The kidney receives blood supply from the renal artery. Approximately 25% of the blood pumped by the heart is always received by the kidneys in humans. The afferent arteriole allows blood to enter the nephron's capillaries. After that, it enters the efferent arteriole via the glomerulus. These arterioles' different sizes contribute to the hydrostatic pressure differential that is necessary for glomerular filtration as well as the stability of renal blood flow and glomerular capillary pressure within the glomerulus. In Figure 1.6, the efferent arteriole is smaller than usual. The glomerular capillary pressure rises as a result.

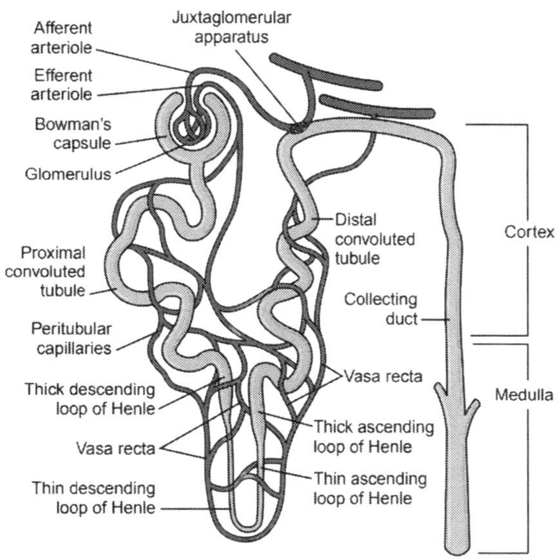

Figure 1.6. *The nephron and its component parts.*

Source: *Susan King Strasinger and Marjorie Schaub Di Lorenzo. Urinalysis and Body Fluids. Fifth Edition. Copyright © 2008 by F. A. Davis Company.*

Blood from the efferent arteriole enters the peritubular capillaries and the vasa recta before slowly passing through the kidney's cortex and medulla near the tubules before returning to the renal vein. The proximal and distal convoluted tubules are surrounded by peritubular capillaries, which allow for the distal convoluted tubule to finalize its adjustment of the urinary composition and the proximal convoluted tubule to immediately reabsorb vital substances from the fluid. In juxtamedullary nephrons, the vasa recta are situated next to the ascending and descending loop of Henle. The main water and salt exchanges in this region occur between the medullary interstitium and the blood. Renal concentration depends on the osmotic gradient, or salt concentration, that is maintained in the medulla by this exchange.

The total renal blood flow is about 1,200 mL/min and the total renal plasma flow is between 600 and 700 mL/min based on an average body size of 1.73 m^2 of surface area. Body size affects normal values for renal blood flow and renal function tests. To ascertain whether the recorded measurements accurately reflect normal function, a correction needs to be computed when working with sizes that deviate significantly from the average 1.73 m^2 of the body surface.

1.2.2. Glomerular Filtration

The afferent arteriole's specialized membranes and high blood pressure cause glomerular filtration to remove the majority of solutes. An independent set of factors that influence systemic blood pressure maintains the blood pressure in the glomerulus. Solutes are easily able to flow through the glomerular capillary network's "leaky" connections between endothelial cells. Everything that is not a macromolecule, such as proteins, diffuses passively through the glomerular capillaries. As the filtration process reaches this point, no energy is needed. A kidney's production of glomerular filtrate per minute is measured by its glomerular filtration rate or GFR. The global functional reserve (GFR) is a crucial measure of kidney health that is regulated by various mechanisms.

A coil of about eight capillary lobes, collectively referred to as the capillary tuft, makes up the glomerulus. It is situated inside

Bowman's capsule, which marks the renal tubule's origin. Many factors affect the actual filtration process, even though the glomerulus acts as a nonselective filter for plasma substances with molecular weights less than 70,000. These include the Bowman's capsule and capillary walls' cellular structure, hydrostatic and oncotic pressures, and the renin-angiotensin-aldosterone system's feedback mechanisms. A diagrammatic view of the glomerular areas affected by these factors is shown in Figure 1.7.

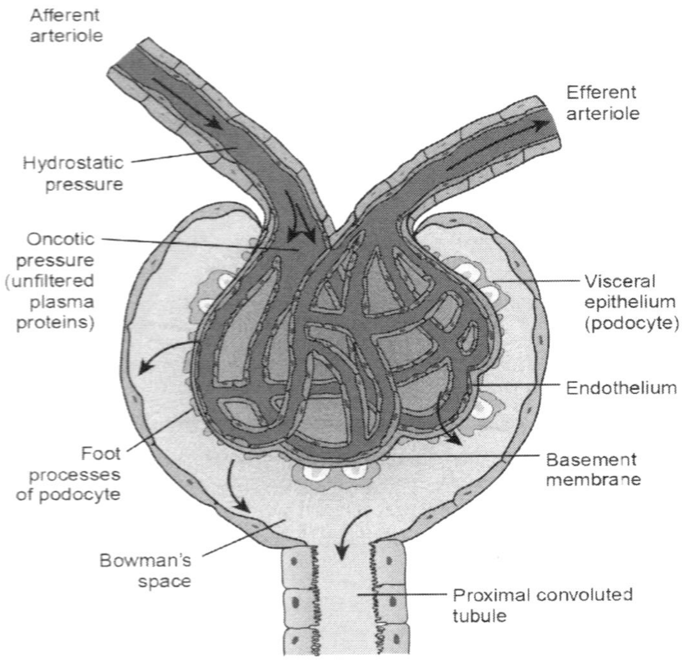

Figure 1.7. *Factors affecting glomerular filtration in the renal corpuscle.*

Source: *Susan King Strasinger and Marjorie Schaub Di Lorenzo. Urinalysis and Body Fluids. Fifth Edition. Copyright © 2008 by F. A. Davis Company.*

1.2.2.1. Cellular Structure of the Glomerulus

The visceral epithelium of Bowman's capsule, the basement membrane (basal lamina), and the capillary wall membrane are the three cellular layers that the plasma filtrate must pass through. The capillary wall's endothelial cells are known as fenestrated because they have pores, setting them apart from those in other capillaries. Although the pores make capillaries more permeable, they prevent blood cells and big molecules from passing through. As the filtrate moves through the basement membrane and the thin membranes covering the filtration slits created by the intertwining foot processes of the podocytes in the inner layer of Bowman's capsule, more restriction of large molecules takes place.

1.2.2.2. Glomerular Pressure

Filtration is improved by the hydrostatic pressure created by the glomerular capillaries and the efferent arteriole's smaller size. This pressure is required to overcome the oncotic pressure of unfiltered plasma proteins in the glomerular capillaries as well as the opposing pressures from the fluid inside Bowman's capsule. An autoregulatory mechanism in the juxtaglomerular apparatus regulates the size of the afferent arteriole to keep the glomerular blood pressure relatively constant despite variations in systemic blood pressure. When blood pressure drops, the afferent arterioles dilate and the efferent arterioles constrict, preventing a significant drop in blood flow through the kidney and an increase in the blood level of toxic waste products. Similar to this, a rise in blood pressure causes the afferent arterioles to constrict to shield the glomerulus from overfiltration or injury.

1.2.2.3. Renin-Angiotensin-Aldosterone System

The regulation of blood flow to and within the glomerulus is carried out by the renin-angiotensin-aldosterone system (RAAS). The juxtaglomerular apparatus, comprising the distal convoluted tubule's macula Densa and the afferent arteriole's juxtaglomerular cells, monitors changes in blood pressure and plasma sodium content, and the system reacts to these changes (Figure 1.8). Low plasma sodium content reduces the circulatory system's ability to retain water, which lowers total blood volume and, in turn, lowers blood pressure. A series of events take place inside the RAAS when the macula Densa detects such alterations (Figure 1.9). The blood-borne substrate angiotensinogen and the enzyme renin, which is produced by the juxtaglomerular cells, combine to form the inactive hormone angiotensin I. Angiotensin converting enzyme (ACE) converts angiotensin I into the active form angiotensin II as it travels through the lungs. The following mechanisms by which angiotensin II corrects renal blood flow are: it causes constriction of the efferent arterioles and vasodilation of the afferent arterioles; it stimulates sodium reabsorption in the proximal convoluted tubules; and it causes the adrenal cortex and hypothalamus to release the hormones that retain sodium, aldosterone and antidiuretic hormone (Table 1.1). Renin secretion declines with increases in systemic blood pressure and plasma sodium content. Consequently, the nephron experiences continuous pressure due to the effects of angiotensin II.

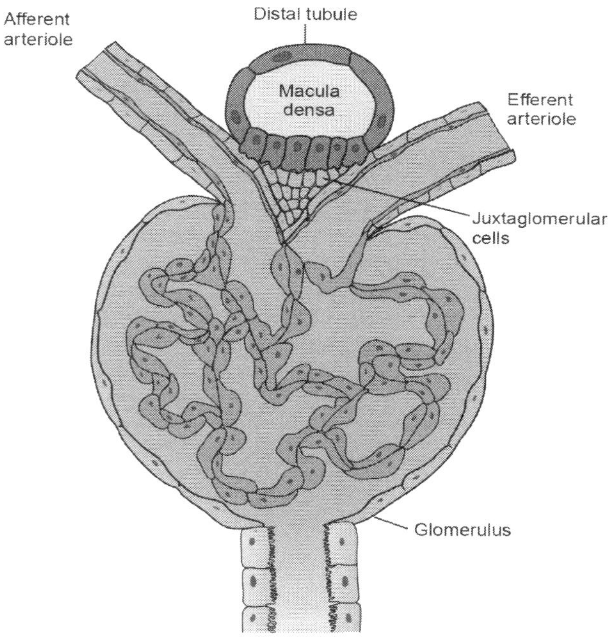

Figure 1.8. *Close contact of the distal tubule with the afferent arteriole, macula Densa, and the juxtaglomerular cells within the juxtaglomerular apparatus.*

Source: *Susan King Strasinger and Marjorie Schaub Di Lorenzo. Urinalysis and Body Fluids. Fifth Edition. Copyright © 2008 by F. A. Davis Company.*

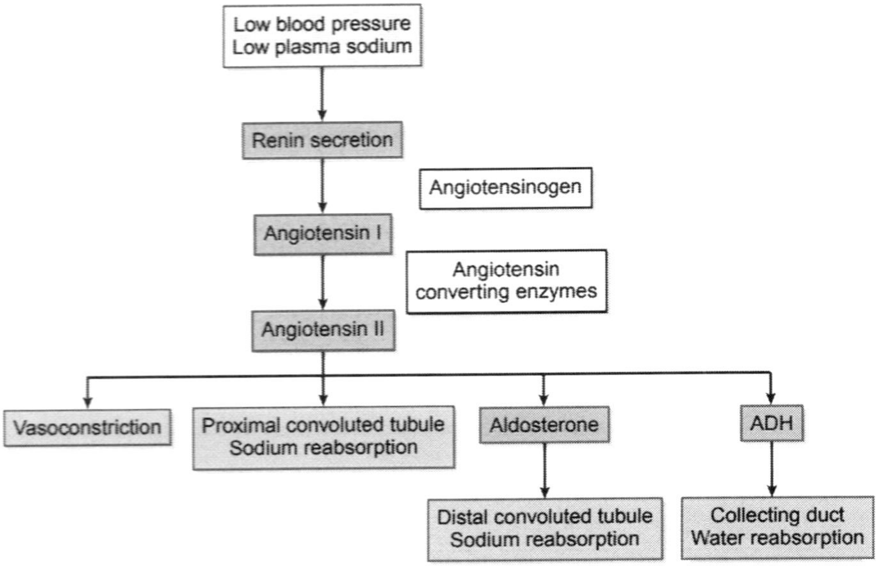

Figure 1.9. *Algorithm of the reninangiotensin-aldosterone system.*

Source: *Susan King Strasinger and Marjorie Schaub Di Lorenzo. Urinalysis and Body Fluids. Fifth Edition. Copyright © 2008 by F. A. Davis Company.*

Table 1.1. Actions of the RAAS

1. Dilation of the afferent arteriole and constriction of the efferent arteriole
2. Stimulation of sodium reabsorption in the proximal convoluted tubule
3. Triggers the adrenal cortex to release the sodium retaining hormone, aldosterone, to cause reabsorption of sodium and excretion of potassium in the distal convoluted tubule and collecting duct
4. Triggers release of antidiuretic hormone by the hypothalamus to stimulate water reabsorption in the collecting duct

Source: *Susan King Strasinger and Marjorie Schaub Di Lorenzo. Urinalysis and Body Fluids. Fifth Edition. Copyright © 2008 by F. A. Davis Company.*

Due to the glomerular mechanisms mentioned above, 2 to 3 million glomeruli filter about 120 mL of low-molecular-weight substances that contain water every minute. The lack of plasma protein, any protein-bound materials, and cells is the only distinction between the compositions of the filtrate and the plasma due to the nonselective nature of this filtration. It is confirmed that the filtrate is chemically an ultrafiltrate of plasma by analysis of the fluid as it exits the glomerulus, which reveals a specific gravity of 1.010. This data offers a helpful starting point for assessing the renal processes that transform the plasma ultrafiltrate into the finished urine product (Maddox & Brenner, 2004; Briggs, Kriz, Schnermann, 2005; Alpern & Hebert, 2008).

1.3. Tubular Function

The high volume of reabsorption that occurs within the renal tubules is demonstrated by the fact that only 1% (or about 1,200 mL) of the initial plasma ultrafiltrate supplied to the tubules is eliminated as urine. Along with this significant volume change, the urine excreted has a drastically different solute makeup than the original ultrafiltrate, highlighting the dynamic processes that the tubules perform. The kidney's ability to regulate the excretion of water and other solutes is what makes it the most significant organ in fluid exchanges. The substances are moved either from the tubular lumen into the peritubular capillary blood and interstitium (reabsorption) or from the peritubular capillary blood and interstitium into the tubular lumen (secretion). The mechanisms causing these changes are the same: tubular reabsorption and tubular secretion.

1.3.1. Transport

The mechanisms of tubular transport (i.e., secretion, and reabsorption) are either passive or active. The passage of a material across a membrane against a gradient is known as active transport. Put another way, the chemical or electrical composition of the compartments divided by the membrane varies. Such transportation necessitates the direct or indirect use of energy.

Direct active transport is the process of actively moving a substance when energy is needed, such as in the potassium-to-sodium exchange facilitated by adenosine triphosphate hydrolysis (the sodium pump). Indirect active transport, also known as cotransport, is the movement of one substance along a gradient accompanied by the movement of another substance (e.g., the proximal tubules' indirect absorption of glucose and sodium).

Certain protein-binding sites that cross the cell membrane are involved in active transport, which happens transcellularly. The steps involved in active transport are as follows: (1) the material attaches to its particular membrane-binding site; (2) it passes through the cell membrane; and (3) it is released either inside or outside the cell when the binding site changes conformation.

The movement of a substance along a gradient, or, to put it another way, from an area of higher concentration to one of lower concentration, is known as passive transport. This type of transport, like that of urea, does not require energy. Transport between cells via junctions and intercellular spaces can be either transcellular or paracellular in nature.

Every solute has a unique transport mechanism. Cellular protein-binding sites can carry multiple solutes, frequently displaying preferential transport of one analyte over another, or they can be specific for a single solute and only carry that solute across the membrane. Furthermore, depending on the location of the tubule, the mode of transportation—passive or active—may change. For instance, chloride is passively reabsorbed in the proximal tubule but actively reabsorbed in the ascending loop of Henle.

Table 1.2. Summary of Tubular Reabsorption of Ultrafiltrate Components

Location	Mode of Reabsorption	Substance
Proximal tubule (convoluted and straight portions)	Passive	H_2O, Cl^-, K^+, urea
	Active	Na^+, HCO_3^-, glucose, amino acids, proteins, phosphate, sulfate, Mg^{2+}, Ca^{2+}, uric acid
Loop of Henle Thin descending limb	Passive	H_2O, urea
U-turn and thin ascending limb	Passive	Na^+, Cl^-, urea
Thick ascending limb (medullary and cortical)	Passive	Urea
	Active	Na^+, Cl^-
Distal tubule (convoluted portion)	Active	Na^+, Cl^-, sulfate, uric acid
	Passive	H_2O
Collecting Tubules Cortical	Passive	H_2O, Cl^-
	Active	Na^+
Medullary	Passive	H_2O, urea

Source: *Nancy A. Brunzel. Fundamentals of Urine & Body Fluid Analysis. Elsevier. ISBN: 978-1-4377-0989-6.*

1.3.2. Reabsorption

Selective tubular function excretes waste products like creatinine and metabolic acids while reabsorbing nutrients like water, salts, glucose, proteins, and amino acids that are essential for maintaining body homeostasis and function. A summary of some significant ultrafiltrate components based on where their tubular reabsorption occurs can be found in Table 1.2. The principal means of transportation for every substance is also listed in the table. Please take note that this summary only covers the primary mode of substance transport; in actuality, multiple mechanisms are involved in the reabsorption of certain solutes. The main interactions between the major solutes and their transport mechanisms are covered in the section that follows.

1.3.3. Secretion

Tubular secretion occurs throughout the nephron, just like tubular reabsorption. The primary functions of the renal secretory process are to: (1) remove waste products from metabolism and substances that aren't typically found in plasma; and (2) modify the body's acid-base balance. These two roles overlap because the body's acid-base balance is directly impacted by the weak acids and bases found in many foreign substances and metabolic byproducts. Some of the significant secreted ultrafiltrate solutes and the tubular secretion locations are compiled in Table 1.3.

Table 1.3. Summary of Tubular Secretion of Important Ultrafiltrate Components

Location	Substance
Proximal tubule	H^+, NH_3, weak acids and bases
Loop of Henle	Urea
Distal tubule	H^+, NH_3, K^+, uric acid (some drugs)
Collecting tubule	H^+, NH_3, K^+ (some drugs)

Source: *Nancy A. Brunzel. Fundamentals of Urine & Body Fluid Analysis. Elsevier. ISBN: 978–1-4377–0989–6.*

Apart from hydrogen ions, ammonia, and potassium, the majority of substances secreted are weak acids or bases. These weak bases and acids come from external or metabolic sources. They are (1) substances that the body has not fully metabolized (e.g., thiamine), (2) chemicals that are secreted unaltered and not at all metabolized (e.g., mannitol and radiopaque contrast media), or (3) materials that aren't typically found in plasma (e.g., salicylate, penicillin). Certain substances are bound to plasma proteins, mainly albumin, which prevents them from excreting through the glomerular filtration barrier (e.g., drugs, unconjugated bilirubin). They consequently have a significant increase in size overall and may lose some of their initial molecular charge. However, tubular secretion offers a way to get rid of them. These comparatively big, protein-bound materials are carried into renal tubular cells, where they interact with endothelium-binding sites before being secreted into the tubular lumen as they pass through the peritubular capillaries.

1.3.4. Regulation of Acid-Base Equilibrium

A basic understanding of the body's endogenous production of bases and acids is necessary to comprehend the function of tubular secretion in maintaining acid-base equilibrium. Normal blood pH in healthy individuals ranges from 7.35 to 7.45, which is alkaline. Nonetheless, the pH can be as high as 7.80 or as low as 7.00 in pathologic disease states. Blood has an alkaline pH, and the endogenous production of acids from regular food metabolism continuously jeopardizes this pH. These endogenous acids are produced in three ways: (1) by the oxidative metabolism of food, which produces carbonic acid, (2) by the breakdown of dietary proteins and phospholipids, or (3) by the production of acids under specific pathologic or physiological conditions, such as lactic acid with exercise or acetoacetic acid in uncontrolled diabetes mellitus.

Three bodily systems—the pulmonary system, the renal system, and the blood-buffer system, which includes hemoglobin, bicarbonate, proteins, and inorganic phosphates—are involved in keeping the blood pH at a level that is conducive to life. While the three systems collaborate to sustain homeostasis, the pulmonary and blood-buffer systems can react promptly to pH variations, albeit to a limited extent. However, the renal system can fully correct deviations in blood pH, even with its relatively slow response.

The kidneys excrete acid or alkali in urine according to blood pH variations. Excess alkali is removed by excreting sodium salts like sodium bicarbonate and disodium phosphate, while excess acids are removed by excreting titratable acids like monosodium phosphate and ammonium salts like e.g., NH_4Cl, $[NH_4]_2SO_4$, etc.

The tubular secretion of H^+ ions is a prerequisite for each of the three secretory mechanisms that regulate blood pH, either directly or indirectly. Renal tubular cells secrete H^+ ions (acids) in exchange for sodium and bicarbonate ions (alkali) in acidotic conditions. Tubular H^+ ion secretion is reduced in alkalotic conditions, aiding in the body's removal of excess alkali.

In the first secretory mechanism, the loss of bicarbonate, an essential part of the blood-buffer system, is directly prevented by the secretion of H^+ ions into the proximal tubular lumen. In Figure 1.10, carbonic acid (H_2CO_3) is formed in the tubular lumen as a result of a reaction between bicarbonate ions (HCO_3^-), which easily cross the glomerular filtration barrier, and the released H^+. However, due to the high concentration of the enzyme carbonic anhydrase found in the brush border of the proximal tubular cells, this carbonic acid is quickly catalyzed to carbon dioxide and water. As the carbon dioxide permeates into the proximal cell, intracellular carbonic anhydrase again converts it to HCO_3^- and H^+. Thus, H^+ ions are once again available for tubular secretion and for the reabsorption of HCO_3^- ions from the lumen of the tubule. Reabsorbed bicarbonate replenishes the blood-buffer system by diffusing into the interstitial fluid and peritubular capillaries.

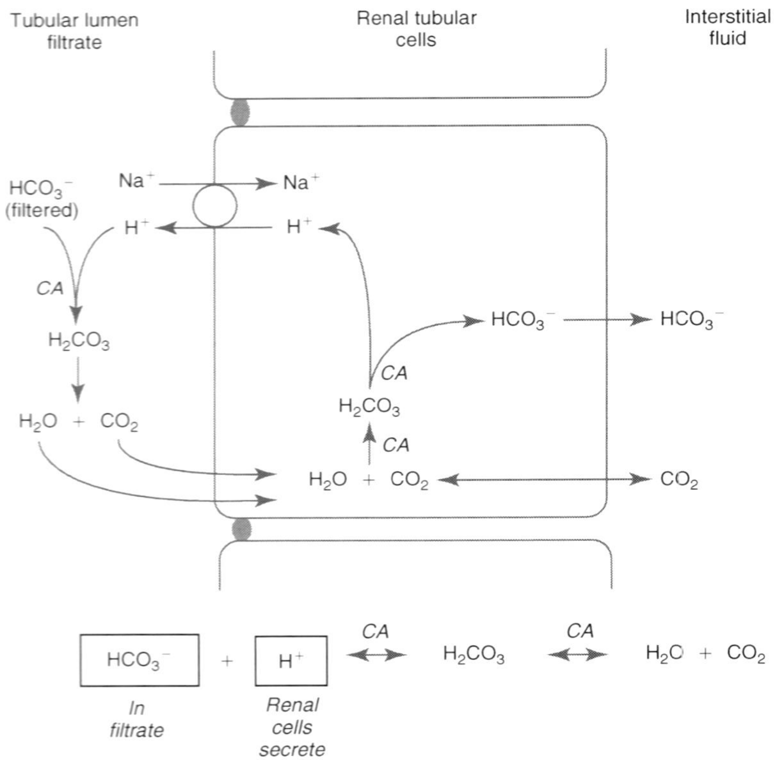

Figure 1.10. *Hydrogen ion secretion and the mechanism of filtered bicarbonate reabsorption in the proximal tube. CA, Carbonic anhydrase.*

Source: *Nancy A. Brunzel. Fundamentals of Urine & Body Fluid Analysis. Elsevier. ISBN: 978-1-4377-0989-6.*

The second secretory mechanism, as seen in Figure 1.11, is contingent upon the ultrafiltrate's phosphate content. The blood quickly transforms phosphoric acids, which are created during food metabolism, into neutral salts (e.g., Na_2HPO_4) and are carried to the renal system. Disodium phosphate (Na_2HPO_4) is converted to monosodium phosphate (NaH_2PO_4) in the tubular lumen of the nephrons by the exchange of secreted hydrogen ions with sodium ions (Equation 1.1). Titratable acids are those monobasic phosphates that are specifically mixed with hydrogen ions and eliminated in the urine. The name derives from the ability to titrate urine to a pH of 7.4 (pH of normal plasma) using a standard base (e.g., NaOH), to determine the amount of acid present as a result of these monobasic phosphates. Note that hydrogen ions combined with other solutes are not measured by this titration.

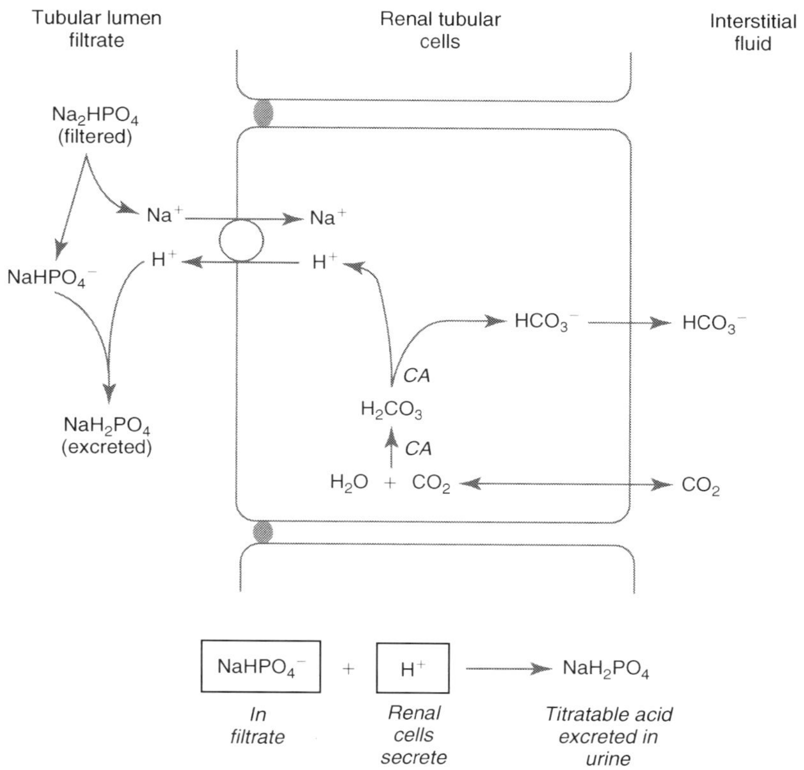

Figure 1.11. *Hydrogen ion secretion and the formation of titratable acids. This is a mechanism of urine acidification in the collecting ducts. CA, Carbonic anhydrase.*

Source: *Nancy A. Brunzel. Fundamentals of Urine & Body Fluid Analysis. Elsevier. ISBN: 978-1-4377-0989-6.*

These phosphates in the ultrafiltrate cause the body to release acid and acidify the urine; additionally, they restore sodium and bicarbonate ions to the blood in the peritubular capillaries.

As seen in Figure 1.12, the third secretory mechanism for acid removal is dependent on the secretion of ammonia and the subsequent exchange of sodium ions for ammonium ions. The renal tubular cells produce ammonia (NH_3) when the enzyme glutaminase reacts with glutamine, which is derived from the blood in the peritubular capillaries. NH_3 is lipid soluble and easily diffuses through tubular cell membranes and into the tubular lumen because it is not ionized. Ammonium ions (NH_4^+) are created when NH_3 quickly combines with H^+ ions inside the lumen. Due to their charge, these ions are essentially nondiffusible; as a result, they stay in the tubular lumen where they may mix with neutral salts like sodium sulfate, a metabolic byproduct, or sodium chloride. Equations 1–3 depict the chemical reactions that take place in the tubular lumen.

$$\begin{array}{ll} \text{In blood} & H_3PO_4 + 6Na^+ \rightarrow 3Na_2HPO_4 \\ \text{In ultrafiltrate} & Na_2HPO_4 + H^+ \rightarrow NaH_2PO_4 + Na^+ \\ & Na^+ + HCO_3^- \rightarrow NaHCO_3 \text{ (reabsorbed)} \end{array} \quad (1)$$

$$\begin{array}{l} NH_3 + H^+ \rightarrow NH_4^+ \\ NH_4^+ + NaCl + HCO_3^- \rightarrow NH_4Cl \text{ (excreted)} + NaHCO_3 \text{ (reabsorbed)} \end{array} \quad (2)$$

$$\begin{array}{l} NH_3 + H^+ \rightarrow NH_4^+ \\ 2NH_4^+ + Na_2SO_4 + 2HCO_3^- \rightarrow (NH_4)_2SO_4 \text{ (excreted)} \\ \qquad + 2NaHCO_3 \text{ (reabsorbed)} \end{array} \quad (3)$$

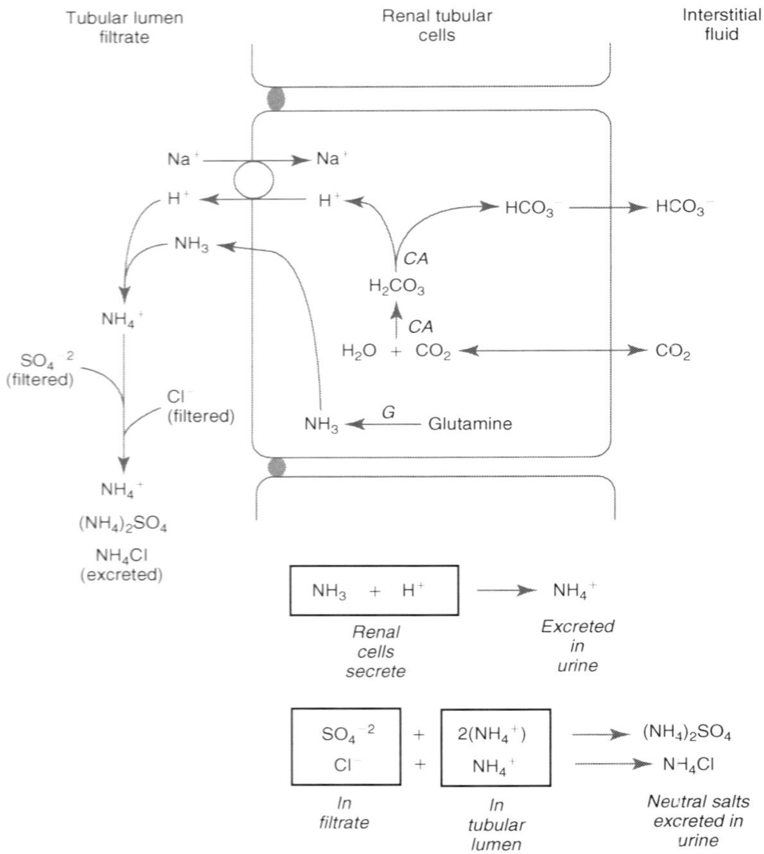

Figure 1.12. *Hydrogen ion secretion and the formation of ammonium ions. This is a mechanism of urine acidification in the collecting ducts. CA, Carbonic anhydrase; G, glutaminase.*

Source: *Nancy A. Brunzel. Fundamentals of Urine & Body Fluid Analysis. Elsevier. ISBN: 978-1-4377-0989-6.*

It should be noted that sodium and bicarbonate are restored and made available for tubular reabsorption in both reactions.

The renal tubules are the main source of ammonia excreted in urine. Ammonia is produced by both the proximal and collecting duct cells, and the collecting ducts are primarily where final urine acidification takes place. However, the body's acid-base status directly affects how quickly ammonia is synthesized. For instance, in acidotic conditions, there is an increase in ammonia production.

In conclusion, the kidney uses three renal secretory mechanisms to control the body's acid-base equilibrium: (1) H^+ ion secretion to recover bicarbonate; (2) H^+ ion secretion to produce urine titratable acids (e.g., monosodium phosphate); and (3) H^+ ion and NH_3 secretion to yield ammonium salts (e.g., ammonium chloride, ammonium sulfate). Through all of these methods, the secretion of hydrogen ions (i.e., the acid loss) causes the reabsorption of sodium or bicarbonate (i.e., the alkali gain). As a result, the kidney adjusts the amount of hydrogen ions and ammonia it secretes based on the body's changing acid-base requirements.

1.3.5. Tubular Transport Capacity

The substance involved determines the renal tubules' capacity for both secretion and reabsorption. For some substances, the rate of tubular reabsorption increases along with the amount of solute presented to the renal tubules, reaching a maximal rate of reabsorption. Even if the solute's concentration rises further, this maximal reabsorptive rate won't change. Urine then contains extra solute that has not been reabsorbed. The maximal tubular reabsorptive capacity refers to this reabsorptive property of the renal epithelium. The amount of solute (milligrams) reabsorbed per minute is indicated by the symbol T_m. The particular solute and additional variables, like the glomerular filtration rate, affect the T_m. Among the solutes with a T_m-limited tubular reabsorptive capacity are glucose, proteins, amino acids, phosphate, sulfate, and uric acid. Additionally, the blood concentration of these solutes has a Tm-specific value known as the renal threshold level. For instance, the glucose T_m is roughly 350 mg/min (corrected to 1.73 m^2 body surface area), meaning that a glucose plasma renal threshold level of 160–180 mg/dL is associated with this value. Put another way, a maximum of 350 mg of glucose can be reabsorbed per minute, independent of the amount of glucose present in the renal tubular lumen. Urine contains glucose excreted when the plasma glucose level surpasses 160 to 180 mg/dL, meaning that the ultrafiltrate glucose concentration surpasses the tubules' capacity to reabsorb (T_m).

Similarly, some solutes secreted by the tubules have a maximal tubular secretory capacity, also denoted T_m (e.g., p-aminohippurate, a weak organic acid). The same designation, T_m, is appropriate because both processes refer to the maximum capacity for the active transport of a substance, and the direction of movement—whether into or out of the tubular lumen—is immaterial.

Conversely, the amount of some solutes that can be reabsorbed is unrestricted (e.g., sodium) or released (e.g., potassium). Several factors, including the tubular flow rate, the duration of the solute's contact with the renal epithelium, the concentrations of other solutes in the filtrate, the presence of transport inhibitors, and variations in hormone levels, all affect the rate of transport for these substances (e.g., ADH).

1.3.6. Proximal Tubular Reabsorption

The proximal tubule reabsorbs over 66% of the filtered sodium, chloride, and water. Furthermore, a cotransport mechanism coupled to sodium essentially reabsorbs all of the proteins, amino acids, and glucose. The proximal tubule is also where other solutes like bicarbonate, phosphate, sulfate, magnesium, calcium, and uric acid are reabsorbed. The proximal tubule fluid exits osmotically unaltered despite these reabsorptive processes drastically reducing the volume and concentrations of particular solutes. To put it another way, even though there is a significant amount of water and solute reabsorption in the proximal tubule, the total number of solute particles (osmoles) in a kilogram of water is still the same as in the original ultrafiltrate, which is the same as the plasma in the peritubular capillaries (assuming it is made protein-free). This filtrate's solute particles also vary greatly (e.g., more chloride and less sodium) compared to those in the initial ultrafiltrate.

In conclusion, the fluid volume has decreased by more than two-thirds as the filtrate exits the proximal tubule; important solutes such as proteins, glucose, and salts have been significantly reabsorbed either actively or passively; and the fluid's osmolality has not changed.

1.3.7. Water Reabsorption

All throughout the nephron, water is reabsorbed, except the thick and thin ascending limbs of the renal medulla's loops of Henle (Figure 1.13). Despite a significant osmotic gradient between the tubular lumen fluid and the medullary interstitium, the tubular epithelium in the ascending limbs is selectively impermeable to water. Water reabsorption in the remaining regions of the nephron is accomplished by osmosis working in concert with the tubular epithelium. The membrane or barrier that prevents water from diffusing into the interstitium (paracellular diffusion) or into the cells themselves (transcellular diffusion) is provided by the epithelium. Throughout the nephron, changes occur in the tubular epithelium's anatomic structure, particularly in the features of its intercellular spaces. The amount of water that is eventually reabsorbed by the nephron, as well as the location and timing of this absorption, are determined by these epithelial properties, which are governed by physiological demands and hormonal regulation.

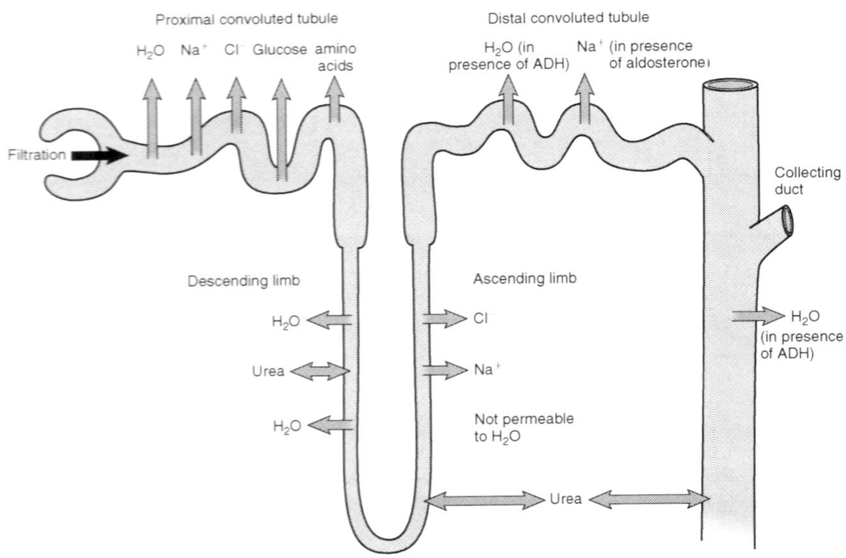

Figure 1.13. *Tubular reabsorption of solutes and water in various segments of the nephron.*

Source: *Nancy A. Brunzel. Fundamentals of Urine & Body Fluid Analysis. Elsevier. ISBN: 978-1-4377-0989-6.*

The transfer of water across a membrane from a solution with a low osmolality to one with a higher osmolality is known as osmosis. Because the cell membrane is semipermeable, some solutes can pass through it while others cannot. A gradient of osmolality (i.e., two regions with different concentrations of solute particles per volume of solvent) causes water to diffuse across the membrane in an effort to achieve an osmotic equilibrium. The massive reabsorption of water by the renal tubules is exclusively the result of this passive mechanism. The renal medulla's high solute concentration, or hypertonicity, is essential to this process because it creates the required osmotic gradient.

1.3.8. Renal Concentrating Mechanism

The body's only tissue that is hypertonic in comparison to normal plasma (i.e., The renal medulla (its osmolality is greater than 290 mOsm/kg). Hypertonicity gradually rises in medullary tissue; it is lowest near the border with the isosmotic cortex and highest in the renal pyramid papillary tips. All the constituents in the medullary interstitium—tissue cells, interstitial fluid, blood vessels, and blood—share this growing hypertonicity. Two countercurrent mechanisms: (1) an "active" countercurrent multiplier mechanism occurring in the loops of Henle, and (2) a "passive" countercurrent exchange mechanism involving the vasa recta, are responsible for establishing and maintaining the gradient hypertonicity of the medullary interstitium. The name "countercurrent mechanism" refers to the perfectly symmetric parallel structures of the vasa recta and the Henle loops, which lie near one another and contain fluid flowing in opposing directions in their ascending and descending segments. The ascending limb of the loop of Henle is practically impermeable to water, actively reabsorbing sodium and chloride into the medullary interstitium (see Figure 1.13). The tonicity of the interstitium rises during this active process, i.e., the lumen fluid's tonicity drops as the solute concentration rises. Water easily enters the interstitium in the descending limb at the same time that solutes—aside from urea—are not reabsorbed. As a result, the osmolality of the fluid in the descending limb and the interstitium equalizes and rises above that of the fluid in the ascending limb (Figure 1.14, A).

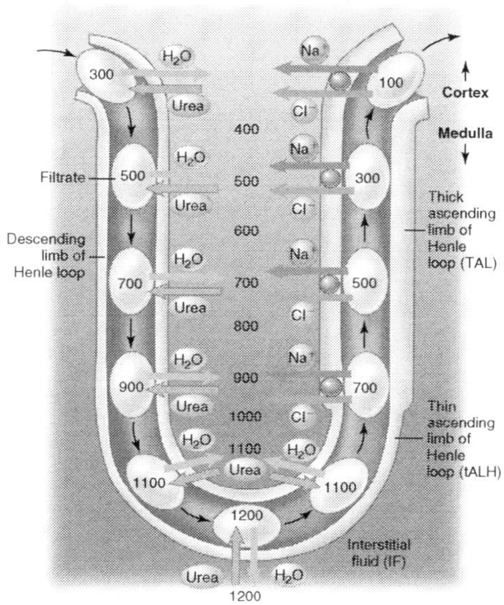

A

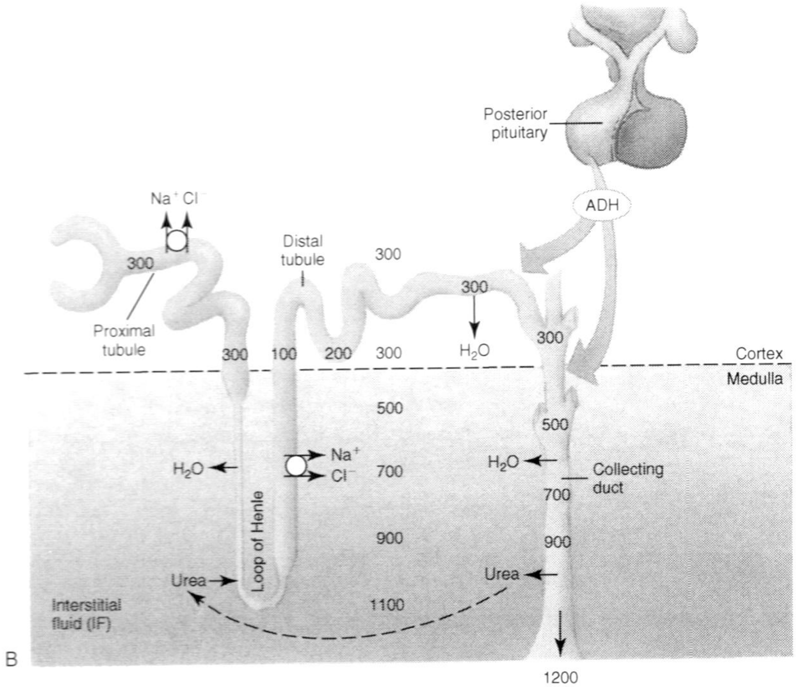

Figure 1.14. *The countercurrent multiplier mechanism and the urea cycle maintain the hypertonicity of the medulla. A: In the loop of Henle, note that the fluid leaving the loop is slightly hypo-osmotic (100) compared with the fluid entering the loop (300). B: Countercurrent mechanisms in an entire nephron.*

Source: *Nancy A. Brunzel. Fundamentals of Urine & Body Fluid Analysis. Elsevier. ISBN: 978–1-4377–0989–6.*

A gradient of hypertonicity forms as a result of this process, with the interstitium and the descending limb fluid getting increasingly more concentrated. Observe that the lumen fluid's intratubular osmolality difference from cortex to medulla is noticeably larger than the difference observed laterally (i.e., in ascending and descending tubules, at the same level). Countercurrent processes, in which sodium and chloride are actively reabsorbed in the ascending limb while water is passively reabsorbed in the descending limb, have essentially "multiplied" the osmotic gradient within the tubule from the cortex to the medulla.

When the lumen fluid in the loop of Henle becomes concentrated in the descending limb and then becomes diluted (by solute removal) in the ascending limb, it seems that the countercurrent multiplier mechanism has not done much at first. Overall, the fluid inside the tubular lumen is somewhat hypotonic compared to what was initially supplied to the Henle loop (Table 1.4). But the main function of the countercurrent multiplier mechanism is to create and preserve the gradient hypertonicity in the medullary interstitium rather than to concentrate the lumen fluid. The lumen fluid then condenses or dilutes to form the final urine when it reaches the collecting tubules, which pass through every part of the renal cortex and the medulla.

Table 1.4. Tubular Lumen Fluid Osmolality throughout the Nephron

Tubule Segment	Osmolality Change
Proximal tubule	Enters: isosmotic Exits: isosmotic
Loop of Henle	Enters: isosmotic
Thin descending limb	Becomes progressively hyperosmotic
U-turn	Maximally hyperosmotic
Thick ascending limb (medullary and cortical)	Becomes progressively hypo-osmotic Exits: slightly hypo-osmotic
Distal tubule (convoluted portion)	Enters: slightly hypo-osmotic Exits: isosmotic
Collecting tubules	Enters: isosmotic Exits: varies, under ADH control; can be hyperisosmotic, hypo-osmotic, or isosmotic

Source: Nancy A. Brunzel. Fundamentals of Urine & Body Fluid Analysis. Elsevier. ISBN: 978-1-4377-0989-6.

The second countercurrent mechanism, on the other hand, is a "passive" exchange process that takes place in the renal medulla's deep vascular bed. Here, water and reabsorbed solutes in the medullary interstitium diffuse into the vasa recta passively. The blood's osmolality increases as it moves toward the papillary tips but gradually decreases as it ascends to the renal cortex, much like the countercurrent mechanism in the tubular lumens. Both the removal of reabsorbed water for distribution throughout the body and the supply of nutrients to medullary tissue are made possible by this vascular countercurrent mechanism. As a result, these activities also keep the renal medulla hypertonic.

The lumen fluid exiting the distal tubules is isosmotic, despite the significant solute and water exchanges occurring in the tubules until this point. The last osmolality change takes place in the collecting tubules (or ducts), the final tubular segment of the nephron; the final urine is either concentrated, diluted, or stays unchanged. It is significant to remember that the tubules selectively avoid reabsorption of water rather than secreting it.

Hormonal control governs the simultaneous processes of solute exchange and water reabsorption in the collecting tubules. Two separate and independent hormonal processes regulate the absorption of water and sodium as the isosmotic lumen fluid enters the cortical collecting tubules. For sodium reabsorption, the renin-angiotensinaldosterone system is in charge. Reduced sodium, blood volume, or blood pressure cause the juxtaglomerular apparatus to release renin into the bloodstream, as illustrated in Figure 1.15. The fast formation of angiotensin II causes the adrenal cortex to release more aldosterone. Aldosterone then causes the distal and cortical collecting tubules to begin reabsorbing sodium.

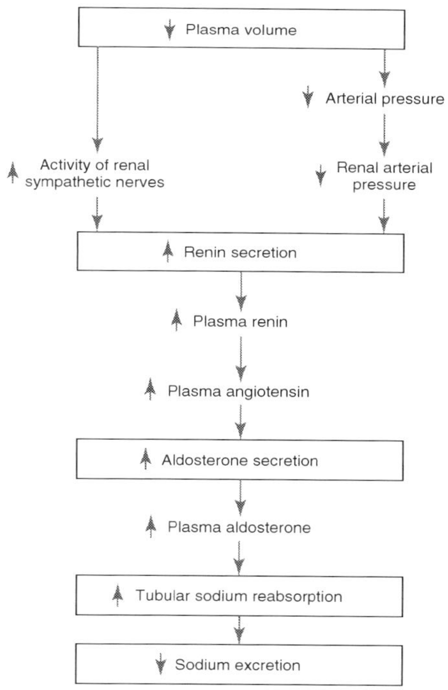

Figure 1.15. *A schematic representation of the renin-angiotensin-aldosterone system and its role in the tubular reabsorption of sodium.*

Source: Nancy A. Brunzel. Fundamentals of Urine & Body Fluid Analysis. Elsevier. ISBN: 978-1-4377-0989-6.

ADH (arginine vasopressin) must be present for the collecting tubules to reabsorb water. The hormone ADH is produced in the hypothalamus and travels to the posterior pituitary (neurohypophysis) via the neuronal stalk, where it is released into the bloodstream. The heart's vascular baroreceptors track arterial blood pressure. The hypothalamus receives a signal when arterial blood pressure rises, which inhibits the release of ADH into the bloodstream. A negative feedback mechanism is the term for this interactive process, which is depicted in Figure 1.16.

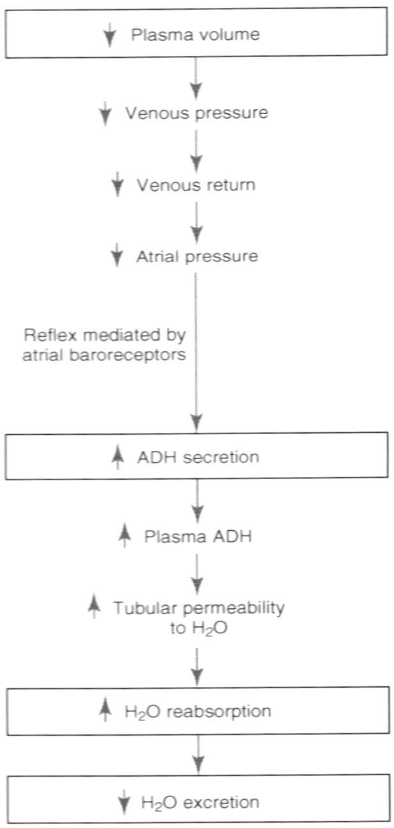

Figure 1.16. *A schematic representation of the mechanism controlling antidiuretic hormone secretion.*

Source: Nancy A. Brunzel. Fundamentals of Urine & Body Fluid Analysis. Elsevier. ISBN: 978-1-4377-0989-6.

The epithelium of collecting tubules changes as the plasma level of ADH drops, which results in a decrease in the amount of water moving from the lumen fluid into the medullary tissue. As a result, water is held in the lumen fluid, which causes the urine to become diluted (hypotonic or hypo-osmotic). On the other hand, ADH release is elevated when baroreceptors detect a drop in blood pressure. ADH stimulation results in changes to the collecting tubule epithelium, increased medullary osmolality that causes increased water reabsorption, and concentrated urine that is either hyperosmotic or hypotonic. Keep in mind that reabsorption of sodium and chloride is unaffected by ADH secretion.-

As the lumen fluid moves deeper into the medulla toward the papillary tips, the osmolality difference between the fluid in the tubules and the medullary interstitium increases. An initial ultrafiltrate osmolality of 290 mOsm/kg in Bowman's space can be concentrated in the final urine to as high as 900 to 1,400 mOsm/kg due to this enormous gradient. Urine osmolality can never be higher than that of the medullary interstitium because the final urine excreted is formed in equilibrium with the renal interstitium.

About half of the solutes concentrated in the renal medulla are normally explained by the countercurrent multiplier mechanism. The urea cycle, which keeps the medullary concentration of urea high, is responsible for half of the solutes present. As a consequence of protein breakdown, urea readily crosses the glomerular filtration barrier and enters the tubules as ultrafiltrate. 40 to 70% of urea is passively reabsorbed into the medullary interstitium, even though it is a metabolic waste product that the body does not need. Subsequently, urea diffuses into the lumen fluid in the Henle loops along its concentration gradient. In the presence of ADH, water is reabsorbed when the lumen fluid enters the cortical collecting tubules, but urea is not. Any additional reabsorption of water helps to concentrate the amount of urea in the lumen fluid. Within the medullary collecting tubules, urea and water (influenced by ADH) easily diffuse into the interstitium when the lumen fluid reaches them. Stated differently, the collecting tubule's cortical epithelium is impervious to urea, while the medullary epithelium is easily permeable. As a result, urea diffuses into the interstitium from the concentrated lumen fluid in the medullary collecting tubules along its concentration gradient until the urea concentration in both of these regions is equal. This urea equilibrium leads to two things happening: (1) the final urine's nonurea solutes are osmotically balanced by the sodium salts in the hypertonic medulla, and (2) urea itself determines the final urine's urea concentration. Urine flow rate is another factor that influences the final urine's urea concentration. More urea is reabsorbed when urine flows slower than 2 mL/min, but urea can still be reabsorbed at constant, minimal flow rates when urine flows faster than 2 mL/min.

In conclusion, the urea cycle and the countercurrent multiplier mechanism cause the medullary interstitium to become hypertonic. The presence of ADH controls the hypertonic medulla, which is created by these two processes and offers a strong osmotic force for water reabsorption from the collecting tubules in response to physiological demands. The concentration of the final urine excreted is ultimately determined by the collecting tubules' regulation of water content, even though solutes like sodium (under aldosterone control) can be selectively reabsorbed or excreted in the distal and collecting tubules. Put another way, solute exchange may take place as isosmotic fluid from the distal tubule enters the collecting tubule; however, the total number of solutes (i.e., osmoles) stays fixed. What changes is the amount of water in which these solutes are expelled? Therefore, whether a concentrated (hypertonic) or diluted (hypotonic) final urine is produced depends on the reabsorption of water by the collecting tubules under ADH control (Maddox & Brenner, 2004; Briggs, Kriz, Schnermann, 2005; Alpern & Hebert, 2008).

1.4. Endocrine Functions of the Kidney

The kidney performs many vital endocrine tasks, such as producing hormones that control fluid balance, blood pressure regulation, red blood cell production, and the body's potassium and calcium balance.

1.4.1. Renin–Angiotensin–Aldosterone System

The kidney is essential for preserving the body's volume and electrolyte balance because it produces renin. A variety of cells, but most notably the granular cells in the juxtaglomerular apparatus, release the proteolytic enzyme renin into the blood in response to sympathetic stimulation and extracellular fluid volume depletion. Angiotensinogen, a globulin the liver forms in the blood, is changed into angiotensin I by renin. ACE then transforms angiotensin I into angiotensin II. ACE is found on blood vessel capillary endothelium, particularly in the brain, kidneys, and lungs. Angiotensin II is an effective vasoconstrictor that works via the AT-1 receptor. Through both direct and indirect mechanisms, angiotensin II increases the kidney's ability to retain Na^+. Through an increase in Na^+/H^+ exchanger activity, angiotensin II improves Na^+ reabsorption in the proximal tubule. In the adrenal cortex, angiotensin II also increases the production of aldosterone. After that, aldosterone stimulates Na^+ reabsorption via the cortical collecting duct in return for K^+ secretion.

Angiotensin II more severely constricts the efferent arteriole in the glomerulus than the afferent arteriole. Maintaining glomerular filtration requires an increase in glomerular hydrostatic pressure. Angiotensin II also causes the release of catecholamines, the stimulation of sympathetic nerve activity, the stimulation of thirst, and the release of ADH.

By inhibiting ACE and preventing the conversion of angiotensin I to II, medications like lisinopril can block the effects of the renin-angiotensin system. We call these medications ACE inhibitors. A comparable result can be achieved by medications (such as losartan) that impede the angiotensin II (AT-1) receptor. Patients with hypertension can effectively lower their blood pressure with the help of either of these agents. These medications also reduce glomerular filtration and glomerular hydrostatic pressure. These medications reduce glomerular hydrostatic pressure, which lessens proteinuria and slows the progressive loss of kidney function in patients with chronic kidney disease.

1.4.2. Erythropoietin

Proximal tubular epithelial cells and cortical interstitial cells in the kidney produce erythropoietin, a glycosylated protein. It promotes the bone marrow's erythrocytes to mature. Anemia is caused by erythropoietin deficiency or underproduction, as chronic kidney disease patients have shown. Patients with chronic kidney disease can effectively treat their anemia with recombinant erythropoietin preparations.

1.4.3. 1,25-Dihydroxyvitamin D_3 (Calcitriol)

The active form of vitamin D, calcitriol, is necessary for the mineralization of bones and the absorption of calcium. A steroid called vitamin D3 is either produced in the skin when exposed to UV light or is consumed through diet. It is transformed into 25-hydroxyvitamin D3 in the liver and then hydroxylated once more into the active metabolite 1,25-dihydroxyvitamin D3 (calcitriol) in the kidney's proximal tubular epithelial cells by the enzyme 1-α hydroxylase. The kidney produces more calcitriol when parathyroid hormone is present because it increases the synthesis of 1-α hydroxylase.

Calcitriol serves the body in many vital ways. Through improved calcium absorption in the gastrointestinal system, it keeps serum calcium levels stable. Through the calcification of osteoid tissue, it encourages the formation of healthy bones. By reducing the synthesis and release of parathyroid hormones, it also directly inhibits the activity of the parathyroid glands. Metabolic bone disease can arise from insufficient calcitriol in patients with chronic kidney disease. For patients with kidney disease, calcitriol and various synthetic vitamin D analogs are now available (Maddox & Brenner, 2004; Briggs, Kriz, Schnermann, 2005; Alpern & Hebert, 2008).

A Closer Look

How Can Kidney Function Be Measured?

To assess someone's kidney function, we would ideally measure their glomerular filtration rate (GFR). This can be done using a radioisotope tracer that is cleared from the blood solely by glomerular filtration, such as Cr-51 EDTA or Tc-99m DTPA. This technique is useful for research and when precise measurements of GFR are required but it is impractical for routine repeated measurements. Routine assessment of kidney function uses the concentration of a substance produced by the body: creatinine, urea or cystatin C. The concentration of these substances is determined by the balance between the rates of their production and excretion. When the rates of production and excretion remain stable, equilibrium is reached.

The rate of excretion of a substance by filtration depends upon the volume filtered per unit of time and the concentration of the substance in the filtrate. If the volume filtered per unit of time—the glomerular filtration rate—is kept constant, the concentration in the blood depends upon the production rate. If the production rate is kept constant, the concentration in the blood depends upon the excretion rate. When production and excretion are stable and in equilibrium, the volume of water in which a substance is dissolved does not affect its concentration. For example, patients who are chronically fluid-overloaded do not have a lower concentration of urea due to dilution. Conversely, the higher concentration of urea found in patients who are dehydrated is due to the reduced excretion of urea, not hemoconcentration.

The ideal substance to be used to measure glomerular filtration would be produced at a constant rate, freely filtered by glomeruli, and neither reabsorbed nor secreted by the tubules. Creatinine fulfills some but not all of these criteria. It is released into the bloodstream at a fairly constant rate from the breakdown of creatine in healthy skeletal muscles and is freely filtered by the glomeruli. However, 10 to 20% of total creatinine excretion is by secretion into the tubules. As GFR declines, tubular secretion keeps the creatinine concentration lower than would otherwise be the case. This is shown by comparing measurements of serum creatinine and GFR (Figure 1.17).

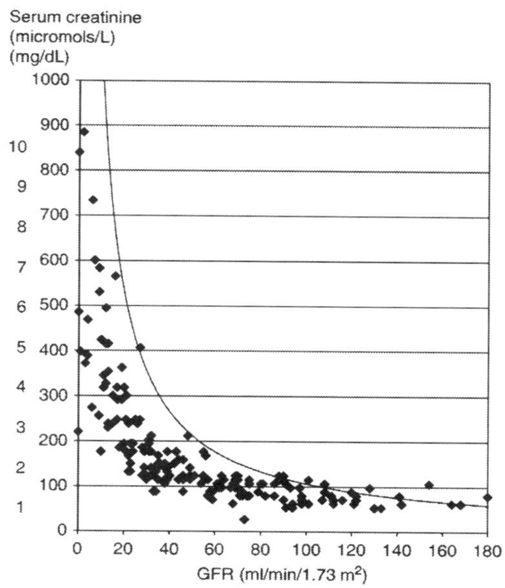

Figure 1.17. *Simultaneous measurements of serum creatinine and GFR (by inulin clearance) in over 100 individuals. The continuous line represents the*

relationship between serum creatinine and GFR that would be found if creatinine was only filtered by glomeruli and not secreted by the tubules.

Source: Hugh C. Rayner, Mark E. Thomas, and David V. Milford. Understanding Kidney Diseases, Second edition. Springer. https://doi.org/10.1007/978-3-030-43027-6.

The curved relationship between creatinine and GFR makes changes in serum creatinine hard to interpret. Figure 1.18 shows a graph of serum creatinine against time in a man with declining kidney function. The shape of the line suggests that the rate of loss of kidney function accelerates over the years.

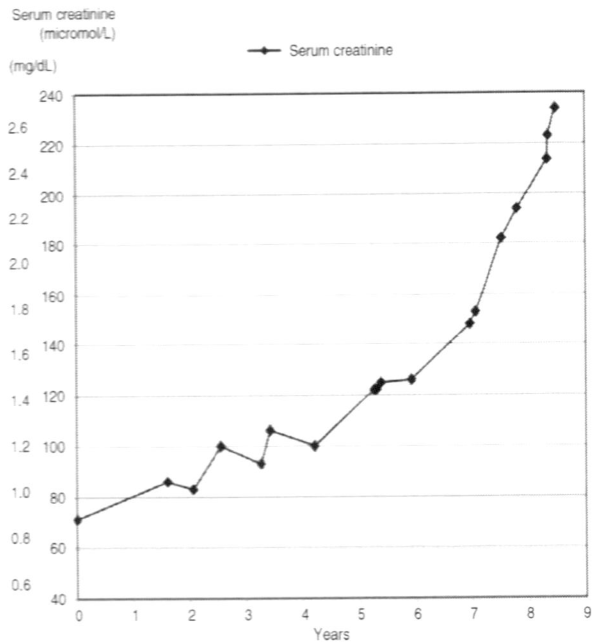

Figure 1.18. *A graph of serum creatinine against time in a man with declining kidney function.*

Source: Hugh C. Rayner, Mark E. Thomas, and David V. Milford. Understanding Kidney Diseases, Second edition. Springer. https://doi.org/10.1007/978-3-030-43027-6.

If we now add in GFR values, it is clear that kidney function has actually declined at a constant rate over the whole period (Figure 1.19).

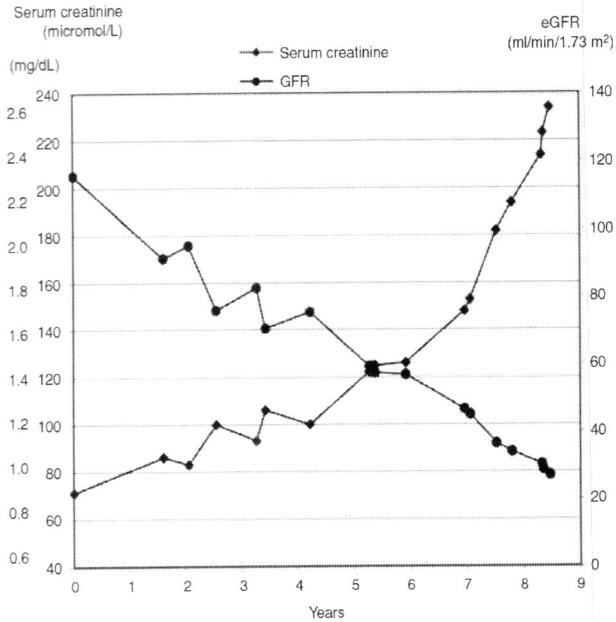

Figure 1.19. *A graph of serum creatinine and GFR against time in a man with declining kidney function.*

Source: Hugh C. Rayner, Mark E. Thomas, and David V. Milford. Understanding Kidney Diseases, Second edition. Springer. https://doi.org/10.1007/978-3-030-43027-6.

Because of the inverse curved relationship between GFR and creatinine, the drop in eGFR from 116 to 60 during the first 5 years causes a smaller increase in serum creatinine than the decline from 60 to 30 over the next 3 years.

Summary

- The kidneys regulate the excretion of excess ingested water, electrolytes, and products of metabolism as well as foreign substances, including drugs and toxins. The kidneys maintain the volume of body fluid as well as its electrolyte composition, pH, and osmolality.
- The kidneys are located behind the peritoneal cavity (retroperitoneal) in the abdomen on either side of the midline. Each kidney weighs approximately 150 g and measures 10 to 12 cm in length. The kidneys are highly vascular organs, receiving 20% of the cardiac output (the greatest amount of blood per 100 g of tissue in the body) via the renal arteries that originate from the abdominal aorta. Each kidney contains 400,000 to 1,200,000 functional units called nephrons.
- The nephron is the functional unit of the kidney, and it consists of a glomerulus and a tubule. Glomeruli are clusters of specialized capillaries contained within the Bowman's capsule in the cortex of the kidney. Blood enters glomeruli through the afferent arterioles and leaves through the efferent arterioles. The urine begins as a glomerular ultrafiltrate (blood minus plasma proteins) that drains from the glomerulus to the tubule.
- Each kidney is usually supplied by a single (at times double) renal artery, which arises from the aorta. The glomerular capillaries are unique in that they are situated between two arterioles: the afferent arteriole, which arises from branches of the renal artery and brings blood to the glomerular capillaries, and the efferent arteriole, which drains the glomerular capillaries. After the glomerulus, the efferent arteriole branches into a cluster of peritubular capillaries that intimately surrounds the tubules.
- Glomeruli are clusters of capillaries that are surrounded by Bowman's capsules and lined with a single layer of epithelial cells called the parietal epithelium. The afferent arteriole supplies the glomerulus, and the efferent arteriole drains it; the proximal tubule drains filtrate from the Bowman's space. Glomerular capillaries are unique in that they are placed between two arterioles
- The tubule of the nephron is divided into several segments. The different segments of the tubules have different structures and play different roles in modifying the content and amount of the final urine that is excreted. The proximal tubule arises from the glomerulus in the cortex. After a convoluted course, the proximal tubule descends into the medulla and becomes the loop of Henle.
- Renal blood flow (RBF) and glomerular filtration rate (GFR) are important aspects of maintaining proper kidney function. RBF is the amount of blood that passes through the kidney's glomeruli, while GFR is the volume of plasma filtered per unit of time. RBF and GFR normally change in parallel, so an increase in RBF causes an increase in GFR.
- The tubular function is selective, reabsorbing the substances necessary for the maintenance of body homeostasis and function, such as water, salts, glucose, amino acids, and proteins, while excreting waste products such as creatinine and metabolic acids.
- The kidney has several important endocrine functions, including the production of hormones that regulate fluid status, the maintenance of blood pressure, red blood cell production, and the body's potassium and calcium balance (Maddox & Brenner, 2004; Briggs, Kriz, & Schnermann, 2005; Alpern & Hebert, 2008).

References

1. Alpern, R. J., & Hebert, S. C. (2008). *Seldin and Giebisch's the Kidney: Physiology and Pathophysiology* (4th ed.). Academic Press/Elsevier.
2. Anderson, S. C., & Cockayne, S. (2003). *Clinical Chemistry: Concepts and Applications.* McGraw-Hill.
3. Bertram, J. F., Douglas-Denton, R. N., Diouf, B., et al. (2011). Human nephron number: Implications for health and disease. *Pediatric Nephrology, 26*(9), 1529–1533.
4. Briggs, J. P., Kriz, W., & Schnermann, J. (2005). Overview of kidney function and structure. In A. Greenberg (Ed.), *Primer on Kidney Diseases* (4th ed., pp. 2–19). National Kidney Foundation.
5. Goldman, L., & Bennett, J. C. (2000). *Cecil Textbook of Medicine* (21st ed.). WB Saunders.
6. Hughson, M., Farris, A. B., III, Douglas-Denton, R., et al. (2003). Glomerular number and size in autopsy kidneys: The relationship to birth weight. *Kidney International, 63*(6), 2113–2122.
7. Keller, G., Zimmer, G., Mall, G., et al. (2003). Nephron number in patients with primary hypertension. *New England Journal of Medicine, 348*(2), 101–108.
8. Longmire, M., Choyke, P. L., & Kobayashi, H. (2008). Clearance properties of nano-sized particles and molecules as imaging agents: Considerations and caveats. *Nanoscience, 3*, 703–717.
9. Luyckx, V. A., & Brenner, B. M. (2005). Low birth weight, nephron number, and kidney disease. *Kidney International Supplements*, S68–S77.
10. Maddox, D. A., & Brenner, B. M. (2004). Glomerular ultrafiltration. In B. M. Brenner (Ed.), *Brenner & Rector's the Kidney* (7th ed., pp. 353–412). Saunders.
11. National Kidney Foundation. (2002). K/DOQI clinical practice guidelines for chronic kidney disease: Evaluation, classification, and stratification. *American Journal of Kidney Diseases, 39*(Suppl 1), S1–S266.
12. Nyengaard, J. R., & Bendtsen, T. F. (1992). Glomerular number and size in relation to age, kidney weight, and body surface in normal man. *Anatomical Record, 232*(2), 194–201.
13. Patton, K. T., & Thibodeau, G. A. (2010). Urinary system. In *Anatomy and physiology* (7th ed.). Mosby/Elsevier.
14. Pincus, M. R., Preuss, H. G., & Henry, J. B. (2001). Evaluation of renal function, water, electrolytes, acid-base balance, and blood gases. In J. B. Henry (Ed.), *Clinical Diagnosis and Management by Laboratory Methods* (20th ed.). WB Saunders.
15. Scheinman, S. J., Guy-Woodford, L. M., Thakker, R. V., & Warnock, D. G. (1999). Genetic disorders of renal electrolyte transport. *New England Journal of Medicine, 340*, 1177–1187.
16. Schrier, R. W., & Gottschalk, C. W. (2001). *Diseases of the Kidney and Urinary Tract* (7th ed.). Lippincott Williams & Wilkins.
17. Stevens, L. A., & Levey, A. S. (2005). Measurement of kidney function. *Medical Clinics of North America, 89*(3), 454–473.

Chapter

2

RENAL PHYSIOLOGY: ACID-BASE BALANCE AND BLOOD PRESSURE REGULATION

Contents

Introduction

Renal physiology is critical to maintaining homeostasis within the body, particularly through the regulation of acid-base balance and blood pressure. The kidneys play a pivotal role in ensuring that the pH levels of blood remain within a narrow range, which is essential for normal cellular function. They achieve this by selectively reabsorbing bicarbonate (HCO_3^-) from the urine and secreting hydrogen ions (H^+) into the urine. This process helps to neutralize excess acids in the body, maintaining the acid-base equilibrium. Additionally, the kidneys produce ammonia, which aids in buffering urine and allows for the excretion of more hydrogen ions.

Beyond acid-base balance, the kidneys are integral in regulating blood pressure. They do this through the renin-angiotensin-aldosterone system (RAAS), a hormone cascade that responds to changes in blood pressure and volume. When blood pressure drops, the kidneys release renin, an enzyme that converts angiotensinogen, a blood protein, into angiotensin I. Angiotensin I is then converted into angiotensin II by the action of the angiotensin-converting enzyme (ACE) primarily in the lungs. Angiotensin II acts as a potent vasoconstrictor, narrowing blood vessels and thus increasing blood pressure. It also stimulates the release of aldosterone from the adrenal cortex, which prompts the kidneys to reabsorb sodium and water, further increasing blood volume and pressure.

The kidneys also influence blood pressure through their regulation of blood volume. By adjusting the volume of urine excreted, the kidneys control the amount of water retained in the body. This ability to conserve or expel water is crucial in response to changes in hydration status or blood pressure. For instance, in conditions of low blood pressure or dehydration, the kidneys will conserve water, producing concentrated urine. Conversely, in states of fluid overload or high blood pressure, the kidneys will excrete more water, producing dilute urine.

Moreover, the kidneys release various hormones that impact cardiovascular health. Erythropoietin (EPO), for example, stimulates the production of red blood cells in response to low oxygen levels, thereby improving oxygen transport and supporting overall circulatory efficiency. Additionally, the kidneys synthesize and secrete prostaglandins and kinins, which have local vasodilatory effects that can influence renal blood flow and systemic blood pressure.

Renal physiology encompasses critical functions that maintain acid-base balance and regulate blood pressure, essential for overall homeostasis. The kidneys' ability to filter blood, reabsorb essential nutrients, secrete waste, and produce hormones underscores their multifaceted role in sustaining life. By meticulously managing the body's internal environment, the kidneys ensure that the physiological conditions remain optimal for the functioning of various organ systems.

Orientation and Directional Terms

Term	Definition	Illustration
Angiotensin-Converting Enzyme (ACE)	Angiotensin-converting enzyme is a central component of the renin–angiotensin system, which controls blood pressure by regulating the volume of fluids in the body. It converts the hormone angiotensin I to the active vasoconstrictor angiotensin II.	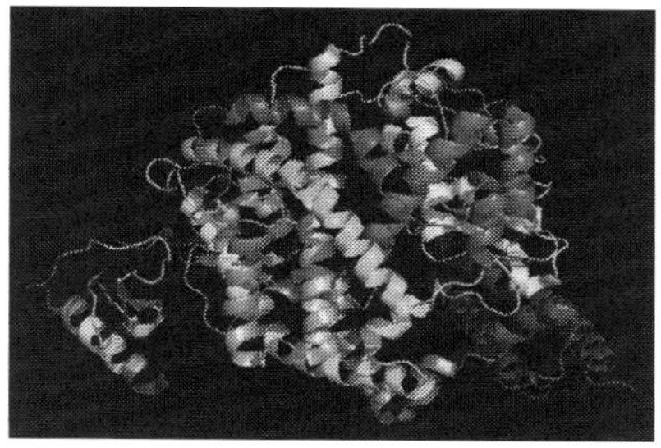
Renin-angiotensin-Aldosterone System (RAAS)	Renin-angiotensin-aldosterone system (RAAS) is a regulator of blood pressure and cardiovascular function. Dysregulated RAAS is implicated in high blood pressure, cardiovascular and kidney conditions, and medications targeting RAAS can improve these conditions.	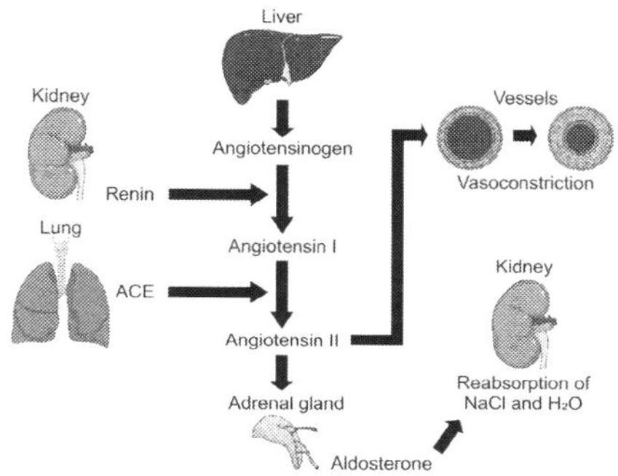
Carbonic Anhydrase (CA)	Carbonic anhydrases form a family of enzymes that catalyze the interconversion between carbon dioxide and water and the dissociated ions of carbonic acid. The active site of most carbonic anhydrases contains a zinc ion. They are therefore classified as metalloenzymes.	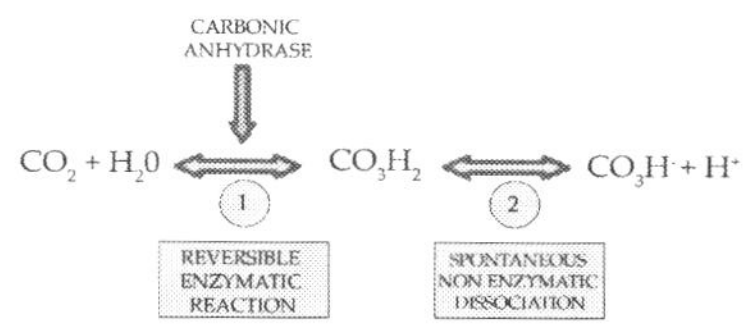
Apical Membrane	Apical membrane of proximal tubular epithelial cells contains numerous microvilli that form the brush border. The brush border contains enzymes that carry out the specialized functions of the proximal tubule. Intracellular enzymes can be released into the urine due to injury either by exocytosis or leakage.	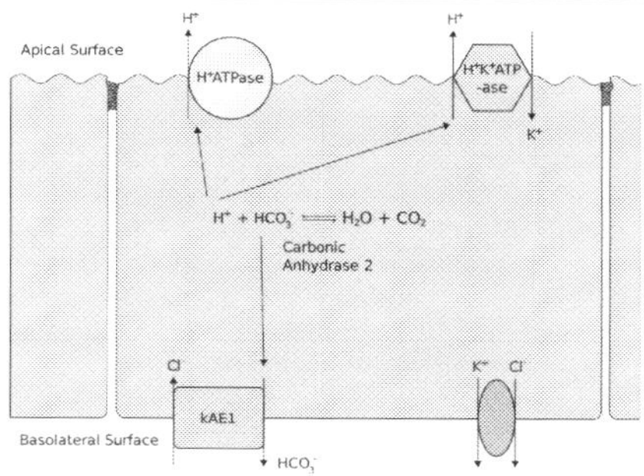

Parathyroid Hormone (PTH)	Parathyroid hormone is directly involved in the bones, kidneys, and small intestine. In the bones, PTH stimulates the release of calcium in an indirect process through osteoclasts which ultimately leads to the resorption of the bones.	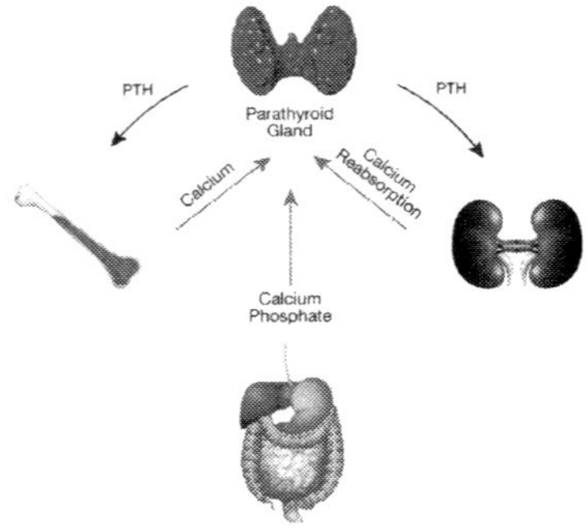
Extracellular Fluid (ECF)	Extracellular fluid (ECF) is the fluid that is not contained within the cells. ECF accounts for around 33% of the body's total water content. Extracellular fluid is made up of interstitial fluid, blood plasma, lymph, and transcellular fluid. Interstitial fluid (IF) is the fluid that surrounds the cells.	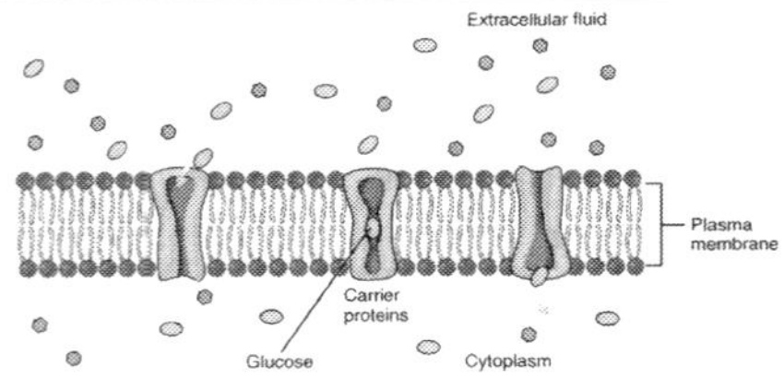
Hormone Aldosterone	Aldosterone (ALD) is a hormone that helps regulate your blood pressure by managing the levels of sodium (salt) and potassium in your blood and impacting blood volume. Having too much or too little aldosterone in your body can cause health issues.	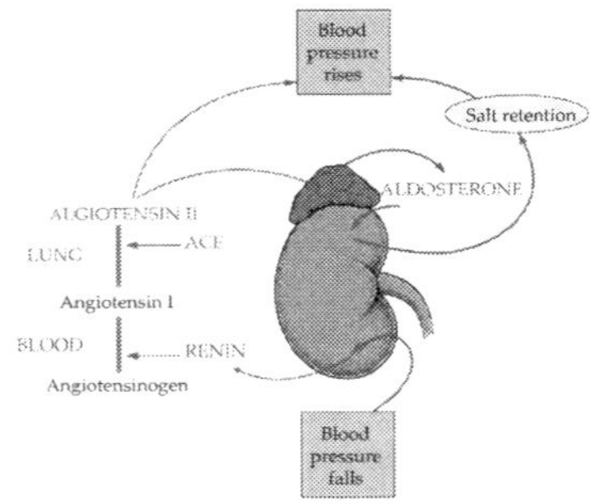

2.1. The Kidney and Acid-Base Regulation

An essential component of homeostasis, the body's acid-base balance, is preserved in large part by the kidneys. Because even small variations in blood pH can have a substantial impact on cellular function and metabolic processes, this regulation is crucial. The function of the kidneys in maintaining the systemic acid-base balance in relation to the lungs. As seen in Figure 2.1, this. The bulk of calories consumed in a normal diet come from fats and carbohydrates. O_2 and insulin are needed for the full metabolism of fats and carbohydrates, which produces CO_2 and H_2O. The 20 mol/day of CO_2 produced is expelled with normal lung function, and the acid-base balance in the body is unaffected. Because of the following reaction:

$$CO_2 + H_2O \leftrightarrow H_2CO_3 \leftrightarrow HCO_3^- + H^+ \quad (1)$$

alterations in ventilation, by changing the Pco_2 of the blood, will alter blood pH (e.g., an increase in Pco_2 produces acidosis, whereas a decrease in Pco_2 produces alkalosis).

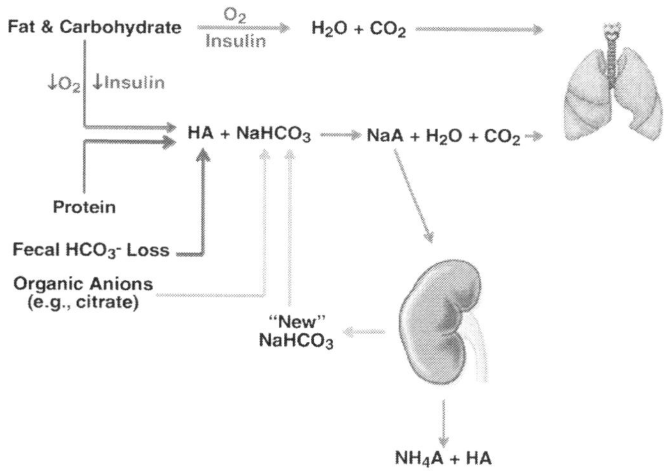

Figure 2.1. *Overview of the role of the kidneys in acid-base balance.*

Source: *https://journals.physiology.org/doi/epdf/10.1152/advan.00054.2009.*

Depending on the particular amino acid, the metabolism of protein can result in the production of acids or alkali. But the breakdown of dietary protein results in the production of net acids (e.g., H_2SO_4 HCl).

$$HCl + NaHCO_3 \rightarrow NaCl + CO_2 + H_2O \quad (2)$$

$$H_2SO_4 + 2NaHCO_3 \rightarrow Na_2SO_4 + 2CO_2 + 2H_2O \quad (3)$$

The lungs expel the CO_2 produced during this buffering process, but the kidneys expel the Na^+ salts of the acids, mostly along with NH_4^+ (NH4Cl and $(NH_4)_2SO_4$). HCO_3^- is produced during the excretion of NH_4^+ and is subsequently added back to the blood to make up for the HCO_3^- lost during the titration of the nonvolatile acid.

Alkali are produced as a result of other food ingredients. For instance, H+ is consumed (i.e., when organic anions are converted to CO_2 and H_2O, HCO_3^- is generated). In terms of nutrition, meat, grains, and dairy products produce acid, while fruits and vegetables produce alkali. Furthermore, the diet might include a variety of acids and alkalis that increase the body's net acid/alkali load when absorbed through the digestive system. Ultimately, every day, the body absorbs an acid load from the HCO_3 lost in the feces. A healthy person eating a "typical Western diet" adds a net amount of acid to their body. This acid produces an equivalent loss of HCO_3^-, which needs to be replaced. This process is known as net endogenous acid production or NEAP. Significantly, the kidneys produce HCO_3^- while excreting acid. Thus, when renal net acid excretion (RNAE) equals NEAP, the systemic acid-base balance is preserved.

RNAE excretion can be quantitated by measuring the excretion of NH_4^+, titratable acid (TA), and HCO_3^- (note that the excretion of H^+ is ignored, since even at a urine pH of 4.0, the concentration of H^+ = 0.1 meq/l):

$$RNAE = U_{NH_4^+} \times V + U_{TA} \times V - U_{HCO_3^-} \times V \quad (4)$$

where V is the rate of urine flow and U is the concentration of urine. When consuming a standard Western diet, NEAP is approximately 1 meq·kg body weight^{-1}·**day**$^{-1}$. RNAE has to be the same as a result. It is imperative that students understand that the nephron's cells transport H+ and HCO_3^-, which facilitates the excretion of RNAE. The kidneys reabsorb the filtered load of HCO_3^-, titrate urinary buffers, excrete NH_4^+, and acidify the urine through the action of different H^+ and HCO_3-transporters (Hamm, Alpern, Preisig, 2008. Hamm & Nakhoul, 2008; Koeppen & Stanton, 2008).

2.1.1. HCO_3^- Reabsorption

The nephron's cells release H+ into the tubular fluid, which allows them to reabsorb the HCO_3^- filtered load. Figure 2.2 illustrates how each nephron segment contributes to this process. The filtered load of HCO_3^- is greater than 4,300 meq/day at a plasma HCO_3^- concentration of 24 meq/l and a glomerular filtration rate of 180 l/day. Proximal tubule reabsorption accounts for about 80% of this filtered load. The distal convoluted tubule and thick ascending limb reabsorb 16% more, with the collecting duct reabsorbing the remaining four percent.

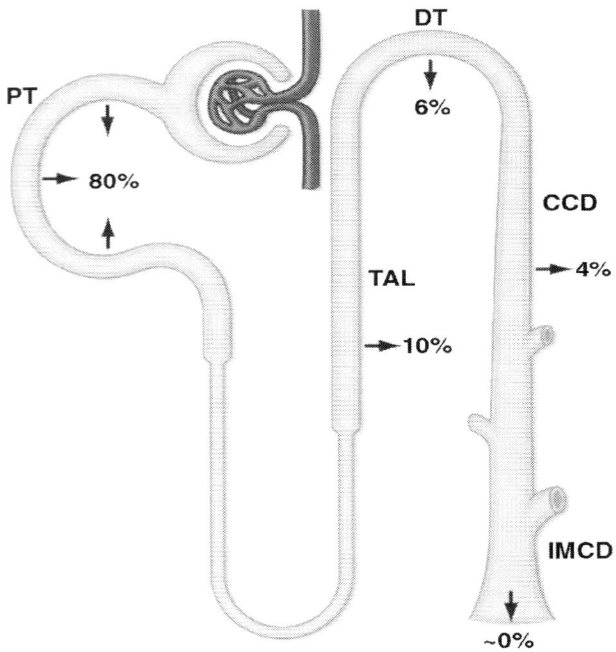

Figure 2.2. *Segmental HCO_3^- reabsorption. The percentage of the filtered load reabsorbed by each segment of the nephron is indicated. PT, proximal tubule; TAL, thick ascending limb of the loop of Henle; DT, distal convoluted tubule; CCD, cortical collecting duct; IMCD, inner medullary collecting duct.*

Source: *https://journals.physiology.org/doi/epdf/10.1152/advan.00054.2009.*

Figure 2.3 illustrates the cellular processes by which H^+ and HCO_3^- are transferred across the proximal tubule's basolateral and apical membranes. There are two ways that H+ is secreted across the apical membrane. Na^+/H^+ antiporter Na^+/H^+ exchanger 3 (NHE3) is the main mechanism. It is estimated that H+ secretion by NHE3 accounts for two-thirds of proximal HCO_3^- reabsorption. Vacuolar H^+-ATPase is accountable for roughly one-third of HCO3- reabsorption and offers an additional pathway for apical H^+ secretion.

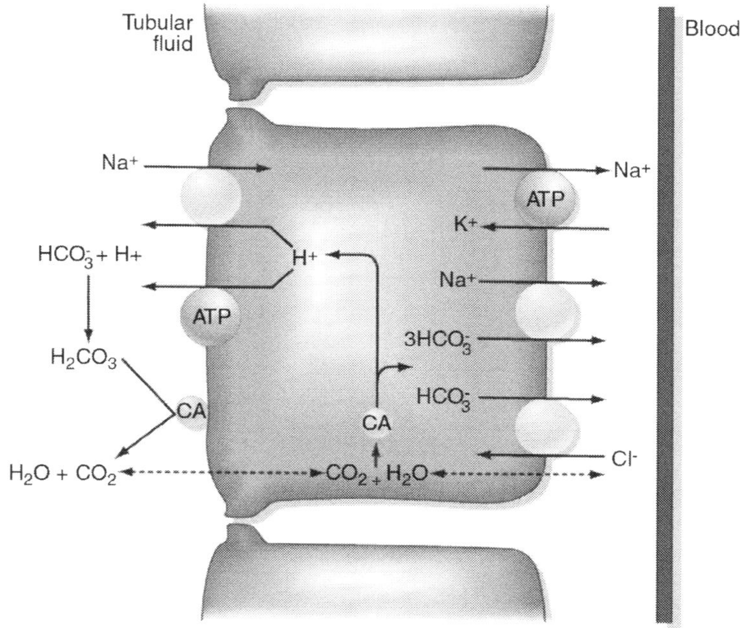

Figure 2.3. *Cellular mechanism for proximal tubule H^+ and HCO_3^- transport. CA, carbonic anhydrase.*

Source: *https://journals.physiology.org/doi/full/10.1152/advan.00054.2009.*

Carbonic anhydrase (CA), as demonstrated in Figure 2.3, is crucial to the H^+ section and HCO_3^- reabsorption processes. CA-II promotes the production of H^+ and HCO_3^- within the cell. The HCO_3^- then exits the cell via the basolateral membrane, while the H^+ is secreted into the tubular fluid through the apical membrane. The conversion of luminal carbonic acid into H_2O and CO_2 is facilitated by membrane-bound CA (CA-IV).

Exit of HCO_3^- from the cell across the basolateral membrane occurs primarily via a $3HCO_3^-$-Na^+ symporter [the electrogenic Na^+-HCO_3^- cotransporter (NBCe1)]. There is also evidence that some HCO_3^- exits the cell in exchange for Cl^-.

The exact same cellular mechanisms that were previously described for the proximal tubule also govern the reabsorption of HCO_3^- by cells in the distal convoluted tubule and the thick ascending limb of the loop of Henle. Nonetheless, there are variations in certain transporter isoforms. One example is the electroneutral Na^+-HCO_3-HCO_3-symporter (NBCn1), which facilitates the exit of HCO_3^- from thick ascending limb cells. Furthermore, a K^+-HCO_3-symporter and an anion exchanger 2 (AE-2) exchange some of the HCO_3-out of these cells for Cl^-. Lastly, the NHE2 isoform may be the apical membrane Na^+/H^+ antiporter in the distal convoluted tubule.

H^+ and HCO_3^- transport in the collecting duct is carried out by intercalated cells (refer to Figure 2.4). Vacuolar H^+-ATPase and H^+-K^+-ATPase are localized to the apical membrane of acid-secreting intercalated cells, and HCO_3^- leaves the cells via the basolateral membrane in exchange for Cl^- (AE-1). Vacuolar H^+-ATPase is located in the basolateral membrane of the less common HCO_3^- secreting cell, while pendrin, a distinct Cl^-/HCO_3^- antiporter, is located in the apical membrane.

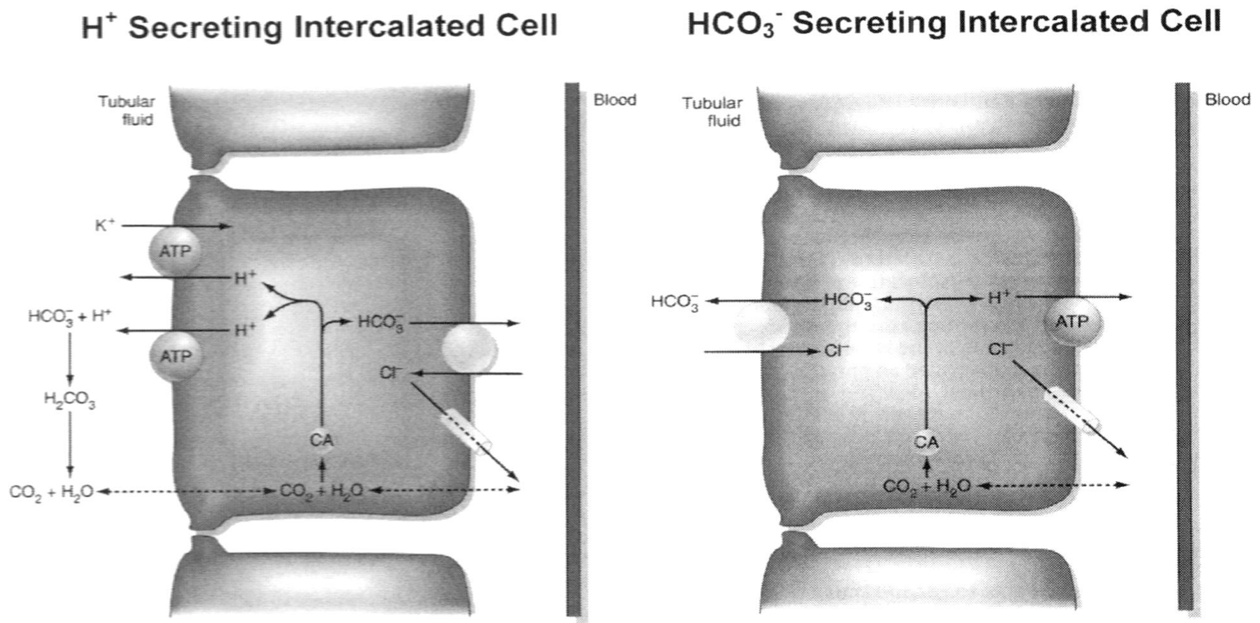

Figure 2.4. *Cellular mechanisms for H^+ and HCO_3^- secretion by intercalated cells of the collecting duct.*

Source: *https://journals.physiology.org/doi/full/10.1152/advan.00054.2009.*

2.1.2. TA

The H^+ secreted into the tubular fluid can drive the reabsorption of the filtered load of HCO_3^- as just described. In addition, the secreted H^+ can combine with other luminal constituents (termed urinary buffers), such as phosphate:

$$HPO_4^{2-} + H^+ \rightarrow H_2PO_4^- \quad (5)$$

In the titration of nonvolatile acids produced in cellular metabolism (NEAP), an HCO_3^- that was previously lost is eventually replaced by a "new HCO_3^-" that is generated within the cell when the secreted H^+ combines with a urinary buffer (see Figure 2.5). The kidney's method of excreting H^+ with urine buffers is referred to as TA. Urine's normally acidic pH is raised to that of blood through alkali titration to quantify this process. Phosphate is the main buffer and accounts for about one-third of RNAE that is caused by TA.

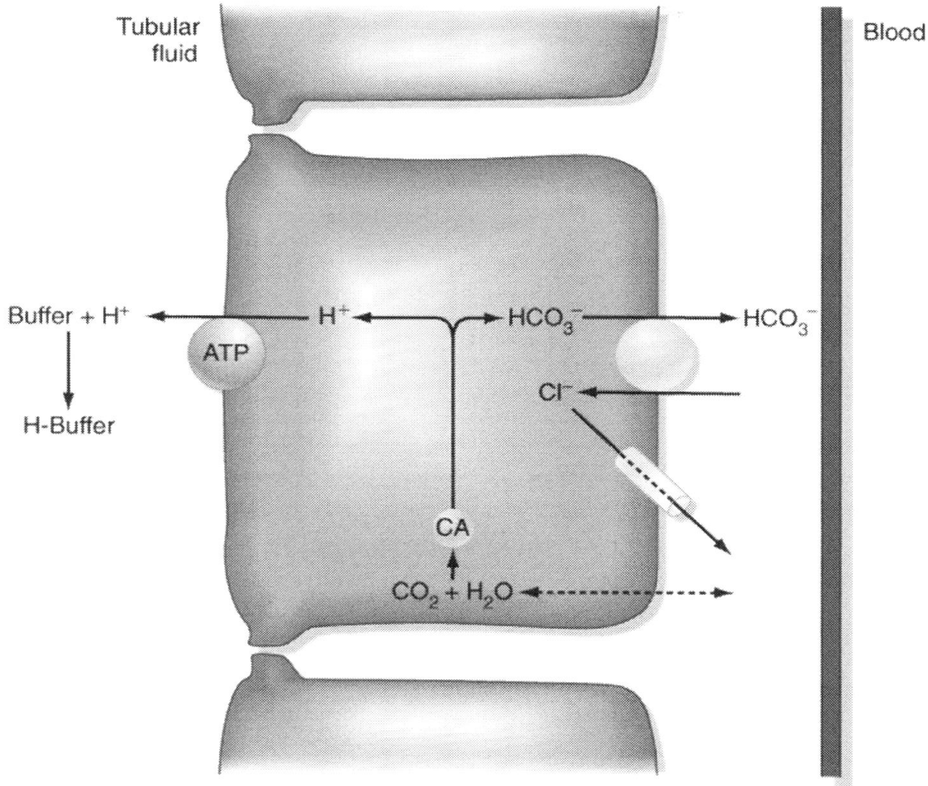

Figure 2.5. *Cellular mechanism for the generation of "new HCO_3^-" through the titration of urinary buffers (titratable acid). See text for details.*

Source: *https://journals.physiology.org/doi/full/10.1152/advan.00054.2009.*

2.1.3. Ammoniagenesis and NH_4^+ Excretion

The synthesis and excretion of NH_4^+, or ammoniagenesis, are crucial processes in renal acid-base physiology. Figure 2.6 illustrates this procedure. The kidney breaks down glutamine into two molecules of HCO_3^- and NH_4^+. Excreted NH_4^+ is disposed of in the urine, while HCO_3^-, or "new HCO_3^-," is added back to the blood to replace the HCO_3^- lost during the nonvolatile acid titration. What happens to the NH_4^+ that is not eliminated in the urine but is instead returned to the blood is also depicted in Figure 2.6. This results in the liver converting the NH_4^+ to urea, which produces H^+ in the process. The process of renal "new HCO_3^-" generation is negated because HCO_3^- buffers this H^+. The NH_4^+ that the kidney produces must therefore be eliminated into the urine and not added back to the blood, according to the theory of renal acid-base physiology. The blood receives back a milliequivalent of fresh HCO_3^- for each milliequivalent of NH_4^+ that is expelled. Approximately two-thirds of RNAE is explained by this process.

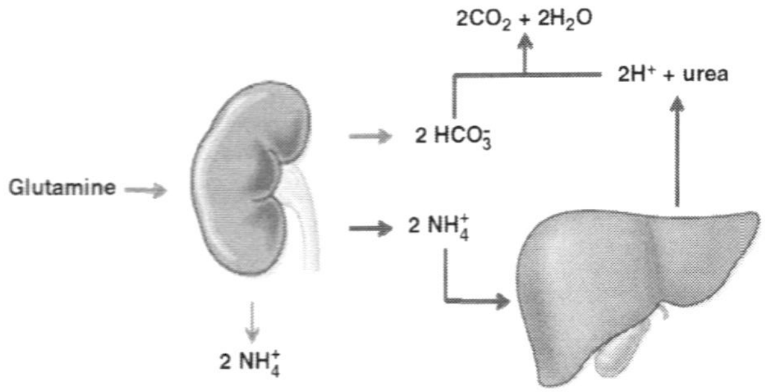

Figure 2.6. *General scheme for the production of HCO_3^- and NH_4^+ from the renal metabolism of glutamine. Also shown is the conversion of NH_4^+ to urea by the liver, which generates and H^+ and thus consumes HCO_3^-.*

Source: *https://journals.physiology.org/doi/full/10.1152/advan.00054.2009.*

Figure 2.7 provides a thorough illustration of the handling of NH_4^+. Proximal tubule cells are involved in the metabolism of glutamine. Each time glutamine is metabolized, two HCO_3^- and two NHC_4^+ are created. The NH_4^+ is secreted into the tubular fluid, while the HCO_3- is returned to the blood as "new HCO_3^-." NHE3 secretes the majority of NH_4^+, which replaces H^+ on the transporter. Furthermore, NH_4^+ may also enter the tubular fluid as NH_3, where it undergoes protonation. Whatever the mechanism, the blood receives a fresh HCO_3^- for each NH_4^+ secreted into the tubular fluid.

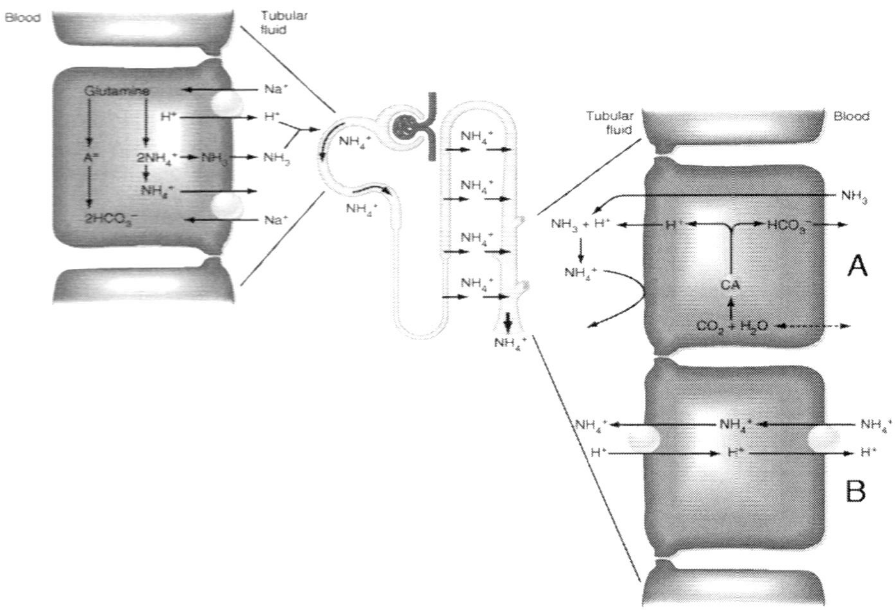

Figure 2.7. *Renal handling of NH_4^+. Two mechanisms for the secretion of NH_4^+ by the collecting duct are shown. A: nonionic diffusion and diffusion trapping of NH_3. B: secretion of NH_4^+ via Rh glycoprotein (RhCG).*

Source: *https://journals.physiology.org/doi/full/10.1152/advan.00054.2009.*

NH_4^+ is reabsorbed in large quantities in the thick ascending limb of the loop of Henle. There are a few different ways that this can be reabsorption, such as when NH_4^+ travels through the paracellular pathway and when it replaces K^+ on the apical membrane Na^+-K^+-$2Cl^-$ symporter (NKCC2). Through K^+ channels, NH_4^+ may be able to leave the cell by crossing the basolateral membrane. The renal medullary interstitium becomes clogged with this reabsorbed NH_4^+. As mentioned previously, the NH_4+ generated by the proximal tubule as a result of glutamine metabolism will be converted to urea by the liver and produce H^+ if it is not eliminated in the urine but rather returns to the blood. Should that happen, the "new HCO_3^-" produced by the metabolism of glutamine is eliminated. It follows that the NH_4^+ that was reabsorbed by the loop of Henle's thick ascending limb must be resecreted into the tubular fluid. The capacity of the collecting duct to acidify the tubular fluid determines how this happens.

The discovery and characterization of Rh glycoproteins have led to an evolution in our understanding of the mechanism of collecting duct NH_4^+ secretion. Rh glycoproteins resemble the NH_4^+ transporters present in bacteria, plants, and yeast. Three Rh glycoproteins in mammals have been found thus far, and research is being done to determine how they contribute to renal NH_3/NH_4^+ transport. RhGB and RhGC have been localized to the kidneys (as well as other organs involved in NH_4^+ transport, such as the liver and gastrointestinal tract), while RhAG is present in erythrocytes. Beginning with the distal convoluted tubule and extending through the inner medullary collecting duct, RhBG is present in distal nephron segments. Compared to principal cells, intercalated cells exhibit higher expression. Similar to RhBG, RhCG is distributed throughout the nephron on both the apical and basolateral membranes. Crucially, prolonged acidosis causes an increase in RhCG expression in the inner and outer medullary collecting ducts as well as the transporter's translocation from an intracellular pool to the apical membrane (note that RhBG expression remains unchanged). In an effort to characterize the nature of NH3/NH4+ transport, functional studies of Rh glycoprotein have produced evidence that is compatible with both electroneutral and electrogenic mechanisms. There is evidence for the Na^+-H^+ antiport as well. The activity of NH_4^+/H^+ antiporters on the apical and basolateral membranes of collecting duct cells, as demonstrated in Figure 2.7B, would account for this pH-dependent NH_4^+ secretion since acidification of the tubular fluid is necessary for NH_4^+ secretion.

The pH dependency of NH_4^+ secretion has traditionally been explained by the process of nonionic diffusion of NH_3 with diffusion trapping of NH_4^+ in the tubular fluid (see Figure 2.7A). It remains to be determined how much of collecting duct NH_4^+ secretion occurs via this mechanism and how much is mediated by RhCG or other NH_3/NH_4^+ transporters.

2.1.4. Renal Response to Acid-Base Disorders

The kidneys react to systemic acid-base disorders by changing RNAE in the right ways. RNAE excretion thus rises during acidosis and falls during alkalosis. The majority of our knowledge about the kidneys' adaptive response to acid-base disorders comes from the use of metabolic acidosis models. Our current understanding of how RNAE increases in this setting is described in the following section. RNAE rises during acidosis. This reaction involves an increase in TA and NH_4^+ excretion as well as a decrease, if not complete elimination, of HCO_3^- from the urine. The stimulation of H^+ and HCO_3-transport along the nephron, elevated ammoniagenesis, and increased availability of urinary buffers (phosphate, for example) are the main components of this response. Renal tubular cells' intracellular pH can be directly lowered by acidosis. It has been demonstrated that this cellular acidosis causes exocytotic insertion of transporters (such as H^+-ATPase and NHE3) into the plasma membrane from intracellular stores, changes transporter kinetics due to altered H^+ gradients across membranes, and stimulates NHE3 activity through allosteric mechanisms. It is unclear if the activation of intracellular regulatory pathways or mechanisms is what triggers these effects of intracellular acidosis, or if pH plays a primary role. Nevertheless, it is now evident that the renal response to acidosis is also mediated by other factors. For instance, it is evident that glucocorticoids and endothelin-1 (ET-1) stimulate renal H^+ and HCO_3^- transport during acidosis.

In reaction to acidosis, both proximal tubule cells and endothelial cells produce ET-1. Both NHE3 and NBCe1 are phosphorylated by acting via the ETB receptor, which causes them to insert into the basolateral and apical membranes, respectively. Acidosis also stimulates the adrenal cortex's release of cortisol. By raising both mRNA levels and translation, cortisol increases the abundance of NHE3 and NBCe1 in proximal tubule cells. Although their effects on distal H+ and HCO3-transport are less well understood, it is likely that ET-1 and cortisol also stimulate important acid-base transporters in these segments. Additionally, acidosis increases parathyroid hormone (PTH) secretion. The proximal tubule is affected by the elevated PTH levels, which prevent phosphate reabsorption. This increases the amount of phosphate that reaches the distal nephron, where it can act as a urinary buffer and help the kidneys excrete more TA. Acidosis stimulates the ammoniagenesis of the proximal tubule. This is a result of both the stimulatory effects of cortisol and intracellular acidosis. As was previously mentioned, acidosis causes an increase in RhCG abundance in the collecting duct, which facilitates NH_4^+ secretion and eventual excretion. As a result, NH_4^+ excretion and ammoniagenesis are increased.

Figure 2.8 illustrates what we currently know about the kidneys' reaction to acidosis. There is an increase in H^+ and HCO_3^-transport along the nephron. This is the result of cortisol and ET-1 effects, as well as a drop in intracellular pH. The production of ammoniagenesis and NH_4^+ collecting duct secretion are induced. In the end, TA is excreted more readily because proximal tubule phosphate reabsorption is inhibited. Overall, RNAE is improved.

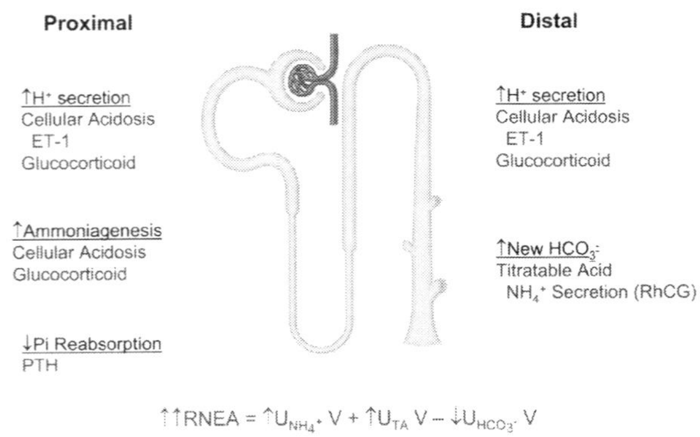

Figure 2.8. *Response of the kidneys to acidosis. ET-1, endothelin-1; PTH, parathyroid hormone; RNAE, renal net acid excretion; U, urine concentration; V, urine flow rate; TA, titratable acid.*

Source: *https://journals.physiology.org/doi/full/10.1152/advan.00054.2009.*

The most important component of the renal response to acidosis is the ability of the kidney to increase ammoniagenesis and NH_4^+ excretion. In the setting of acidosis, it is often useful to calculate the urinary net charge (UNC):

$$UNC = ([Na^+] + [K^+]) - [Cl^-] \quad (6)$$

As urinary HCO_3^- excretion is nearly zero, the principal urine anion in this context is Cl^-, according to the UNC concept, which also assumes that the principal urine cations are Na^+,

K^+, and NH_4^+ (not evaluated). Acidosis causes the excretion of NH_4^+, which is why UNC, as determined by Equation 6, should be negative. Certainly, in this configuration, a value of zero or a positive value would suggest a problem with NH_4+ excretion. Few research studies have been conducted on the kidneys' reaction to alkalosis. Without a doubt, decreased excretion of NH_4^+ and TA and increased HCO_3^-excretion lead to RNAE reduction. Generally, this reaction is said to indicate a decrease in the factors that are known to promote ammoniagenesis, H^+ and HCO_3^-transport, and the reaction to acidosis.

2.1.5. Alterations in RNAE

While RNAE can be changed by other factors, they do not aim to preserve the acid-base balance. Instead, as Table 2.1 shows, they may cause acid-base disturbances to arise. Factors that modify renal Na^+ transport, such as adjustments to the volume of extracellular fluid (ECF), can have secondary effects on RNAE because H^+ and HCO_3^-transport are connected to Na^+ in specific areas of the nephron. The renin-angiotensin-aldosterone system, for instance, is activated in response to a decrease in ECF volume, and this activation is mediated by ANG II. Additionally, ANG II may stimulate HCO_3- reabsorption in the thick ascending limb and distal convoluted tubule. Furthermore, by increasing the excretion of NH_4^+ and titrating urine buffers like phosphate, aldosterone promotes the secretion of H^+ from intercalated cells, which in turn produces new HCO_3^-. An increase in ECF volume would have the opposite effect (Hamm, Alpern, & Preisig, 2008; Hamm & Nakhoul, 2008; Koeppen & Stanton, 2008).

Table 2.1. Some Factors that Alter RNAE

Factor	Principle Nephron Site of Action
Increased RNAE	
ECF volume contraction	
ANG II	Proximal and distal tubules
Aldosterone	Distal tubule and collecting duct
Hyperaldosteronism	Distal tubule and collecting duct
Hypokalemia	Proximal tubule and intercalated cells
Decreased RNAE	
ECF volume expansion	Proximal and distal tubules and collecting duct
Hypoaldosteronism	Distal tubule and collecting duct
Hyperkalemia	Proximal tubule

Source: https://journals.physiology.org/doi/full/10.1152/advan.00054.2009.

Hyperkalemia has the opposite effect of hypokalemia on proximal tubule HCO_3^-reabsorption and ammoniagenesis, while hypokalemia stimulates both. Changes in intracellular pH may be associated with the mechanisms involved, although they are not entirely clear. Moreover, intercalated cells of the collecting duct with hypokalemia express more H^+-K^+-ATPase, which in turn promotes H^+ secretion.

2.2. Regulation of Renal Function and Blood Pressure Control by P2 Purinoceptors in the Kidney

The maintenance of normal, healthy kidney function is crucial for blood pressure regulation. Roughly one in three adult Americans, or 67 million, suffer from high blood pressure. Every 20 mmHg increase in systolic blood pressure doubles the risk for renal and cardiovascular disease. Blood pressure control is essential from a clinical, financial, and social perspective because treating high blood pressure costs the country about 48 billion dollars annually.

The mechanism regulating blood pressure is intricate and multifaceted. Guyton created a computer model in 1961 that predicted the kidney would serve as the focal point for long-term blood pressure management. "The kidneys are primarily responsible for the long-term regulation of mean arterial pressure," he said. 1969 saw Guyton et al. continued to demonstrate the critical molecular relationship, known as the "pressure natriuresis relationship," between long-term sodium excretion and blood pressure regulation. This link between blood pressure, sodium excretion, and renal perfusion pressure was characterized by Guyton's model as a crucial mechanism for controlling circulatory volume. By balancing the amounts of sodium and water in the blood, the kidneys maintain extracellular fluid volume (ECFV) homeostasis and thus regulate circulatory volume. To put it simply, drinking more water and sodium causes an increase in ECFV, which raises blood volume. Systemic blood pressure rises as a result of increased cardiac output and increased venous return to the heart, which causes atrial stretch. The phenomenon known as "pressure natriuresis" occurs when arterial pressure rises because the nephron increases sodium and water excretion and decreases sodium and water reabsorption to bring blood pressure and ECFV back to normal. On the other hand, when blood pressure drops, the nephron increases the absorption of salt and water, which raises ECFV and raises blood pressure. The discovery that several P2 receptor subtypes are expressed along renal vascular and tubular structures has highlighted the significance of renal P2 purinoceptors, or P2 receptors. Similar to the renin-angiotensin-aldosterone system or sympathetic nervous activity, the renal P2 purinoceptor system is important for controlling blood pressure and preserving cardiovascular health. P2 receptors are widely dispersed throughout the kidney, where they regulate tubular reabsorption, autoregulation, and renal vascular resistance.

2.2.1. P2 Receptor Function in the Renal Vasculature

While one study suggested that $P2Y_1$ receptors are on both the afferent and efferent arterioles, other studies have demonstrated that $P2X_1$ receptors are located on the afferent arteriole. The activation of P2X1 receptors controls glomerular filtration rate, glomerular capillary pressure, and renal blood flow through autoregulatory control of renal vascular resistance. With the preparation of the juxtamedullary nephron, Inscho et al. found that when renal perfusion pressure was raised, $P2X_1$ receptor blockade with NF279 prevented pressure-mediated vasoconstriction, which was consistent with a compromised autoregulatory response. Additionally, they reported that in $P2X_1$ receptor knockout mice ($P2X_1^{-/-}$), afferent arteriole autoregulatory behavior was significantly blunted when compared to wild type controls. Osmond and associates found that rats given the $P2X_1$ receptor antagonist IP5I had impaired renal blood flow autoregulation throughout their entire kidneys (Figure 2.9A). During the course of treatment with the A1 receptor antagonist DPCPX, whole kidney autoregulation of renal blood flow remained unchanged (Figure 2.9B). According to these findings, $P2X_1$ receptors are critical for whole kidney autoregulation and afferent arteriole. Lately, Schnermann and associates... examined how P2X receptors mediate the preglomerular resistance modifications that tubuloglomerular feedback signaling triggers. They found that P2 receptor blockade had no effect on the tubuloglomerular feedback responses in mice, indicating that P1 and adenosine receptors may be involved in the in vivo tubuloglomerular feedback-induced vasoconstriction. These findings imply that the functions of P1 and P2 receptors in controlling renal microvascular function may differ significantly.

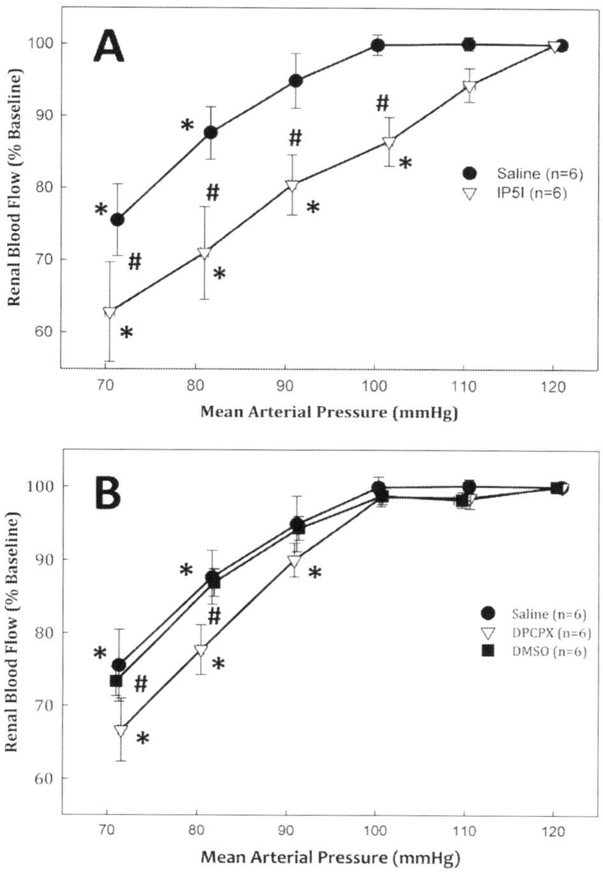

Figure 2.9. *Percent change of baseline renal blood flow (RBF) in response to decreasing renal perfusion during $P2X_1$ receptor antagonism. Percent change from baseline RBF in response to decrements in renal perfusion pressure with (open triangles) and without (closed circles) $P2X_1$ receptor antagonism by IP5I. Panel B: percent change from baseline RBF in response to decrements in renal perfusion pressure with A1 receptor inhibition by DPCPX (open triangles) and during DMSO vehicle infusion (closed squares) and saline experiments (close circles).*

Source: *https://www.ncbi.nlm.nih.gov/pmc/articles/PMC5515225/#:~:text=The%20kidneys%20regulate%20circulatory%20volume,in%20turn%20increases%20blood%20volume.*

Menzies along with others found that "selective" blockade of P2X7 receptors with Brilliant Blue G resulted in lower blood pressure and renal vascular resistance, indicating a potential link between increased renal vascular resistance and P2X7 receptor activation. As a result, abnormal increases in glomerular capillary pressure may be allowed by compromised vascular P2 receptor activation, which could compromise renal autoregulatory control and result in glomerular injury (Hamm, Alpern, Preisig, 2008. Hamm & Nakhoul, 2008; Koeppen & Stanton, 2008).

Vasodilation or vasoconstriction can result from P2Y receptor activation in the renal vasculature. Research employing the juxtamedullary nephron preparation revealed that afferent arterioles are vasoconstrictor when $P2Y_1$ (2 methlythio-ATP) or $P2Y_{2,4}$ receptors (UTP) are stimulated. Eltze et al. used isolated perfused kidneys. demonstrated that at low concentrations, P2Y receptor agonists (ATP, ADP, UTP, and ATPγS) produced vasodilation and at high concentrations, vasoconstriction. Vasodilation induced by "selective" P2Y receptor agonists appears to be independent of prostaglandins and to be related to endothelial factors such as nitric oxide (NO) or endothelium-derived relaxing factor. Research employing $P2Y_2$ receptor knockout mice ($P2Y_2^{-/-}$), which showed elevated renal vascular resistance in comparison to wild-type controls, has revealed evidence for P2Y2 receptor-dependent vasodilation. This implies that the renal vasculature is subject to basal vasodilatory influence by $P2Y_2$ receptors. Additionally, Rieg et al. demonstrated that deletion of $P2Y_2$ receptors ($P2Y_2$-/-) raises systemic blood pressure and $P2Y_2$ receptor activation lowers blood pressure in wild-type mice. These findings demonstrate the vasodilatory effect of P2Y receptors, which lowers systemic blood pressure. Consequently, $P2X_7$ and $P2Y_2$ receptors could offer new therapeutic targets for controlling blood pressure in the system. Renal vascular resistance, glomerular capillary pressure, and whole kidney autoregulation are all regulated by the activation or inhibition of renal vascular P2 receptors. These processes in turn affect the regulation of renal function and systemic blood pressure.

2.2.2. P2 Receptor Activation in Renal Tubular Segments

Modulating sodium transport along the nephron regulates the sodium balance and ECFV. Renal perfusion pressure to the kidney is increased by an increase in systemic blood pressure. Even though autoregulation is effective, it is not flawless; this can result in a slight rise in glomerular capillary pressure and a slight rise in glomerular filtration rate, which can raise the rate at which fluid flows through the tubular epithelium, stimulate the release of ATP, which can then activate P2 receptors and decrease epithelial sodium transport. Therefore, P2-receptor-mediated control of the nephron's salt and water reabsorption contributes to the regulation of ECFV.

2.2.2.1. Proximal Tubule

Renal tubule P2 receptor activation can prevent the kidneys from transporting sodium. It appears that P2Y receptors are more common in the proximal tubule. Inhibiting sodium and bicarbonate reabsorption, activation of $P2Y_2$ receptors lowers the activity of the Na^+/H^+ exchanger and Na^+/K^+ ATPase. In the proximal tubule lumen, $P2Y_1$ receptor agonists microperfusion inhibits the Na^+/H^+ exchanger 3 in vivo and decreases Na^+ reabsorption. The filtered load that the proximal tubule receives increases as a result of a slight increase in glomerular filtration rate brought on by increases in renal perfusion pressure. Through autocrine and paracrine processes, this causes the proximal tubule to experience increased shear stress, which causes a local release of ATP and activates the P2Y receptors in the tubule. P2Y receptor activation lowers sodium reabsorption from the proximal tubule, increases the delivery of solutes and water to the distal nephron, and aids in the pressure natriuresis response, which lowers blood pressure and ECFV (Figure 2.10A).

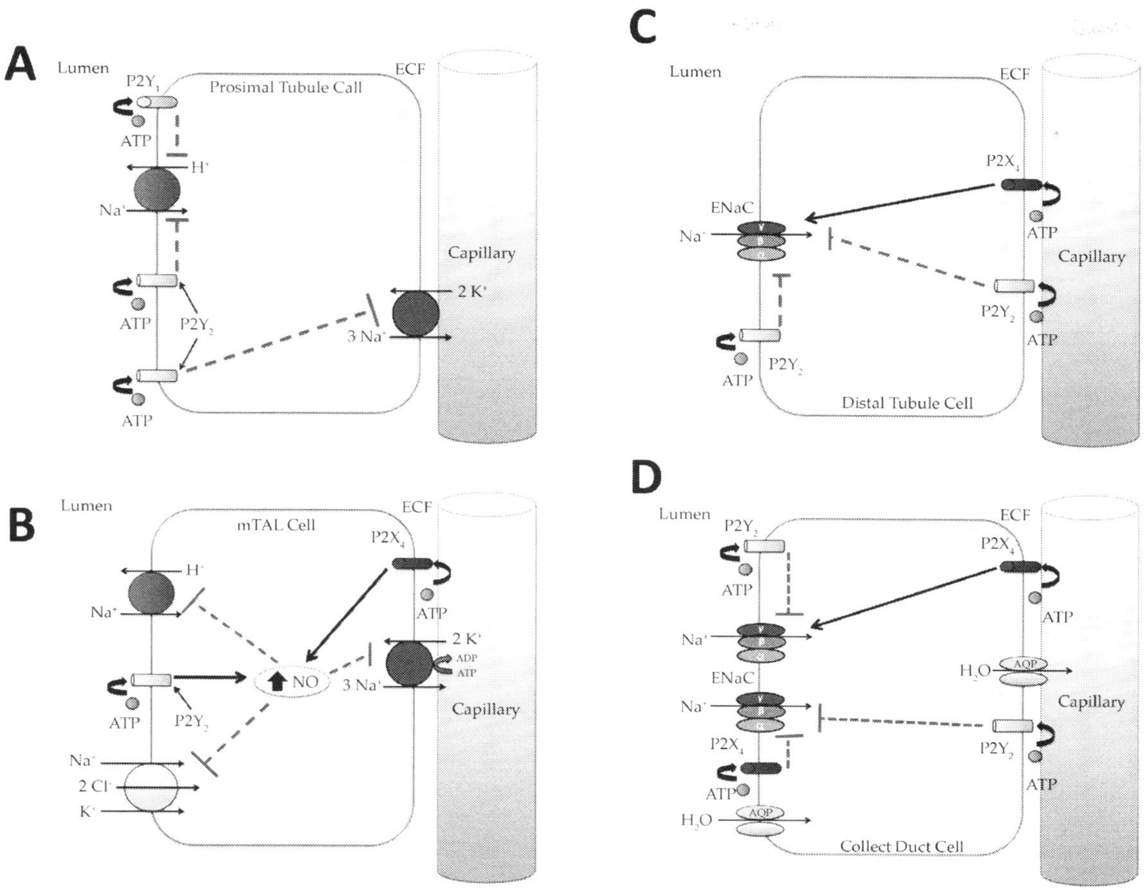

Figure 2.10. *A summary of P2 receptor regulation of sodium transport throughout major segments of the nephron.*

Note: A (Proximal Tubule): Activation of apical $P2Y_1$ and $P2Y_2$ receptors by luminal ATP inhibits the activity of the Na^+/H^+ exchanger. $P2Y_2$ receptor activation can also inhibit Na^+/K^+ ATPase in the basolateral membrane. B (Medullary thick ascending limb): Basolateral $P2X_4$ and apical $P2Y_2$ receptor stimulation by ATP causes an increase in intracellular nitric oxide, that reduces sodium reabsorption through mechanisms of inhibiting the Na^+/H^+ exchanger, $N^+/K^+/2Cl^-$ co-transporter, and the Na^+/K^+ ATPase. C (Distal Tubule): P2 receptors in the distal tubule cause both an inhibition and stimulation of epithelial sodium channel (ENaC) activity. Activation of basolateral and apical $P2Y_2$ receptors reduces sodium transport through inhibition of ENaC activity. $P2X_4$ receptor stimulation by ATP causes an increase in sodium reabsorption through mechanisms associated with ENaC channel activity. D (Collecting Duct): P2 receptor activation by ATP causes a reduction or stimulation in sodium reabsorption in a collecting duct cell. Apical and basolateral $P2Y_2$, and basolateral $P2X_4$ receptor, at high levels of ATP, activity inhibits ENaC activity, reducing sodium transport. Low levels of ATP may stimulate ENaC activity through mechanisms linked to $P2X_4$.

Source: https://www.ncbi.nlm.nih.gov/pmc/articles/PMC5515225/#:~:text=The%20kidneys%20regulate%20circulatory%20volume,in%20turn%20increases%20blood%20volume.

2.2.2.2. Loop of Henle

A rise in the flow rate of tubular fluid through the Henle loop causes the release of ATP, which in turn triggers the autocrine/paracrine activation of P2 receptors. Garvin along with others showed that in rat medullary thick ascending limb (mTAL) cell suspensions, ATP and UTP boost intracellular nitric oxide (NO) production. This ATP-mediated rise in NO synthesis in mTAL inhibits the activity of Na^+/K^+ ATPase and Na^+/H^+ exchanger. Marques along with others. stated that by increasing intracellular NO through $P2X_4$ receptor stimulation, the apical $Na^+/K^+/2CL-$ (NKCC2) co-transporter was inhibited. Vallon's group demonstrated an increase in NKCC2 co-transporter protein in a study involving $P2Y_2^{-/-}$ mice, indicating that $P2Y_2$ receptors have an inhibitory effect on sodium reabsorption and NKCC2 transporter expression in mouse mTAL. According to these findings, tubular fluid flow rate increases trigger the release of ATP, which in turn activates the basolateral and apical P2 receptors in the Henle loop, enhancing intracellular NO production and decreasing sodium reabsorption. Increases in glomerular filtration rate cause the proximal tubule's tubular fluid flow rate to rise, which in turn promotes the activation of P2 receptors in the loop of Henle and the release of ATP from the tubular epithelium. In this segment, P2 receptor activation potentiates the pressure natriuresis response and lowers blood pressure by inhibiting Na^+/K^+ ATPase, Na^+/H^+ exchanger, and NKCC2 co-transporter, thereby reducing sodium transport (Figure 2.10B).

2.2.2.3. Distal Tubule

The distal tubule's P2 receptors' functional aspects have only been studied in studies utilizing cultured cell lines. Zhang and colleagues conducted a study has demonstrated that basolaterally adding 2-methylthio-ATP to A6 (Xenopus kidney) cells increases the activity of the epithelial sodium channel (ENaC), presumably through the activation of $P2X_4$ receptors. In cultured rabbit connecting tubule cells, extracellular ATP inhibited the absorption of calcium and sodium and increased intracellular Ca^{2+} concentration, most likely through the activation of $P2Y_2$ receptors. These results suggest that distal tubule P2 receptors may modulate ENaC activity in this segment to regulate sodium transport (Figure 2.10C).

2.2.2.4. Collecting Duct

The apical expression of ENaC is the rate-limiting step in sodium reabsorption in the collecting duct. The inhibition of ENaC by ATP was initially observed in primary and immortalized mouse cell cultures. Work by Sipos and Associates implies that the pressure natriuretic response is influenced by the inhibition of ENaC activity in the collecting duct caused by the release of ATP from the collecting duct epithelium into the tubular fluid. Through $P2Y_2$ receptor activation, ATP lowers the open probability of ENaC in isolated split open cortical collecting ducts of $P2Y_2^{-/-}$ and WT mice, according to patch clamp studies. Pochynyuk along with others. It was also reported that the lack of ENaC inhibition caused $P2Y_2^{-/-}$ mice to develop salt-sensitive hypertension. Wildmann along with others found that while low extracellular sodium concentration levels (50 mM) enhanced ENaC activity, high extracellular sodium concentration levels (145 mM) elicited a $P2X_4$ receptor-mediated inhibition of ENaC in the rat collecting duct. In comparison to their WT littermates, $P2X_4^{-/-}$ mice on a low Na^+ diet had a lower mean arterial pressure. All of these findings point to the possibility that when tubular fluid flow rate rises, ATP is released into the tubular lumen and P2X and P2Y receptors in the collecting duct are activated. P2 receptor activation influences urinary sodium excretion and systemic blood pressure by suppressing or, in certain cases, stimulating ENaC activity and sodium reabsorption (Figure 2.10D) (Hamm, Alpern, Preisig, 2008. Hamm & Nakhoul, 2008; Koeppen & Stanton, 2008).

2.2.3. The Kidneys and Their Influence on Blood Pressure

An essential part of controlling arterial blood pressure is the kidneys. Renal control of extracellular volume and renal perfusion pressure are closely linked to the maintenance of arterial circulation and blood pressure, according to a substantial body of experimental and physiological evidence. Renal artery perfusion pressure affects the activity of several vasoactive systems, including the renin-angiotensin-aldosterone (RAS) system, and directly controls sodium excretion, a process known as pressure natriuresis. Blood viscosity is one of the main factors influencing resistance and, consequently, blood pressure, along with vessel morphology. The renin-angiotensin system, also known as the renin-angiotensin-aldosterone system (RAAS), is a hormone system that controls blood pressure and water balance. It is a major modulator of blood viscosity.

The blood pressure in the body depends upon:

- The force by which the heart pumps out blood from the ventricles of the heart – and this is dependent on how much the heart muscle gets stretched by the inflowing blood into the ventricles.
- The degree to which the arteries and arterioles constrict-- increases the resistance to blood flow, thus requiring a higher blood pressure.
- The volume of blood circulating around the body; if the volume is high, the ventricles get more filled, and the heart muscle gets more stretched.

The kidney influences blood pressure by:

- Causing the arteries and veins to constrict
- Increasing the circulating blood volume

A section of the distal tubule near and in the wall of the afferent arteriole contains specialized cells known as macula Densa. While the arterial cells (juxtaglomerular cells) sense blood pressure, these cells sense the Na in the filtrate. The quantity of filtered Na decreases along with a drop in blood pressure. The macula Densa cells transmit the decrease in Na concentration to the arterial cells, which in turn transmits the drop in blood pressure. Then, an enzyme known as renin is released by the juxtaglomerular cells. Angiotensinogen is a peptide or derivative of an amino acid that is changed into angiotensin-1 by renin. The lungs' angiotensin-converting enzyme (ACE) then transforms angiotensin-1 into angiotensin-2. Blood vessel constriction is induced by angiotensin-2, and these constrictions increase blood pressure. Renin is directly secreted into circulation by kidney arterial cells when blood volume is low. The liver's release of angiotensinogen is subsequently converted to angiotensin-1 by plasma renin. Subsequently, the lungs' angiotensin-converting enzyme transforms angiotensin-1 into angiotensin-2. Blood vessels constrict as a result of the powerful vasoactive peptide angiotensin-2m, raising blood pressure. Additionally, the hormone aldosterone is secreted from the adrenal cortex in response to angiotensin-2.

The kidney's tubules reabsorb more water and salt into the blood when aldosterone is present. As a result, the body retains more fluid, which raises blood pressure. An overactive renin-angiotensin-aldosterone system will result in excessively high blood pressure. Numerous medications obstruct various stages within this system to reduce blood pressure. One of the main methods for managing hypertension, heart failure, kidney failure, and the negative effects of diabetes is with these medications. Angiotensin-2 is the main bioactive substance, with angiotensin-1 possibly having some trace activity. Angiotensin-2 is a powerful vasoconstrictor of arterioles with a range of physiological effects.

2.2.4. How the Kidneys Increase Circulating Blood Volume

The hormone aldosterone is also secreted by the adrenal glands in response to angiotensin-2 stimulation. In the distal tubule, aldosterone promotes increased Na reabsorption, which results in the reabsorption of water as well. Urine output is decreased and blood volume is increased due to the distal tubule's increased reabsorption of Na and water. Blood pressure rises as a result of the heart muscle being stretched and producing more force with each beat due to the increased blood volume. The heart muscle's stretch directly relates to the volume of blood in circulation.

The kidney's functions to control blood pressure are particularly crucial in the event of a traumatic injury when maintaining blood pressure and preventing fluid loss are imperative. In addition to keeping the amount of calcium in the blood steady, the body stores calcium in the bones. The parathyroid glands in the neck release a hormone known as parathyroid hormone when the blood calcium level drops. To raise the blood calcium level again, parathyroid hormone increases calcium reabsorption from the nephron's distal tubule. In addition to encouraging the release of calcium from bone, parathyroid hormone also causes the intestines to absorb calcium.

The body also needs vitamin D to promote the kidney and intestines' absorption of calcium. Dairy products contain vitamin D. Cholecalciferol, a precursor to vitamin D, is produced in the skin and metabolized in the liver. The proximal tubule of the nephron is where the final step in the transformation of an inactive form of cholecalciferol into active vitamin D occurs. Once activated, vitamin D increases blood calcium levels by stimulating the intestine's and the proximal tubule's absorption of calcium. Abnormalities known as kidney stones are typically brought on by issues with the kidneys' capacity to metabolize calcium. Furthermore, the disease osteoporosis, which affects many elderly people, particularly women, is influenced by the kidney's function in regulating blood calcium levels.

The kidneys therefore function in the body to:

- Control the composition of the blood and eliminate wastes by filtration/reabsorption/secretion
- Influence blood pressure by renin secretion
- Help regulate the body's calcium by vitamin D activation

Renal dialysis techniques, also known as artificial filtration techniques, are the only option available to help a patient survive if their kidneys stop working for whatever reason. They work by cleaning the blood. This is particularly important if both kidneys fail.

2.2.5. Mechanisms of Blood Pressure Control by the Kidneys

2.2.5.1. Intra-Renal Actions of the Renin-Angiotensin System in Blood Pressure Control

Renin-angiotensin system (RAS) dysregulation leads to hypertension, as the RAS is a powerful blood pressure modulator. In a significant number of hypertensive patients, pharmacological blockade of the RAS with renin inhibitors, angiotensin-converting enzyme (ACE) inhibitors, or angiotensin receptor blockers effectively lowers blood pressure, indicating the critical role that RAS activation plays in the development of hypertension in humans. While overexpression of RAS genes results in hypertension, RAS gene deletion lowers blood pressure in rodents.

While the arterial cells (juxtaglomerular cells) sense blood pressure, the distal tubule cells (macula Densa) sense the Na in the filtrate. Research has demonstrated that a shift in the pressure-natriuresis relationship results in hypertension when low doses of angiotensin II are continuously infused directly into the kidney. Additionally, it is thought that the kidney's local and independent regulation of RAS activity affects blood pressure regulation and sodium excretion. According to this theory, elevated levels of angiotensin II in the bloodstream are linked to the build-up of angiotensin peptides in the kidney, elevated expression of the main RAS substrate, angiotensinogen, in the proximal tubule epithelium, and elevated excretion of angiotensinogen and angiotensin peptides in urine. Through the use of type 1 angiotensin (AT1) receptors in the kidney, angiotensin II stimulates the RAS locally and increases the amount of angiotensin II produced in the renal tubule lumen. This feed-forward pathway leads to the autocrine and paracrine stimulation of epithelial transporters.

In the context of RAS activation, recent research supporting this theory has confirmed the essential need of ACE within the kidney to fully manifest stimulation of sodium transporter expression, renal sodium reabsorption, and hypertension (Figures 2.11 and 2.12) (Samuel, Francis, & Anthony, 2018).

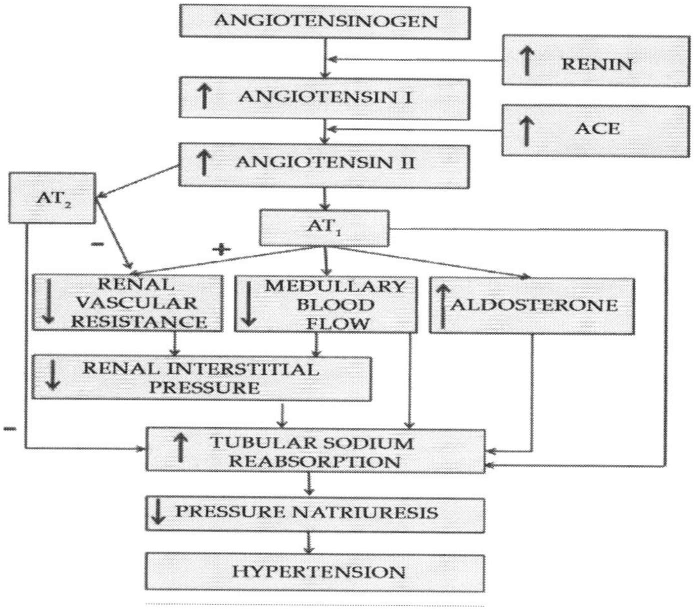

Figure 2.11. *Renal mechanism whereby activation of the renin-angiotensin system reduces pressure natriuresis relationship and leads to hypertension.*

Source: *Samuel SA, Francis AO, Anthony OO. Role of the Kidneys in the Regulation of Intra- and Extra-Renal Blood Pressure. Ann Clin Hypertens. 2018; 2: 048–058. DOI: 10.29328/journal.ach.1001011.*

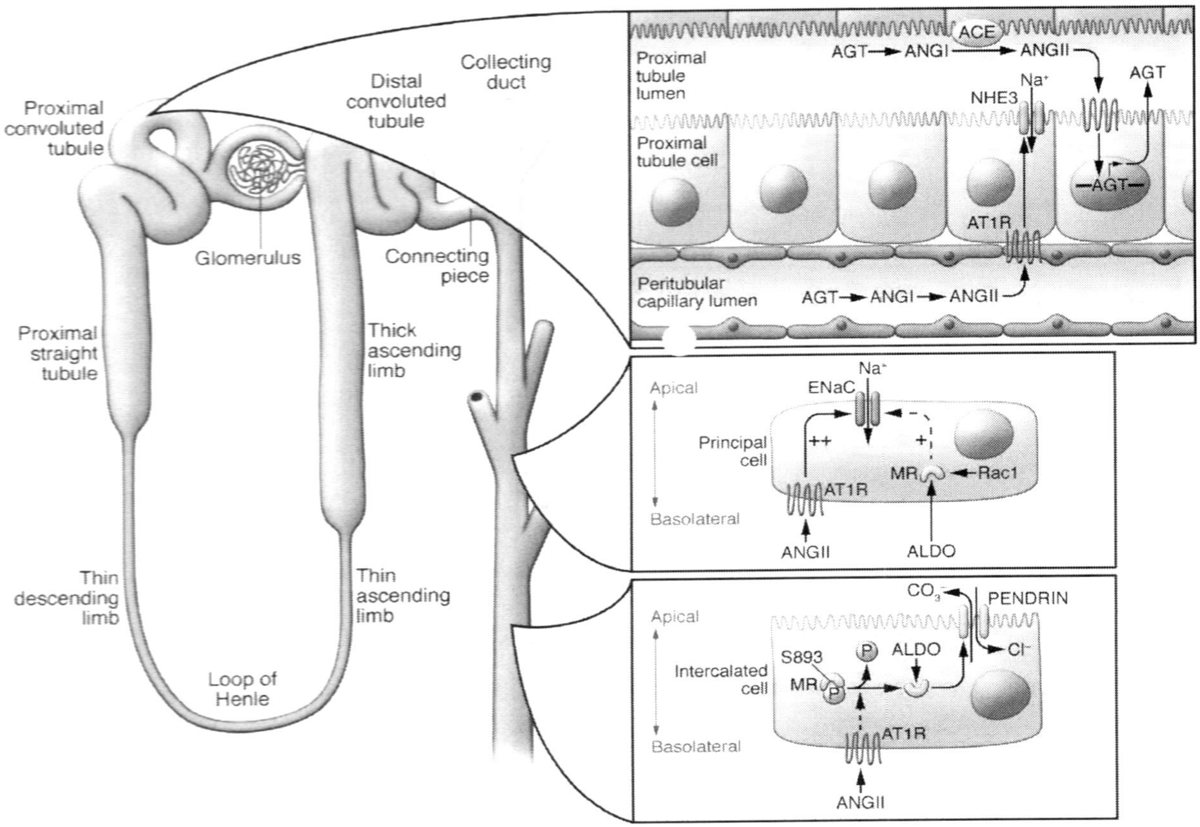

Figure 2.12. *A model for local control of RAS activity within the kidney- High levels of angiotensin II (ANGII) in circulation, derived from angiotensinogen (AGT) generated primarily by the liver, are associated with; increased ANGII in the kidney, up-regulation of AGT in the proximal tubule epithelium, increased levels of AGT in the tubular lumen, generation of ANGII requiring angiotensin-converting enzyme (ACE) expression in the brush border of the proximal tubule (PT), and increased excretion of AGT and ANG peptides in urine.*

Source: *Samuel SA, Francis AO, Anthony OO. (2018). Role of the kidneys in the regulation of intra- and extra-renal blood pressure. Ann Clin Hypertens., 2, 048–058. DOI: 10.29328/journal.ach.1001011.*

2.2.5.2. Novel Control Mechanisms and Sites of Action for Aldosterone in Hypertension

Aldosterone is a downstream effector of the RAS because AT1 receptors in the adrenal gland's zona glomerulosa stimulate aldosterone release. In aldosterone-sensitive nephron segments, activation of the mineralocorticoid receptor (MR) promotes the assembly and translocation of the ENaC subunits. Liddle's syndrome is caused by mutations in ENaC subunits that hinder its degradation. This leads to an increase in membrane density and the likelihood that the channels will open. The condition is characterized by severe, early-onset hypertension that resembles hyper-aldosteronism, but with low aldosterone levels. Similarly, activating mutations in the MR gene also result in hypertension, which is made worse by changes in steroid hormones during pregnancy. These syndromes might draw attention to the kidney's ability to promote hypertension through dysregulation of the MR/ENaC signaling pathway.

Aldosterone stimulates the reabsorption of sodium and also encourages the secretion of potassium into the urine. Studies by Shibata et al. have demonstrated that the kidney's aldosterone responses are modulated by the MR's regulated phosphorylation. They demonstrated that ligand binding is inhibited when S843 on the MR is phosphorylated. This type of MR is limited to intercalated kidney collecting duct cells, where hyperkalemia and volume depletion differentially regulate its phosphorylation. For instance, during volume depletion, intercalated cells' MR is dephosphorylated, potentiating the absorption of sodium and chloride and enabling a unique response to volume depletion. Even in the case of suppressed aldosterone levels, new research indicates that the small GTPase Rac1 may promote hypertension through an MR-dependent pathway, despite the fact that aldosterone is the classical activator of the MR (Figure 2.13).

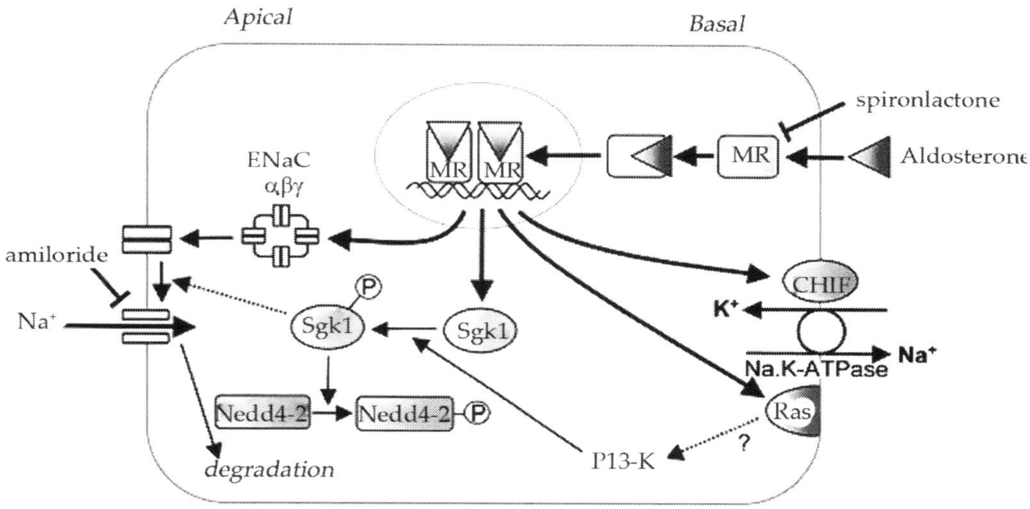

Figure 2.13. *Representation of an aldosterone-responsive epithelial cell. The proteins encoded by aldosterone-induced genes are discussed in the text: ENAC α, β, and γ, CHIF, SGK, and RAS are indicated are their known or putative functions.*

Source: *Samuel SA, Francis AO, & Anthony OO. (2018). Role of the kidneys in the regulation of intra- and extra-renal blood pressure. Ann Clin Hypertens., 2, 048–058. doi: 10.29328/journal.ach.1001011.*

2.2.5.3. The WNKs: Novel Pathways Regulating Renal Solute Transport

The genetic basis of almost all known Mendelian disorders linked to aberrant blood pressure phenotypes in humans has been determined by credible evidence suggesting the kidney plays a major role in blood pressure regulation. These mutations affect fluid and sodium reabsorption along the nephron in each instance. Mutations in the genes encoding WNK1 (without lysine [K]) kinase and WNK4 have been found to be the cause of several disorders, including pseudo-hypo-aldosteronism type II (PHAII), a Mendelian syndrome characterized by the unusual combination of hypertension and hyperkalemia. The identification of roles for WNK1 and WNK4 in the regulation of sodium and potassium flux in the distal nephron resulted from the intensive study of these special kinases that followed this discovery. The thiazide-sensitive Sodium (Na) Chloride Cotransporter (NCC) and/or the Renal Outer Medullary Potassium (K) channel (ROMK) are the primary mechanisms through which these actions are mediated. Effective and commonly used antihypertensive medications called thiazide diuretics target the NCC, a significant pathway for sodium reabsorption in the distal nephron. Thiazides are a cornerstone of PHAII treatment, in line with research showing that NCC hyperactivity is a major characteristic of the illness. It is noteworthy that although WNK4's actions to suppress ROMK activity have been consistent throughout these studies, its effects on NCC activity have varied, possibly as a result of the different concentrations of WNK4 in different experimental systems. Here, endogenous WNK4-accumulating mutations increase NCC activity, possibly via phosphorylating STE20/SPS-1-related proline-alanine-rich protein kinase (SPAK). On the other hand, intentional overexpression of WNK4 seems to direct NCC toward lysosomal degradation (Figure 2.14).

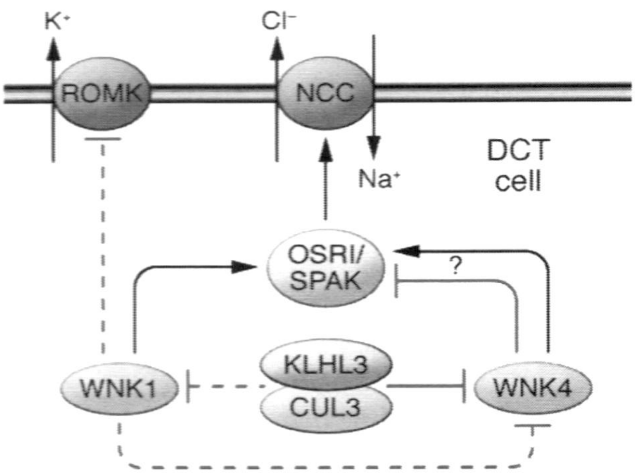

Figure 2.14. *Mechanisms regulating sodium and potassium flux in the distal nephron.*

Source: *Samuel SA, Francis AO, & Anthony OO. (2018). Role of the Kidneys in the Regulation of Intra- and Extra-Renal Blood Pressure. Ann Clin Hypertens., 2, 048–058. DOI: 10.29328/journal.ach.1001011.*

In the kidney's distal convoluted tubule (DCT) cells, WNK family kinases regulate the activity of the sodium chloride cotransporter (NCC) and the renal outer medullary potassium channel (ROMK). NCC-dependent sodium transport is facilitated by WNK1's phosphorylation and stimulation of the protein kinases oxidative stress-responsive kinase 1 (OSR1) and SPS1-related proline/alanine-rich kinase (SPAK). WNK1 might obstruct ROMK as well. Although WNK4 inhibits ROMK, depending on the experimental setup, it has also been shown to have both stimulating and inhibitory effects on NCC. The activity of the cullin 3-KLHL3 ubiquitin ligase, which has also been proposed to modulate WNK1, controls the levels of WNK4 (Samuel, Francis, & Anthony, 2018).

2.2.5.4. How Sodium and Potassium Flux in the Distal Nephron is Regulated

In several situations, increased NCC activity via WNK modulation appears to be the last common pathway leading to the development of hypertension. For instance, WNK4 suppression and increased NCC activity are the ways in which β-adrenergic stimulation raises blood pressure. Furthermore, hypertension is a common side effect of calcineurin inhibitors, which are often used to treat autoimmune diseases and prevent transplant rejection. According to recent research by Ellison et al., the use of calcineurin inhibitors is linked to hypertension through a mechanism that involves NCC stimulation via WNK3 upregulation. Although much information about kidney physiology has been gained from the ongoing delineation of WNK functions, only a small portion of PHAII patients have mutations in WNK genes. Lifton's group used exome sequencing to identify mutations in the cullin 3 (CUL3) and kelch-like 3 (KLHL3) genes in PHAII patients. Furthermore, in about 80% of cases of PHAII, the disease was caused by mutations in these two genes. KLHL3 belongs to a group of over 50 kelch proteins that are tramtrack, broad-complex, bric-a-brac complex-containing (BTB-containing), and are distinguished by having six-bladed, β-propeller domains that are used to bind particular target proteins. The complex, which consists of BTB-domain proteins like KLHL3 and a RING domain protein that acts as an E3 ubiquitin ligase and targets particular protein substrates for ubiquitination, is scaffolded by CUL3 (Figure 2.15).

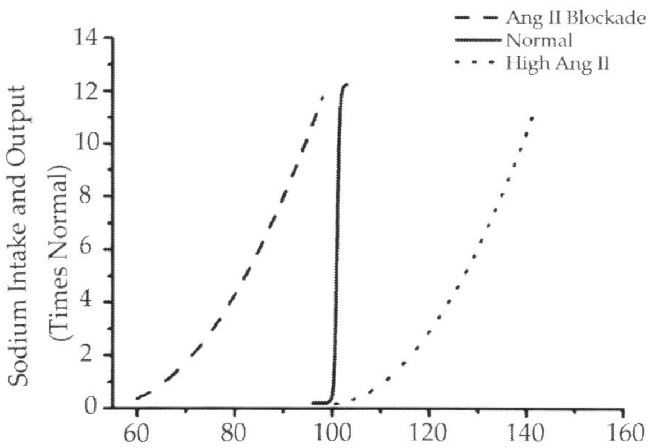

Figure 2.15. *Effect of changes in mean arterial pressure during chronic changes in sodium intake after angiotensin-converting enzyme (ACE) inhibition, or when angiotensin II was infused at a constant low dose (5 ng/ kg/min) to prevent angiotensin II from being suppressed when sodium intake was raised.*

Source: Samuel SA, Francis AO, & Anthony OO. (2018). Role of the kidneys in the regulation of intra- and extra-renal blood pressure. Ann Clin Hypertens., 2, 048–058. DOI: 10.29328/journal.ach.1001011.

2.2.5.5. Salt Homeostasis

Salt sensitivity is a relatively common condition that is defined as an exaggerated change in blood pressure in response to extremes in dietary salt intake. It is linked to an increased risk of developing hypertension. According to traditional Guytonian theories, the cause of salt sensitivity is a malfunction in the kidney's excretion of sodium. When a person consumes a lot of salt, their extracellular fluid volume expands, which raises blood pressure. This model assumes equilibrium between the two primary extracellular volume components found in the intravascular and interstitial spaces. Therefore, to maintain iso-osmolality, sodium accumulation would be accompanied by corresponding retention of water, which would proportionally increase the intravascular volume. Still, research by Titze et al. revealed that sodium handling is more intricate than this traditional two-compartment model; the skin's interstitium may serve as a sodium reservoir, reducing the effect of sodium buildup on blood pressure and intravascular volume. In the subdermal interstitium, sodium builds up at hypertonic concentrations in complexes with proteoglycans during high-salt feeding. When sodium builds up in excess of water, macrophages infiltrating the interstitial space sense hypertonicity, which causes TonEBP, a transcription factor that controls the expression of osmo-protective genes, to be expressed. Vascular endothelial growth factor-C (VEGF-C), a strong inducer of lymph angiogenesis, is one of the genes downregulated by TonEBP. Titze's group discovered robust lymphatic vessel hyperplasia in the dermal interstitium as a reaction to high-salt feeding. This pathway is crucial for the extrarenal regulation of sodium and fluid volumes, as evidenced by the prevention of lymphatic vessel hyperplasia and the elevation of sodium-dependent hypertension caused by depletion of macrophages, cell-specific deletion of TonEBP from macrophages, or selective blockade of VEGF-C. Patients with refractory hypertension showed elevated plasma levels of VEGF-C, suggesting that this system may be disturbed in the human condition. Preclinical models, however, indicate that lower VEGF-C levels would encourage hypertension. However, since human chronic hypertension is a complicated condition, the elevated VEGF-C levels seen here are probably the result of tissue resistance to VEGF-C or even a compensatory mechanism.

2.2.5.5.1. Hypertensive Kidney Injury and the Progression of Chronic Kidney Disease

The primary cause of end-stage renal disease (ESRD) is primarily diabetic nephropathy, with hypertensive target organ damage to the kidney being the second most common site. Furthermore, it has been demonstrated that the existence of chronic kidney disease (CKD), including hypertension-related CKD, is a potent independent risk factor for unfavorable cardiovascular outcomes. Major components of clinical hypertensive renal disease, such as the marked individual variability in susceptibility to hypertensive renal damage and the seemingly inconsistent reno-protective efficacy of antihypertensive classes, are still poorly understood. According to studies, there is a consistent increase in the risk of incident CKD above an SBP of 120 mmHg, and time-varying SBP has been linked to incident CKD. A faster decline in renal function was linked to time-weighted SBP. The greatest risk factor for incident CKD was diabetes, and worse glycemic control and a faster rate of kidney function decline were linked to higher risk. These findings support the role of blood pressure and other established risk factors, such as diabetes, in the development and progression of kidney function decline in hypertensive patients with normal kidney function at baseline (Samuel, Francis, & Anthony, 2018).

A Closer Look

Renin-Angiotensin-Aldosterone System (RAAS)

The renin-angiotensin-aldosterone system (RAAS) is a critical hormonal cascade that plays a fundamental role in regulating blood pressure, fluid, and electrolyte balance, thus maintaining cardiovascular homeostasis. It is activated in response to low blood pressure, low blood volume, or low sodium concentration, primarily detected by the juxtaglomerular cells in the kidneys. The cascade begins with the release of renin, an enzyme produced by these juxtaglomerular cells. Renin then cleaves angiotensinogen, a precursor protein synthesized by the liver, converting it into angiotensin I. This relatively inactive peptide undergoes further conversion by the angiotensin-converting enzyme (ACE), predominantly in the lungs, into angiotensin II, a potent bioactive octapeptide.

Angiotensin II serves as the primary effector molecule of the RAAS and exerts multiple physiological actions to restore blood pressure and volume. It is a powerful vasoconstrictor, narrowing blood vessels, which increases systemic vascular resistance and, consequently, elevates blood pressure. Additionally, angiotensin II stimulates the secretion of aldosterone from the adrenal cortex. Aldosterone acts on the distal tubules and collecting ducts of the nephron in the kidneys, promoting the reabsorption of sodium and water while excreting potassium. This reabsorption increases blood volume and blood pressure, enhancing the circulatory system's ability to deliver oxygen and nutrients efficiently.

Furthermore, angiotensin II stimulates the release of antidiuretic hormone (ADH) or vasopressin from the posterior pituitary gland. ADH enhances water reabsorption in the kidneys' collecting ducts, contributing to increased blood volume and pressure. Angiotensin II also has direct effects on the heart and blood vessels, contributing to cardiac remodeling and vascular hypertrophy. These changes can improve the heart's pumping efficiency in the short term but may lead to pathological conditions such as hypertension and heart failure if the RAAS is chronically overactivated.

The regulation of RAAS is finely tuned, involving feedback mechanisms that prevent excessive activation. For instance, increased blood pressure and blood volume resulting from RAAS activation can inhibit further renin release through negative feedback. Additionally, natriuretic peptides, which are released by the heart in response to increased blood volume and pressure, counteract the effects of the RAAS by promoting natriuresis (sodium excretion) and vasodilation, thereby reducing blood pressure and volume.

Pharmacological intervention targeting the RAAS is a cornerstone in the management of hypertension, heart failure, and chronic kidney disease. ACE inhibitors, angiotensin II receptor blockers (ARBs), and aldosterone antagonists are commonly used to disrupt various points of the RAAS pathway. These medications help to lower blood pressure, reduce fluid overload, and minimize adverse cardiovascular and renal remodeling. By attenuating the effects of angiotensin

II and aldosterone, these drugs alleviate the burden on the heart and kidneys, improving clinical outcomes for patients with cardiovascular and renal disorders.

In conclusion, the renin-angiotensin-aldosterone system is a vital hormonal network that ensures blood pressure stability and fluid balance. Through a series of enzymatic conversions and hormonal actions, the RAAS modulates vascular tone, sodium and water reabsorption, and systemic vascular resistance. Its precise regulation is essential for maintaining cardiovascular health, and its dysregulation is implicated in various pathological states. Understanding the intricate mechanisms of the RAAS has paved the way for effective therapeutic strategies, highlighting its significance in medical science and clinical practice.

Summary

- The kidneys play a crucial role in maintaining the body's acid-base balance, a key aspect of homeostasis. This regulation is essential because even slight deviations in blood pH can significantly affect cellular function and metabolic processes.
- All acid-base disturbances result in compensation that tends to normalize the pH. Metabolic acid-base disorders result in respiratory compensation (change in PCO_2); respiratory acid-base disorders result in metabolic compensation (change in HCO_3^-).
- Acidosis also stimulates the secretion of parathyroid hormone (PTH). The increased levels of PTH act on the proximal tubule to inhibit phosphate reabsorption. In this way, more phosphate is delivered to the distal nephron, where it can serve as a urinary buffer and thus increase the capacity of the kidneys to excrete TA.
- $P2X_1$ receptor activation regulates renal vascular resistance and confers autoregulatory control of renal blood flow, glomerular capillary pressure and thus glomerular filtration rate.
- Activation of P2Y receptors in the renal vasculature can produce either vasoconstriction or vasodilation. Studies using the juxtamedullary nephron preparation demonstrated that stimulation of either $P2Y_1$ (2 methlythio-ATP) or $P2Y_{2,4}$ receptors (UTP) vasoconstricts afferent arterioles.
- Activation of P2 receptors in renal tubules can inhibit renal sodium transport. P2Y receptors seem to predominate in the proximal tubule. Activation of $P2Y_2$ receptors inhibits sodium and bicarbonate reabsorption by decreasing the activity of the Na^+/H^+ exchanger and Na^+/K^+ ATPase activity.
- The kidneys play a central role in the regulation of arterial blood pressure. A large body of experimental and physiological evidence indicates that renal control of extracellular volume and renal perfusion pressure are closely involved in maintaining the arterial circulation and blood pressure.
- Angiotensin-2 also stimulates the adrenal gland to secrete a hormone called aldosterone. Aldosterone stimulates more Na reabsorption in the distal tubule, and water gets reabsorbed along with the Na.
- The renin-angiotensin system (RAS) is a potent modulator of blood pressure and dysregulation of the RAS results in hypertension.
- Reliable evidence implicating a predominant role of the kidney in the regulation of blood pressure has defined the genetic basis of virtually all of the known Mendelian disorders associated with abnormal blood pressure phenotypes in humans.
- Salt sensitivity, defined as an exaggerated change in blood pressure in response to extremes in dietary salt intake, is relatively common and is associated with an increased risk for the development of hypertension.
- Macrophages infiltrating the interstitial space sense hypertonicity caused by this accumulation of sodium in excess of water, triggering the expression of TonEBP, a transcription factor regulating the expression of osmo-protective genes.

- The kidney remains a major site for hypertensive target organ damage which is second only to diabetic nephropathy as a primary cause of end-stage renal disease (ESRD).

References

1. Boron, W. (2006). Acid-base transport by renal proximal tubule. *Journal of the American Society of Nephrology, 17*, 2368–2382.
2. Breton, S., & Brown, D. (2007). New insights into the regulation of V-ATPase-dependent proton secretion. *American Journal of Physiology-Renal Physiology, 292*, F1–F10.
3. Curthoys, N. P. (2008). Renal ammonium ion production and excretion. In R. J. Alpern & S. C. Hebert (Eds.), *Seldin and Giebisch's the Kidney* (4th ed., pp. [specific page numbers]). Academic Press.
4. Guyton, A. C., & Coleman, T. G. (1999). Quantitative analysis of the pathophysiology of hypertension. *Journal of the American Society of Nephrology, 10*(10), 2248–2258.
5. Guyton, A. C., Coleman, T. G., & Granger, H. J. (1972). Circulation: Overall regulation. *Annual Review of Physiology, 34*, 13–46.
6. Guyton, A. G. (1961). Physiologic regulation of arterial pressure. *The American Journal of Cardiology, 8*(3), 401–407.
7. Hamm, L. L., & Nakhoul, N. L. (2008). Renal acidification. In B. M. Brenner (Ed.), *Brenner & Rector's The Kidney* (8th ed., pp. [specific page numbers]). Saunders.
8. Hamm, L. L., Alpern, R. J., & Preisig, P. A. (2008). Cellular mechanisms of renal tubular acidification. In R. J. Alpern & S. C. Hebert (Eds.), *Seldin and Giebisch's the Kidney* (4th ed., pp. [specific page numbers]). Academic Press.
9. Heidenreich, P. A., Trogdon, J. G., Khavjou, O. A., Butler, J., Dracup, K., Ezekowitz, M. D., Finkelstein, E. A., Hong, Y., Johnston, S. C., Khera, A., Lloyd-Jones, D. M., et al. (2011). Forecasting the future of cardiovascular disease in the United States: A policy statement from the American Heart Association. *Circulation, 123*(8), 933–944.
10. Inscho, E. W. (2001). P2 receptors in regulation of renal microvascular function. *American Journal of Physiology-Renal Physiology, 280*(6), F927–F944.
11. Koeppen, B. M., & Stanton, B. A. (2007). *Renal Physiology* (4th ed.). Mosby.
12. Koeppen, B. M., & Stanton, B. A. (2008). *Berne and Levy Physiology* (6th ed., pp. 638–640, 642–643). Mosby.
13. Lewington, S., Clarke, R., Qizilbash, N., Peto, R., & Collins, R. (2002). Age-specific relevance of usual blood pressure to vascular mortality: A meta-analysis of individual data for one million adults in 61 prospective studies. *Lancet, 360*(9349), 1903–1913.
14. McCormick, J. A., & Ellison, D. H. (2011). The WNKs: Atypical protein kinases with pleiotropic actions. *Physiological Reviews, 91*(1), 177–219.
15. Menzies, R. I., Unwin, R. J., Dash, R. K., Beard, D. A., Cowley, A. W. Jr, Carlson, B. E., Mullins, J. J., & Bailey, M. A. (2013). Effect of P2X4 and P2X7 receptor antagonism on the pressure diuresis relationship in rats. *Frontiers in Physiology, 4*, 305.

16. Oh, M. S., & Carroll, H. J. (2008). External balance of electrolytes and acids and alkalis. In R. J. Alpern & S. C. Hebert (Eds.), *Seldin and Giebisch's the Kidney* (4th ed., pp. [specific page numbers]). Academic Press.

17. Osborn, J. W., Fink, G. D., & Kuroki, M. T. (2011). Neural mechanisms of angiotensin II-salt hypertension: Implications for therapies targeting neural control of the splanchnic circulation. *Current Hypertension Reports, 13*, 221–228.

18. Parker, M. D., & Boron, W. F. (2008). Sodium-coupled bicarbonate transporters. In R. J. Alpern & S. C. Hebert (Eds.), *Seldin and Giebisch's the Kidney* (4th ed., pp. [specific page numbers]). Academic Press.

19. Rieg, T., Gerasimova, M., Boyer, J. L., Insel, P. A., & Vallon, V. (2011). $P2Y_2$ receptor activation decreases blood pressure and increases renal Na^+ excretion. *American Journal of Physiology-Regulatory, Integrative and Comparative Physiology, 301*(2), R510–R518.

20. Samuel, S. A., Francis, A. O., & Anthony, O. O. (2018). Role of the kidneys in the regulation of intra- and extra-renal blood pressure. *Annals of Clinical Hypertension, 2*, 048–058. https://doi.org/10.29328/journal.ach.1001011.

21. Sebastian, A., Frassetto, L. A., & Morris, R. C. Jr. (2008). The acid-base effects of the contemporary western diet: An evolutionary perspective. In R. J. Alpern & S. C. Hebert (Eds.), *Seldin and Giebisch's the Kidney* (4th ed., pp. [specific page numbers]). Academic Press.

22. Shibata, S., Zhang, J., Puthumana, J., Stone, K. L., & Lifton, R. P. (2013). Kelch-like 3 and Cullin 3 regulate electrolyte homeostasis via ubiquitination and degradation of WNK4. *Proceedings of the National Academy of Sciences U S A, 110*(20), 7838–7843.

23. Stewart, A. K., Kurschat, C. E., & Alper, S. L. (2008). The SLC4 anion exchanger gene family. In R. J. Alpern & S. C. Hebert (Eds.), *Seldin and Giebisch's the Kidney* (4th ed., pp. [specific page numbers]). Academic Press.

24. Vallon, V., Stockand, J. D., & Rieg, T. (2012). P2Y receptors and kidney function. *Wiley Interdisciplinary Reviews: Membrane Transport and Signaling, 1*(6), 731–742.

25. Weiner, I. D., & Hamm, L. L. (2007). Molecular mechanisms of renal ammonium transport. *Annual Review of Physiology, 69*, 317–340.

Chapter 3

URINE FORMATION AND CONCENTRATION MECHANISMS

Contents

Introduction

Urine is a liquid or semi-solid mixture of waste that is produced by animals and humans as a result of physiological processes. It also contains toxic substances that are released by excretory organs during fluid circulation. Urine is a common way for the human body to expel waste. Our kidneys have a vital function in the excretion process.

Both organic and inorganic materials can be found in urine. Urine can contain organic substances such as urea, creatinine, and uric acid. Among the inorganic solutes are chloride, sodium, and potassium. Its acidic pH of about 6 is caused by the presence of proteins. In healthy individuals, urobilin is primarily responsible for the color of their urine. As old blood cells undergo apoptosis, heme is broken down from hemoglobin, producing urobilin as a byproduct.

Adult humans produce between 1–2 liters (L) of urine on average per day, depending on their weight, activity level, environment, and overall health. Urine production that is either excessive or insufficient needs medical attention. Excessive urine production (> 2.5 L/day) is known as polyuria. Anuria (less than 100 mL per day) and oliguria (less than 400 mL per day) are conditions involving low urine output.

The kidneys' initial stage of producing urine is blood filtration. The percentage of cardiac output that reaches the kidney in a healthy person ranges from 12 to 30%, with an average of 20%, or 1.25% L/min.

The nephron is the fundamental structural and functional unit of the kidney. Its main job is to filter blood, reabsorb what's needed, and excrete the remainder as urine to control the concentration of water and soluble substances like sodium.

Bowman's capsule filters blood entering the tubules from the circulatory system in the first segment of the nephron. Filtration through a semipermeable membrane is facilitated by gradients in osmotic and hydrostatic pressure. Water, ions, and tiny molecules that easily flow through the filtration membrane make up the filtrate. Larger molecules, like proteins and blood cells, can't pass through the filtration membrane, though. The glomerular filtration rate, or GFR, is the volume of filtrate produced per minute and is equivalent to 180 liters per day. As this filtrate moves through the nephron, about 99% of it is reabsorbed, with the remaining 1% turning into urine.

The ability of land-dwelling mammals, including humans, to produce urine that is more concentrated than plasma is vital to their survival. The body loses water all the time through a variety of processes, such as evaporation into the expired air in the lungs, feces in the gastrointestinal tract, sweating and perspiration on the skin, and urine excretion by the kidneys.

Although the body needs to replace this lost fluid, the kidneys create concentrated urine by increasing water reabsorption, decreasing the volume of urine produced, and continuing to excrete solutes. A maximum urine concentration of 1,200–1,400 mOsm/L, or four–five times the osmolarity of plasma, can be produced by the human kidney. Urine concentrations in some desert animals can reach 10,000 mOsm/L, like in the case of the Australian hopping mouse. Because of this, the mouse can survive in the desert without drinking water because it can get enough water from the food it eats and the water it produces during its metabolism.

Orientation and Directional Terms

Term	Definition	Illustration
Urobilin	Urobilin is the chemical primarily responsible for the yellow color of urine. It is a linear tetrapyrrole compound that, along with the related colorless compound urobilinogen, are degradation products of the cyclic tetrapyrrole heme.	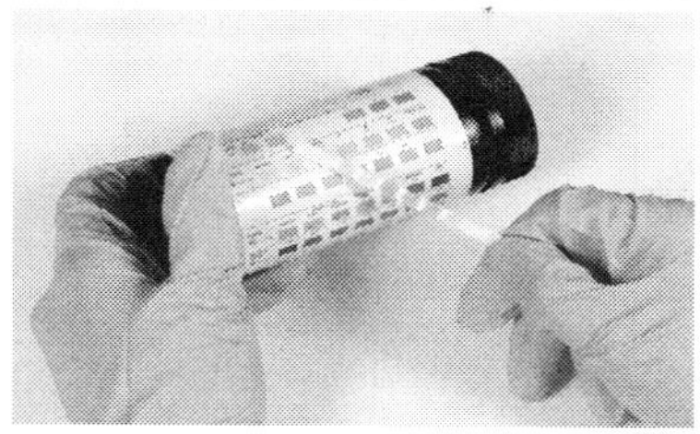
Uremia	Uremia is a clinical condition associated with declining renal function and is characterized by fluid overload, electrolyte imbalances, metabolic abnormalities, and physiological changes. The term "uremia" literally means "urine in the blood," which develops most commonly in chronic and end-stage renal disease.	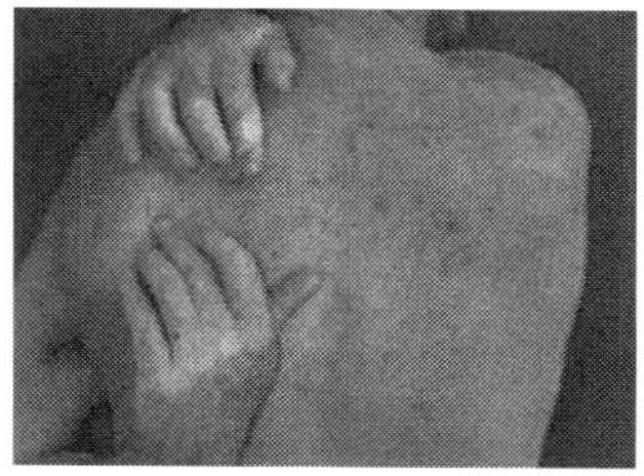
Uromodulin	Uromodulin is a zona pellucida-like domain-containing glycoprotein that in humans is encoded by the UMOD gene. Uromodulin is the most abundant protein excreted in ordinary urine.	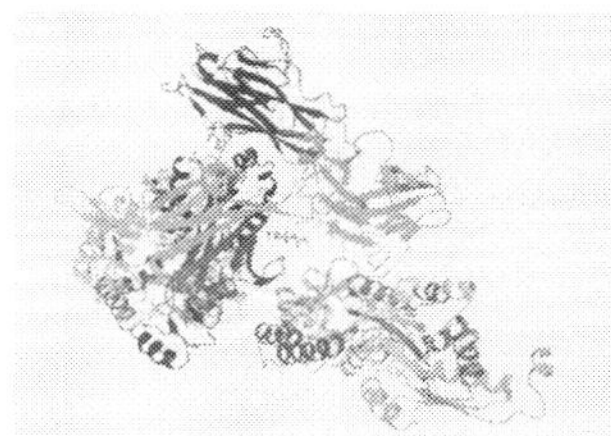
Nephron	The nephron is the minute or microscopic structural and functional unit of the kidney. It is composed of a renal corpuscle and a renal tubule.	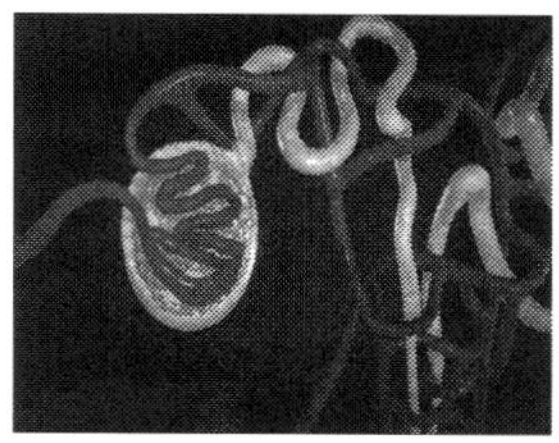
Glomerulus	The glomerulus is the filtering unit of the kidney, and each glomerulus consists of several capillary loops. Blood enters the glomerulus through the afferent arterioles and exits via the efferent arterioles; the glomerular capillaries are located between these two arteriolar systems.	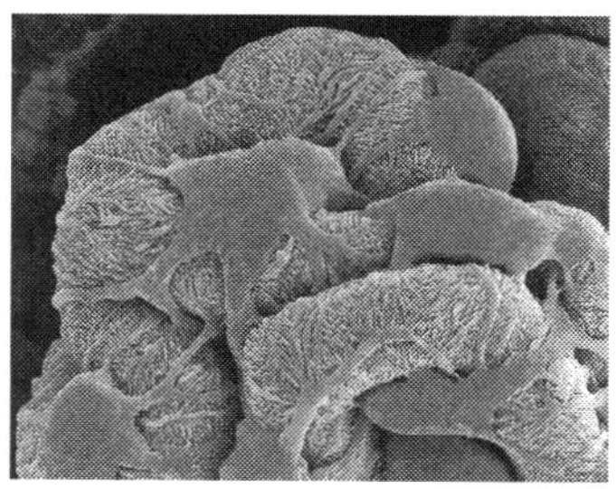

3.1. The Urine Formation

The formation of urine is an intricate process that involves excretion, tubular resorption, and glomerular ultrafiltration.

3.1.1. Glomerular Filtration

Every day, 180 liters of plasma are filtered through the glomerular capillaries, resulting in the production of 120 ml of ultrafiltrate per minute. The glomerular filter acts as though it is made up of pores with a diameter of 10 nm, allowing substances with a molecular weight of less than 70,000 Daltons to appear in the filtrate based on their molecular configuration. Globulins with a molecular weight of around 90,000 Daltons are not filtered, while small amounts of albumin (with a molecular weight of 69,000 Daltons) are filtered and reabsorbed in the proximal tubules. The process of glomerular filtration is similar to filtration at the arterial end of capillaries throughout the body. The driving force behind ultrafiltration is the hydrostatic pressure of blood generated by the heart. Unlike capillaries in striated muscles, the permeability of glomerular capillaries is 400 times greater and the pressure is significantly higher, but ultrafiltration of blood plasma does not require local energy supply. The effective filtration pressure is determined by the hydrostatic blood pressure, the oncotic pressure of plasma proteins, and the pressure inside the Bowman's capsule. It typically measures around 3.3 kPa (25 torr). The ultrafiltrate, or primary urine, contains minimal proteins (maximum of 150 mg/l), low molecular weight non-electrolyte substances (such as glucose, amino acids, and urea), and monovalent ions (like sodium, potassium, and chlorides) at similar levels to plasma. Diffusion of plasma proteins does not occur, and instead, the distribution of monovalent diffusible ions follows Gibbs-Donnan principles. Minor variations in ion concentration are due to the Gibbs-Donnan effect, with cation levels in ultrafiltrate around 5% lower and anion levels around 5% higher than in plasma. In conditions like severe paraproteinemia and hyperlipidemia, the concentration of low-molecular substances in ultrafiltrate can exceed that of plasma. Divalent ions like calcium and magnesium, as well as organic acids and bases that bind to plasma proteins, are significantly lower in concentration in ultrafiltrate compared to plasma.

Should a substance pass from blood into the primordial urine it has to cross three barriers:

1. The endothelial layer with pores-fenestrations on the inner surface of glomerular capillaries
2. Three layers make up the basement membrane. The appropriate filtering membrane is in the middle layer. It is made up of minuscule collagenous fibers woven into a three-dimensional network and embedded in a uniform matrix made possible by pores ranging in size from 30 to 60 nm.
3. The layer of glomerular capillary outer wall is made up of epithelial cells called podocytes, which have multiple foot processes. A layer of acid mucopolysaccharides, or glycocalyx, covers the surface of podocytes and fills in the spaces between them. Both electric charge and the makeup of the particles leaking into the ultrafiltrate have an impact on the permeability of capillaries.

Glomerular filtration is crucial for the metabolism of fluid and electrolytes. This can be inferred from the fact that kidneys filter four times the volume of fluid in the entire body, 15 times the volume of extracellular fluid, and 60 times the volume of blood plasma every day.

Glomerular filtration is affected by the following factors:

1. Changes of systemic arterial pressure or anatomically restrained blood supply for glomeruli (e.g., in renovascular diseases)
2. Changes of intrarenal tissue pressure (in obstructions of ureters, in edema of kidneys, in perinephritis)
3. Changes in oncotic pressure of plasma (e.g., in dehydration)
4. Reduction of filtration surface (involution of glomeruli, partial nephrectomy)

Glomerular filtration is dependent upon the age, body surface, and state of hydration. Renal functions are lowered in the first four days following delivery. Glomerular filtration in adults is limited to only 25–50% of the filtration values. The newborn typically has lower plasmic pH and bicarbonate values due to decreased concentration ability, excretion of water, NaCl, phosphates, and ammonia formation. The tubular apparatus has decreased formation of ADH, which makes it less sensitive and less efficient. Even though a baby's or suckling's kidney function is limited, it is still adequate in most situations, particularly when the baby is breastfed. The glomerular filtration in men is higher in relation to the body surface. As one ages, glomerular filtration decreases. This discovery provides broad insights into an individual's biological age. Additionally, glomerular filtration varies by up to 30% throughout the day.

3.1.1.1. Measurement of Glomerular Filtration Rate

A healthy kidney carries out its many tasks by filtering blood through a procedure called glomerular filtration. The glomerular filtration rate is a key indicator of kidney function (GFR). The rate at which filtered fluid passes through the kidney is known as the glomerular filtration rate. The volume of blood plasma cleared of creatinine per unit of time is known as the creatinine clearance rate (C^{Cr} or CrCl), and it is a useful metric for estimating GFR. Because creatinine secretion can be inhibited by cimetidine, creatinine clearance surpasses GFR. GFR and C_{Cr} can be reliably determined by comparing the amounts of different substances in the blood and urine, or they can be estimated using formulas that only require the results of a blood test (eGFR and eC_{Cr}). The outcomes of these examinations are used to evaluate the kidneys' excretory capacity. The causes of kidney disease, albuminuria, and GFR categories are taken into consideration when staging chronic kidney disease.

- **Creatinine:** GFR is, however, measured in clinical practice using serum creatinine level-based estimates of creatinine clearance or creatinine clearance itself. The body naturally produces creatinine, which is a byproduct of the breakdown of creatine phosphate, which is present in muscle. It is actively secreted by the peritubular capillaries in very small amounts and is freely filtered by the glomerulus. As a result, creatinine clearance overestimates the actual GFR by 10 to 20%. Considering how simple it is to measure creatinine clearance, this margin of error is acceptable. Since creatinine is already at a steady-state concentration in the blood, measuring creatinine clearance is far less laborious than precise GFR measurements that require continuous inulin infusions. Nevertheless, there are restrictions on creatinine-based GFR estimations. The 24-hour creatinine excretion rate, which is a highly variable function of muscle mass, is the basis for all of the estimating equations. The Cockcroft and Gault equation is one of the equations that does not account for race. For any given rate of clearance, serum creatinine will be higher in people with greater muscle mass.

- **Inulin:** By injecting inulin or its inulin-analog sinistrin into the bloodstream, the GFR can be ascertained. Since the kidneys do not reabsorb or secrete inulin or sinistrin following glomerular filtration, the rate at which these substances are excreted is directly correlated with the rate at which water and other solutes are filtered through the glomerular filter.
One major source of error in the measurement of inulin clearance is incomplete urine collection. When it comes to comparing different methods of estimating glomerular filtration rate, the "gold standard" for measuring kidney function is inulin. Inulin and sinistrin-based products were taken off the market by the French pharmacovigilance agency in 2018 after some patients experienced hypersensitivity reactions that resulted in death. As a result, the contrast agents iohexol and iothalamate have gained popularity as GFR alternatives since they are thought to exhibit adequate accuracy.
- **Radioactive Tracers:** Chromium-51 and technetium-99m, two radioactive substances, can be used to measure GFR accurately. These are more practically measured with a small number of urine or blood samples, but they are nearly identical to the ideal properties of inulin (undergoing only glomerular filtration). In Europe, renal or plasma clearance measurements of ^{51}Cr-EDTA are commonly performed; in the US, however, this is not possible; instead, ^{99}mTc-DTPA may be utilized. It has been demonstrated that ^{51}Cr-EDTA renal and plasma clearance is accurate when compared to the gold standard, inulin. In UK guidelines, the use of ^{51}Cr-EDTA is regarded as a reference standard measure. (Henriksen et al. 2015).
- **Cystatin C:** Issues with creatinine (differentiating muscle mass, recent meat consumption—much less reliant on diet than urea) have prompted the assessment of substitute agents for GFR estimation. Among these is cystatin C, a widely distributed protein that is secreted by the majority of body cells and functions as an inhibitor of cysteine protease.

The glomerulus freely filters cyclostatin C. Cystatin C is catabolized and reabsorbed by tubular epithelial cells following filtration, with only trace amounts excreted in the urine. Thus, the bloodstream rather than urine is used to measure cystatin C levels.

There are now developed equations that relate serum cystatin C levels to the estimated GFR. Recently, adjusted cystatin C and creatinine have been combined with variables for age, race, and sex in some proposed equations. The most accurate is adjusted cystatin C (based on age, race, and sex), which is followed by adjusted creatinine (based on age, race, and sex) and cystatin C alone (which differs slightly from adjusted creatinine) (Pallone et al, 2003; Sands & Layton, 2008).

3.1.2. Tubular Functions

Urine's final volume and composition are adjusted by changes in the tubules to conform to the organism's requirements. The tubular function is to retain the beneficial substances while excreting harmful and unnecessary substances. Complex reabsorption and secretion processes carry out the tubular functions.

3.1.2.1. Mechanisms of Tubular Absorption

Pinocytosis is the process by which filtered proteins are absorbed. Through the cellular membrane, protein molecules can enter tubular cells. There are stereospecific receptors on the cell surface that can capture a portion of the filtered proteins. Other substances travel across chemical and electrical gradients by active transport as well as passive diffusion in their direction. During active transport, oxygen is consumed (aerobic oxidation). The presence of carriers is required for both active and passive transport mechanisms.

Most solutes found in ultrafiltrate and absorbed in tubules are electrolytes, either strongly or weakly charged electrically. Both their size and the transtubular electrical potential are significant factors in the absorption of these substances.

Without requiring an instant energy source, water, chlorides, and urea move passively in the direction of an electrical gradient.

Na^+, K^+, PO_4^-, amino acids, glucose, creatine, sulfate, uric acid, and ketonic substances are all actively absorbed. It was discovered that there are various transporting systems for individual amino acids.

3.1.2.2. Mechanisms of Tubular Secretion

Substances are transported by the kidneys from tubular fluid into the interstitium as well. Transport of substances from peritubular fluid into the tubules happens in the kidneys during the intricate process of excreting substances from the body. Tubular secretion is the term for this process. Tubular secretion plays a significant role in maintaining isotonia and controlling the acid-base balance.

The tubular secretion can be accomplished:

1. actively with limited transport maximum (Tm)
2. actively with transport capacity limited by gradient and time
3. passively

Active mechanisms limited by Tm or by gradient and time require energy for substance transport from blood into urine. Passive secretion does not need direct energy, but relies on concentration and electric gradients, both of which require energy. The mechanism of para-aminohippuric acid (PAH) excretion, particularly with limited Tm, has been extensively studied. Its excretion through glomerular filtration and tubular secretion increases in proportion to its plasma concentration. Once a certain level is surpassed, tubular secretion remains consistent and unaffected by plasma concentration. This is why PAH clearance is used to measure renal blood flow.

Weak acids and bases (ammonia, salicylic acid, phenobarbital, penicillin), as well as potassium, are secreted into the urine through the tubules. An active mechanism that is limited by gradient and most likely by time secretes hydrogen ions. Hydrogen ions are secreted in large quantities in the proximal tubule against a low concentration gradient and in small quantities against a high concentration gradient in the collecting tubules.

3.1.2.3. Maintenance of Extracellular Milieu Stability

Kidneys create ideal conditions for the intracellular milieu by preserving the stability of the extracellular milieu.

Since sodium accounts for 80–90% of the osmotic active substances in plasma and interstitial fluid, its concentration predetermines the extracellular fluid volume.

In this way, kidneys serve an essential role in the body by eliminating excess sodium and, conversely, storing it when necessary. Mineralocorticoids are produced in the suprarenal cortex and work in tandem with the endocrine system to accomplish this function. Aldosterone is the primary "representative" of mineralocorticoids, as it ensures the renal sodium economy and, consequently, the regulation of body fluid volume.

Throughout the entire nephron, multiple cells have aldosterone receptors. The cells of collecting tubules are most likely where aldosterone receptors are found in the greatest quantity. Aldosterone promotes potassium excretion and sodium reabsorption in collecting tubules. It's called the potassium excretion and sodium resorption dependent on aldosterone. This process mostly takes place in the collecting tubular medullar region. The aldosterone effect is only temporary and only acts in response to the body's demands. The renin-angiotensin-aldosterone system controls the secretion of aldosterone.

The kallikrein-kinin system is another important hormonal system that impacts renal functions. Kallikrein is produced in distal tubule cells, where the highest activity of kallikrein-synthetase is found. Kallikrein converts plasmatic kininogens into kinins (such as bradykinin, lysyl-bradykinin, and methionyl-lysyl bradykinin) through proteolysis. Interestingly, the same enzyme that converts angiotensin I to angiotensin II also breaks down kinins. Kinins have a contrasting effect to angiotensin, acting as potent vasodilators in the kidneys and stimulating the release of prostaglandins (PGE2). They counteract the vasoconstrictive and antidiuretic actions of angiotensin, dilating both the afferent and efferent vessels.

Glucocorticoids, specifically cortisol, have an impact on sodium secretion (but also progesterone). In contrast to mineralocorticoids, glucocorticoids improve sodium reabsorption and raise glomerular filtration. In the absence of glucocorticoids, the glomerular ultrafiltrate volume decreases, and the excretion of excess water is reduced due to the increased permeability of distal tubules to water under water loading. Aldosterone's tubular effects are countered by progesterone. It uses the spironolactone mechanism to increase the excretion of sodium. It directly lessens the effect of aldosterone in the renal tubules.

In the proximal tubule, sodium reabsorption, along with chloride ions (Cl^-), occurs first, followed by the reabsorption of water due to the permeability of the epithelium. Sodium salts make up 80% of the solutes in the ultrafiltrate, serving as a pumping system for transporting other substances. Around 60 to 75% of the sodium filtered in the proximal tubule is reabsorbed along with chloride and bicarbonate ions, resulting in an isoosmotic process with an equivalent volume of water. This process keeps the tubular fluid in the proximal tubule isonatremic and isoosmotic with plasma, with a sodium concentration of 140 mmol/l and an osmolality of about 300 mosm/l. If poorly resorbable but osmotically active substances such as mannitol enter the tubular fluid, the reabsorption of sodium and water continues but some water may be retained to maintain isoosmotic conditions with the interstitial fluid. This can lead to a reduction in the sodium concentration in the tubular fluid, sometimes by half.

Reabsorption of the filtered sodium load occurs in tubules concurrently. This compensation is typically insufficient during more significant changes in glomerular filtration (glomerulo-tubular dissociation). As was previously mentioned, sodium is transported from tubules passively and without the need for metabolic energy; its active transport is reliant on the availability of energy. Proximal tubule cells are functionally polarized, meaning that passive sodium flow from the tubular lumen into the cell is more permeable through the luminal membrane portion of the cell. There is less permeability in the area of the cell membrane that faces the intracellular space and the interstitium. This is where the sodium pump's active sodium transport actually takes place.

Because of the electrochemical gradient between tubule and tubular cell, passive sodium transport across the luminal membrane of proximal tubule cells precedes active transtubular sodium transport. Sodium can be carried either alone or in combination with the HCO^{-}_{3} anion, amino acids, phosphates, glucose, uric acid, and other materials. Certain substances can cross the luminal membrane even in the presence of a concentration gradient thanks to the cotransport of sodium, which increases their cellular concentration. By passive transport, they subsequently travel in the direction of the concentration gradient, entering the peritubular space and peritubular capillaries. The sodium pump, which is the enzyme Na^{+}–K^{+}–ATP-ase, is responsible for the decreasing Na^{+} gradient between the tubule and the tubular cell. It converts the high-energy binding of inorganic phosphorus in ATP to an electrochemical gradient. Three Na^{+} and two K^{+} are moved into and out of the cell by the hydrolysis of one ATP molecule. In light of the sodium concentration in the tubule (chemical gradient) and the high concentration of K+ that exits the cell under the same chemical gradient, the cell maintains a low cellular sodium ion concentration. As a result, the cell inside becomes electronegative (-70 to -90 mV) in relation to its surroundings.

Through the sodium transtubule and pertinent anion transport (Cl–, HCO^{-}_{3}, amino acids, etc.) into the peritubular labyrinth and the intercellular space, the so-called stationary osmotic gradient is formed. However, it is quickly disrupted by water diffusing into the peritubular space and retrograde diffusion occurring through intracellular space into the tubule. The osmotic concentration in the tubule or peritubular space remains constant because an appropriate volume of water is reabsorbed after the primary active solute reabsorption. Because of the buildup of water, the hydrostatic pressure in the peritubular space increases. The peritubular capillaries receive the fluid that is absorbed from the peritubular space. The hydrostatic and colloidal osmotic pressure ratios are necessary for this process to occur.

In the proximal tubule, the filtered potassium is nearly entirely reabsorbed. Additionally, active reabsorption of other substances (such as calcium, magnesium, glucose, amino acids, etc.) occurs in the proximal tubule.) and, from a pharmacological perspective, the location of significant acid and base carrier mechanisms.

In the proximal tubule, the filtered potassium is nearly entirely reabsorbed. In addition, the proximal tubule is the location of significant acid and base carrier mechanisms from a pharmacological perspective as well as the site of active resorption of other substances, including calcium, magnesium, glucose, and amino acids.

The same locations as sodium reabsorption—primarily in the proximal tubule—also host calcium reabsorption. Only about 50% of plasmatic calcium can be filtered out and dissolved; the remainder is bound to plasmatic proteins. Calcium and sodium ion ratios are kept equal in both plasma and ultrafiltrate.

The concentration of calcium in plasma is between 2,25 and 2,75 mmol/l. Proteins bind to some of it, while other parts are diffusible and exist as free Ca^{2+} ions and their compounds, such as phosphates, citrates, and bicarbonates. Urine excretes between 0.5 and 5.0% of the filtered calcium loading. It is necessary for filtered calcium loading for tubular reabsorption. Ca^{2+}–Na^{+}–ATP-ase actively transports calcium across the peritubular membrane. The distal tubule's reabsorption is improved by parathormone. Calcium reabsorption is inhibited by cortisol and thyrocalcitonin. A parathyroidectomy causes the excretion of calcium in the urine to increase. Hypercalciuria is brought on by thyroxine stimulating the metabolism of bone tissue.

In proximal tubules, approximately 90% of filtered phosphate is reabsorbed under physiological conditions. By preventing phosphate from being reabsorbed, parathormone increases phosphate excretion. Under 15% of phosphates may be reabsorbed as a result of increased parathormone secretion. Phosphate reabsorption in proximal tubules is gradually reduced to achieve optimal phosphate excretion. The primary factor regulating phosphate excretion is an increase in parathormone release accompanied by a decrease in the number of nephrons. Despite perfect regulation, there is a brief increase in plasmatic phosphates, which results in a slight decrease in the level of ionized calcium and an increase in the release of parathormones. Once equilibrium is reached, an increase in plasmatic phosphate levels disturbs it once more. The level of parathormone increases almost permanently as a result of this repeated process. Parathormone degradation in the kidneys is insufficient as a result of progressive nephron loss. And lastly, if the glomerular filtration rate is less than 25 ml/min. the organism starts to hold onto the phosphates. A secondary parathyroidism that is linked to renal osteodystrophy occurs. The breakdown of the functioning renal parenchyma affects the metabolism of phosphate, calcium, and bone.

The process of converting vitamin D into its active metabolites is significantly aided by the kidneys. The skin synthesizes the precursors of vitamin D active form, or dietary intake provides them, and the liver hydroxylates them to form 25-hydroxycholecalciferol. Kidneys carry out additional hydroxylation, which forms l, 25-dihydroxycholecalciferol. This active form of vitamin D promotes bone resorption as well as the intestinal absorption of calcium and phosphate. It is likely that 1,25-dihydroxycholecalciferol prevents parathormone's phosphaturic effect in renal tubules. Renal disorders may have an impact on the hydroxylation of vitamin D (Pallone et al, 2003; Sands & Layton, 2008).

Magnesium concentration in plasma is between 0.7 and 0.9 mmol/l. Approximately one-third of this quantity is in an undiffusible state. Free magnesium ions, or Mg^{2+}, make up the diffusible portion. Urine excretes 3 to 6% of the filtered load. Glucocorticoids, parathormone, calcitonin, and vitamin D all increase the excretion of magnesium.

When a substance's glomerular supply does not surpass a threshold, it is classified as a threshold substance because it has been fully reabsorbed in the proximal tubule. Phosphates, glucose, and amino acids are a few of them. There are no truly true threshold drugs or truly true substances without a renal threshold. One common threshold substance is glucose. In the proximal tubule, it is almost quantitatively reabsorption. If the tubular load and, consequently, the plasmatic concentration of glucose do not surpass the renal glucose threshold, glucose is almost entirely reabsorbed, leaving no trace. At a normal glucose plasmatic concentration of 90 mg%, or roughly 5 mmol/l, approximately 110 mg (0,6 mmol) of glucose is reabsorbed every minute.

GFPg, the glucose concentration in plasma, and the glomerular ultrafiltrate volume can be used to calculate the amount of reabsorbed glucose. If every nephron is functioning to its full potential, tubular cells can reabsorb up to three times as much. The first half of the proximal tubule is where the majority of glucose is reabsorbed. The glucose threshold, also known as the maximum amount that a tubule could reabsorb and return to the blood, is known as the transport maximum (Tmg). The difference between the amount of filtered glucose and the amount of glucose expelled by urine can be used to calculate it.

$$T_{mg} = (GF.Pg) - (V.Ug)$$

V is the urine volume per minute, GF is the amount of glomerular ultrafiltrate, and Pg and Ug are the glucose concentrations in plasma and urine, respectively.

The total functional capacity of tubular cells to transport glucose is provided by T_{mg}. Technically speaking, T_{mg} determination is challenging since maintaining such a high glucose concentration is necessary to prevent glycosuria. Renal threshold is directly correlated with T_{mg} and indirectly correlated with glomerular filtration. In the proximal tubule, there is a linear relationship between sodium reabsorption and glucose transport. This relationship is also evident in the reabsorption of specific amino acids. The proximal tubule's sodium reabsorption is primarily dependent on glomerular filtration rather than glucose reabsorption. The proximal tubule reabsorbs more sodium when the tubular sodium load is higher. As previously stated, because tubules have such a large capacity for reabsorption, the tubular load needs to be greater than three times the filtrated load to fully saturate the tubular reabsorption capacity and prevent the excess glucose from leaking into the urine. A portion of the maximum glucose transport is influenced by the reabsorption of water and sodium. Reabsorption of sodium, water, and glucose rises in tandem with glomerular filtration. However, even when compared to sodium and water reabsorption, tubular glucose absorption increases significantly if the tubular glucose load rises noticeably due to the elevated plasmatic glucose level. However, the excretion of glucose into the urine starts if the T_{mg} is reached. It is unclear exactly how glucose excretion works. The most likely method would be active transportation. This assumption may be supported by the observation that cyanides, acidosis, and hypoxia inhibit the transport of glucose.

Even though uric acid makes up only 5% of the products of the global metabolism of nitrogenous substances, kidneys are crucial to the excretion of uric acid. In hyperuricemic syndrome, excretion of uric acid is particularly significant. As with other organic acids, uric acid is freely filtered in glomeruli. Additionally, it is partially reabsorbed after being secreted in the proximal tubule. The clearance of uric acid is low, only 12 ml/min, when compared to the clearance of creatinine and inulin. (Creatine has a clearance rate of roughly 120 ml/min.). The fact that undissociated uric acid is poorly soluble is significant from a practical standpoint. Acidosis decreases uric acid's solubility. 98% of uric acid is in dissociated form at pH 7.4. A pH of 4 or lower causes only 5% of uric acid to dissociate. Under these circumstances, uric acid may go through the process of crystal nucleation and form urate stones. Greater sodium concentrations facilitate the easier formation of uric acid into urate crystals or calculi. Water diuresis can stop or inhibit the precipitation of uric acid.

Urea is the most significant byproduct of protein metabolism. In and of itself, urea is not very toxic to living things. Its level during uremia is a sign of concurrently retained hazardous byproducts of metabolism. Generally speaking, the amount of food protein consumed and its metabolic turnover determine how stable its plasmatic level is. The plasmatic urea level can normally range from twice the physiological value (4,5 mol/l) to higher values. In healthy subjects, the amount of urea that is cleared is between 50 and 60% of the filtered amount. It is clear that both the rate of tubular fluid flow and glomerular filtration affect the clearance of urea. Due to decreased diuresis brought on by dehydration, urea clearance increases significantly more than inulin clearance. Because of this, abnormalities in renal function may be roughly indicated by the urea clearance. However, it is unable to differentiate between disorders that are caused by hemodynamics and renal disturbances. The mechanism of retrograde diffusion or solvent drag is used to explain the urea reabsorption, which is thought to be a passive process. In addition to tubular fluid concentration and transtubular retrograde water diffusion, tubular permeability to urea and tubular fluid volume also play a role in urea reabsorption. The primary contributing factor is most likely the urea concentration gradient between the surrounding interstitium and tubular fluid. When tubular cellular membranes are unbroken, urea and water diffuse isoosmotically. It's likely that the same mechanism applies to other substances as well.

3.1.2.4. Na^+ and Cl^- Reabsorption in the Loop of Henle by Counter-Current Multiplication System

The concentration of urine is primarily driven by the descending and ascending limbs of Henle's loop, the collecting tubule, and vasa recta. The active transport of sodium from the ascending limb of Henle's loop into the surrounding interstitium is the key force behind this process. Water cannot diffuse with sodium in this segment of the nephron, as it is impermeable to it. However, the descending limb of Henle's loop becomes permeable to water in the presence of ADH. With a concentration gradient in place, water is drawn into the interstitium. The osmotic gradient between the ascending and descending limbs, as well as the interstitium, only accounts for a small portion of the overall concentration gradient between plasma and final urine. Despite a low osmotic gradient, water continuously diffuses from the ascending limb into the interstitium, which remains slightly more hyperosmotic. This is maintained through constant water diffusion and an increase in the osmolality of tubular fluid towards the papilla. Conversely, the fluid within Henle's loop's ascending limb consistently has a slightly higher osmolality than the interstitium around it. This fact encourages the transport of sodium into the interstitium. Since the counter-current system multiplies many of these partial effects, a concentration difference develops that progressively increases toward the loop's bend and achieves multiple values of individual partial effects. From a thermodynamic perspective, this is an incredibly energy-efficient process that uses less energy than the kidneys would use to concentrate urine to its final concentration in a single step.

The fluid at the end of Henle's loop's ascending limb returns to being hyposmotic, with a sodium concentration that is 100 mmol/l lower than that of the plasmatic concentration (140 mmol/l). This fluid enters the distal tubule and causes the wall to become permeable to water once more, allowing for the achievement of osmotic balance, or the equilibration of osmotic concentration gradients between the tubular fluid and the isomotic interstitium at the distal tubule's end. When compared to the volume in the Henle loop, the tubular fluid volume decreases by half as a result of water diffusion and additional sodium reabsorption. Next, tubular fluid travels through areas of the interstitium where the concentration of sodium is increasing as it flows in collecting ducts towards the papilla. When ADH is present, this hyperosmotic environment suctions water out of the collecting tubule until osmotic balance manifests.

In addition to the counter-current exchange system, the vasa recta aids in the kidneys' concentrating and diluting processes. The descending section of these capillaries experiences a water transfer (shift) from the lumen into the interstitium because their wall is permeable to water and osmotically active substances. Water and osmotically active substances move in the opposite direction during their ascending phase. The vasa recta experiences a reduction in counter-current diffusion as the medullar blood flow increases. The administration of medications that cause medullar vessel vasodilation may result in this condition. This is also seen in shock, where there is a decrease in glomerular filtration, but there is no change in medullar blood flow. In a physiological setting, a decrease in the osmotic concentration gradient between the renal cortex and medulla can reduce the effectiveness of counter-current diffusion in the vasa recta.

The exchange of H^+ for Na^+ most likely happens throughout the tubule. This process, which produces bicarbonate reabsorption, urine acidification, and the excretion of fixed anions in combination with $NH4^+$ rather than Na^+, is extremely significant for maintaining homeostasis. On the luminal poles of cells, tubular cells secrete hydrogen ions, which are concurrently exchanged for other cations. One sodium ion enters the cells for every hydrogen ion. Every day, approximately 4,000 mmol of H+ are secreted from the proximal tubules, and 500 mmol of hydrogen ions are likewise secreted from the distal tubules. This excess amount of hydrogen ions is secreted every day. Its pH would drop to 1.4 if 60 mmol of free acids in 1.5 l were eliminated every day. Urine never has a pH lower than 4.5.

The kidneys play a vital role in the resorption of bicarbonate. The majority of filtered bicarbonates are actively reabsorbed in the proximal tubules. The bicarbonate renal threshold matches their plasma concentration, which is typically 22 to 25 mmol/l under normal conditions. In the tubular cell, carbonic acid is responsible for exchanging hydrogen ions for sodium ions.

It is formed by the following reactions:

$$H_2O + CO_2 \rightleftharpoons H_2CO_3 \rightleftharpoons H^+ + HCO_3^-$$

A significantly higher rate of CO_2 hydration is needed to supply the exchange reaction with a sufficient supply of hydrogen ions than occurs during the reaction's spontaneous course. The carbonic anhydrase enzyme keeps the cell at the proper rate of hydration.

H^+ and Na^+ are switched during the bicarbonate reabsorption process. Na^+ conjugates with $HCO^-{}_3$ in the tubular cell and returns to the blood as $NaHCO_3$.

Urine containing hydrogen ions reacts with $HCO^-{}_3$, producing H_2CO_3, which breaks down quickly into CO_2 and water. Rediffusion of CO_2 from urine occurs, and it is either exhaled by the lungs or utilized by tubular cells to form H_2CO_3. Even after all of the bicarbonate has been used, hydrogen ions and sodium ions are still exchanging.

Phosphoric acid is created during metabolic processes and neutralized to produce neutral salts. Phosphate excretion in the form of neutral salts may cause sodium depletion, which in turn may cause a decrease in $HCO^-{}_3$ Urine contains hydrogen ions that react with the buffer system, primarily converting Na_2HPO_4 to NaH_2PO_4. When Na^+ and $HCO^-{}_3$ react within the cell once more, the organism's alkali reserve rises.

When bicarbonate and phosphate buffers are not present, H^+ is substituted for Na^+ in a neutral salt (mostly NaCl). The hydrogen ion transport can only overcome a maximum difference of approximately three pH units, so the HCl formed would acidify urine (raise the hydrogen ion concentration) to the point where further exchange is impossible. But then something else starts to work. Ammonia is mostly synthesized by the renal cells from glutamine and amino acids. Ammonia readily penetrates the cell membrane because it is soluble in lipids. Through the process of non-ionic diffusion, it enters the tubular fluid and forms here with H^+ ammonium NH_4^+. Because ammonium ions are poorly liposoluble, urine excretes them instead of them undergoing rediffusion. As a result, both H^+ and NH_3 vanish from urine, and additional hydrogen ion exchange for sodium ion as well as additional NH_3 diffusion into the urine are once more feasible. In this manner, a significant amount of Na^+ from neutral urine salts is reabsorbed by the renal cells and returned to the blood as bicarbonate. Strong acid anions in tubular fluid are expelled as ammonium salts, sparing sodium and bicarbonates in the process (Pallone et al, 2003; Sands & Layton, 2008).

3.2. Countercurrent Mechanism – Urine Formation and Steps

Urine concentration is the kidney's countercurrent mechanism. An osmotic gradient is produced by the filtrate flowing in opposing directions through the two limbs of the loop of Henle. The kidneys can reabsorb water from the filtrate and generate concentrated urine because of this gradient.

3.2.1. Countercurrent Mechanisms

The kidneys' ability to recycle salts and water to concentrate urine is known as the countercurrent mechanism.

The kidney uses this mechanism to produce hypertonic urine from isotonic nephric filtrate. The nephron's loop of Henle and Vasacounter-current recta is where this process occurs. The descending and ascending limbs make up the Henle loop. In these two limbs, the filtrate flows in the opposite direction, producing a counter-current (counter-opposite counter-current, Current – flow). The capillaries known as vasa recta run parallel to the Henle loop. Additionally, blood flows in the opposite direction in the vasa recta. Osmolarity is maintained by the loop of Henle and the vasa recta being close to one another.

There are three types of counter-exchange systems:

- **Countercurrent Exchange:** In this scenario, the fluid flows in the opposite direction of the original flow.
- **Current Exchange:** The fluid flows in the same direction as the starting flow during the current exchange.
- **Contra-current Exchange:** This kind of exchange is comparable to countercurrent exchange, as the name suggests, in that fluid is transferred in the opposite direction. The term might imply a more inclusive meaning that encompasses both countercurrent and current exchange.

3.2.2. Where Does the Counter-Current Mechanism of Urine Formation Occur?

The kidneys exhibit this process. Nephrons are the functional units that make up the kidney. Nephrons can be classified into two types according to where the glomerular capsule is located.

They are:

- Superficial Cortical nephrons that make up 70–80% of nephrons.
- Juxtamedullary nephrons making up to 20% of nephrons.

Nephrons can be categorized based on their function and structural makeup. The proximal tubule, distal tubule, loop of Henle, collecting duct, and glomerulus are some of these sections. A thin ascending limb that continues into a thick ascending limb makes up the Loop of Henle. A thin descending limb also forms part of it. This has a hairpin-like shape to it. The inner medulla of the kidney is deeply penetrated by the Loop of Henle of juxtamedullary nephrons.

Urine concentration depends on the development of the osmotic gradient, which is primarily brought about by countercurrent multiplication in the Henle loops of juxtamedullary nephrons. Additional concentration adjustments take place in the distal convoluted tubule, where fluid drains into collecting tubules after leaving the ascending limb of the loop of Henle. The ureter then carries the urine to the bladder.

3.2.3. Steps in Countercurrent Mechanism

- **Step 1:** Assume that the concentration of 300 mOsm/L that exits the proximal tubules fills Henle's loop.
- **Step 2:** The Henle's loop thick ascending limb active ion pump raises the interstitial concentration while lowering the tubule's internal concentration.
- **Step 3:** The lower limb's tubular fluid and the interstitial fluid quickly reach osmotic equilibrium as a result of the descending limb's osmosis of water.
- **Step 4:** Extra fluid enters Henle's loop from the proximal tubule, allowing the hyperosmotic fluid created in the descending limb to enter the ascending limb.
- **Step 5:** Up until an osmotic gradient of 200 mOsm / L was established, more ions were pumped into the interstitium while the water in the tubular fluid was still present.
- **Step 6:** Once more, the fluid in the descending limb and the hyperosmotic interstitial medullary fluid come into equilibrium. The more solute that is continuously drained from the tubules and deposited in the medullary interstitium, the more the hyperosmotic tubular fluid from the descending limb flows into the ascending limb.
- **Step 7:** By repeating these steps repeatedly, more and more water-soluble substances are added to the medulla. Over time, this cycle multiplies the concentration gradient created by the active pumping of ions from the thick ascending limb, gradually trapping the solutes in the medulla and raising the interstitial fluid's osmolarity to 1,200–1,400 mOsm / L (Figure 3.1).

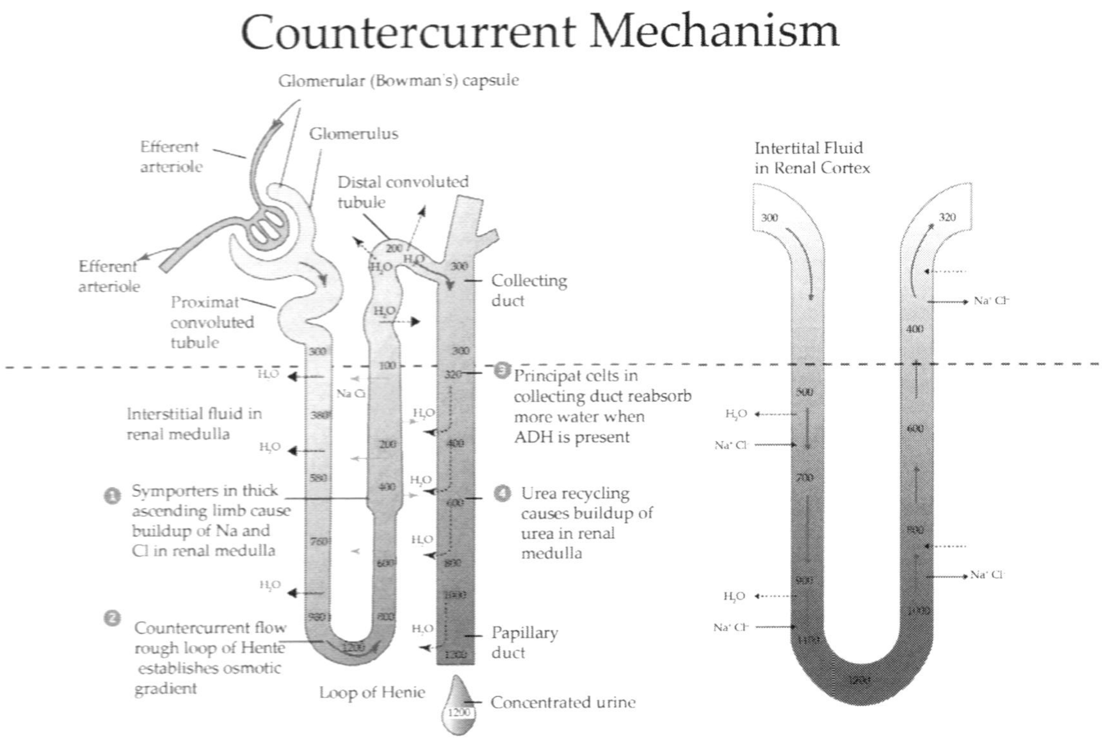

Figure 3.1. *Countercurrent mechanism.*

Source: https://www.geeksforgeeks.org/countercurrent-mechanism-urine-formation/.

3.2.4. Countercurrent Exchange Multiplication

Primarily, countercurrent multiplication takes place in the kidney's nephrons, more precisely in the hairpin-shaped loop of Henle. The kidney uses this process to help produce concentrated urine. During this process, the reabsorption of water causes the filtrate to become concentrated as it passes through the descending limb of the Henle loop. Active transport mechanisms eliminate solutes in the ascending limb, resulting in a hypertonic interstitial environment.

This gradient promotes the formation of concentrated urine in the collecting duct by encouraging additional water reabsorption in the descending limb and diluting the filtrate in the ascending limb.

3.2.5. How is Concentrated Urine Produced?

The following steps are carried out to form concentrated urine:

- NaCl is transported to the descending limb of the vasa recta through the ascending limb of Loop of Henle.
- This leads to the formation of a concentration gradient that extends from 300 mm in the cortex to 1,200 mm in the medulla.

- The space that lies between the vasa recta and the loop of Henle is known as the interstitium.
- The descending limb of the loop of Henle carries urea to the interstitium.
- Urine encounters increasing solute concentrations in the interstitium as it travels lower in the collecting tubule. It thus keeps losing water as a result of osmosis.
- Absorbent water is reintroduced into the circulation through the vasa recta. Because blood flow in these capillaries is extremely slow, any reabsorbed solutes have time to diffuse back into the interstitial fluid, preserving the gradient in solute concentration in the medulla.
- The antidiuretic hormone, or ADH, helps the kidneys conserve water by controlling the concentration of urine. Its main impact on the renal tubules is to raise the osmotic gradient by making the late distal tubule and collecting ducts more permeable to water. Moreover, it improves urea recycling and countercurrent multiplication and raises sodium chloride active transport in the thick ascending limb of the loop of Henle.

3.2.6. Importance of Counter-Current Mechanism

Kidney countercurrent mechanism occurs. The process by which the kidneys reabsorb water from the tubular fluid and produce concentrated urine is known as osmotic gradient generation, and it is powered by energy.

1. **Concentration of Urine:** Enables the production of concentrated urine, crucial for water conservation and maintaining hydration.
2. **Efficient Solute Exchange:** Enhances the exchange of ions like sodium and chloride, optimizing the reabsorption of essential substances.
3. **Energy Efficiency:** Achieves water reabsorption with minimal energy expenditure, contributing to metabolic efficiency.
4. **Adaptation to Fluid Intake:** Allows kidneys to adapt urine concentration based on varying fluid intake levels.
5. **Prevention of Water Loss:** Helps prevent excessive water loss by reabsorbing water from the tubular fluid
6. **Maintenance of Homeostasis:** Crucial for overall fluid balance and electrolyte regulation, ensuring systemic homeostasis (Pallone et al, 2003; Sands & Layton, 2008).

3.3. Physiology of Urinary Concentration

Through mechanisms that separately control sodium and water excretion, the mammalian kidney maintains nearly constant blood plasma concentration and blood plasma osmolality. Since many mammals do not always have access to water, the capacity to regulate the excretion of water can be crucial for survival. The main osmotic components of blood plasma are sodium and its anions, and stable electrolyte concentrations are also necessary, so mechanisms that dissociate water excretion from sodium excretion are needed to control it. The excretion of sodium and water is fundamentally regulated by the urine-concentrating mechanism. Urine that is more concentrated than blood plasma is produced when water intake is so small that blood plasma is concentrated, and vice versa when water intake is large enough to dilute blood plasma. Both the total excretion rate of solutes in the urine and the excretion rate of sodium in the urine are small and typically vary within narrow bounds.

Urine osmolality fluctuates greatly in response to variations in water intake, in contrast to solute excretion. Human urine osmolality can increase to approximately 1,200 mOsm/kg H_2O after several hours without water intake, such as during sleep. This is approximately 4 times higher than plasma osmolality, which is approximately 290 mOsm/kg H_2O. On the other hand, after consuming a lot of water, as is normal during breakfast, urine osmolality can drop quickly, down to about 50 mOsm/kg H_2O in humans and other mammals. The majority of physiological research pertaining to the mechanism of urine concentration has been carried out on animals with higher maximum urine osmolalities than humans. Rats can concentrate to about 3,000 mOsm/kg H_2O, mice and hamsters to about 4,000 mOsm/kg H_2O, rabbits to about 1,400 mOsm/kg H_2O, and chinchillas to about 7,600 mOsm/kg H_2O, for instance.

The osmotic gradient in the kidneys of all mammals increases from the cortico-medullary boundary to the papillary tip, the tip of the medulla. Even during diuresis, this osmotic gradient persists, albeit at a lower magnitude than during antidiuresis. The main components of the osmotic gradient in the outer medulla are NaCl, whereas the main components in the inner medulla are NaCl and urea. The inner medullary (papillary) tip is hypertonic to plasma and has an osmolality similar to urine during antidiuresis, whereas the cortex is almost isotonic to plasma. The main solutes in the urine are potassium, sodium, and urea, along with univalent anions; urea typically predominates in the urine during a strong antidiuresis.

Most of the mechanisms responsible for the autonomous regulation of sodium and water excretion are found in the renal medulla. The anatomic relationships between the medullary nephron segments and vasa recta are intricate and distinct, involving both the arrangement of the segments in three dimensions and their connections to one another. The medullary nephron segments and vasculature interact intricately to produce concentrated urine. The thick ascending limbs of the Henle loops actively reabsorb NaCl in the outer medulla. This performs two essential tasks: it dilutes the luminal fluid and supplies sodium chloride (NaCl) to raise the osmolality of the descending limbs, pars recta, medullary interstitium, vasculature, and collecting ducts. This countercurrent arrangement of the nephron segments and vessels makes it easier for a medullary osmolality gradient to form along the cortico-medullary axis. Osmolality in the inner medulla keeps rising, but it's still unclear where the concentrating effect originates. The passive reabsorption of NaCl from the thin ascending limbs of the loops of Henle, above solute secretion, is still the most widely recognized mechanism.

Numerous theories regarding the production of concentrated urine have their roots in perfused tubule studies. Further understanding of the urine-concentrating mechanism has been made possible by the cloning of numerous proteins that mediate the transport of urea, sodium, and water in nephron segments that are crucial for urine concentration and dilution. As a whole, the highly specific urea, sodium, and water transport proteins seem to rule out a molecular basis for solvent drag; this implies that the reflection coefficients ought to be 1 (Sands et al., 2008).

3.3.1. General Features of the Concentrating Mechanism

3.3.1.1. Countercurrent Multiplication

The process by which a small osmolality difference between fluid flows in the ascending and descending limbs of the loops of Henle is multiplied by the countercurrent flow configuration at each level of the outer medulla to establish a large axial osmolality difference is known as countercurrent multiplication. Because of its distribution along the cortico-medullary axis, this axial difference is commonly referred to as the cortico-medullary osmolality gradient. The countercurrent multiplication principle is shown in Figure 3.2.

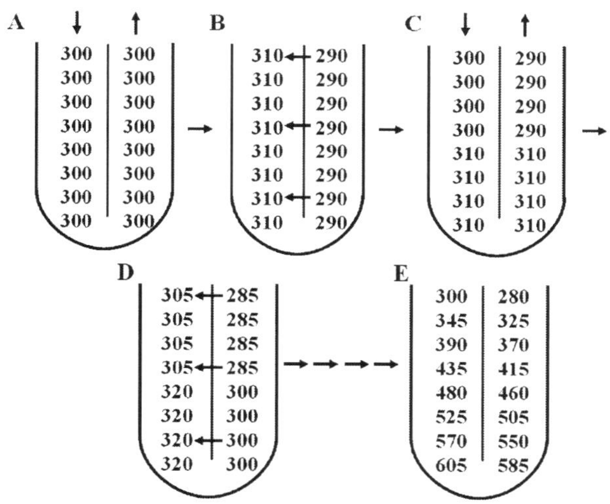

Figure 3.2. *Countercurrent multiplication of a single effect in a diagram of the loop of Henle in the outer medulla.*

Panel A: process begins with isosmolar fluid throughout both limbs. Panel B: active solute transport establishes a 20 mOsm/kg H_2O transverse gradient (single effect) across the boundary separating the limbs. Panel C: fluid flows half-way down the descending limb and up the ascending limb. Panel D: active transport reestablishes a 20 mOsm/kg H_2O transverse gradient. Note that the luminal fluid near the bend of the loop achieves a higher osmolality than loop-bend fluid in panel B. Panel E: as the processes in C and D are repeated, the bend of the loop achieves a progressively higher osmolality so that the final axial osmotic gradient far exceeds the transverse 20 mOsm/kg H_2O gradient generated at any level.

Source: https://www.ncbi.nlm.nih.gov/pmc/articles/PMC2709207/.

A schematic of a brief loop of Henle is depicted in the figure panels; the thick ascending limb is represented by the right channel, and the descending limb by the left. Two channels are divided by a barrier that is impermeable to water. The left channel flows down, and the right channel flows up, as indicated by vertical arrows. Left-directed horizontal arrows show that there is active solute transport from the right channel to the left channel. The numbers within the channels indicate the osmolality of the local fluid. The multiplication process's time course is depicted in successive panels.

The schematic loop in Figure 3.2's panel A begins with an isosmolar fluid. An active transport mechanism in panel B has pumped enough solute to create an osmolality difference of 20 mOsm/kg H_2O between the ascending and descending flows at each level. The term "single effect" refers to this tiny osmolality difference that is transverse to the flow. Panel C shows the osmolality values half way down the left channel and halfway up the right channel after the fluid has converted the solute. The luminal fluid close to the loop's bend has reached a higher osmolality than in panel A, and the active transport mechanism has restored a 20 mOsm/kg H_2O osmolality difference in panel D. By repeating this process, a higher osmolality is reached at the loop bend over time. As seen in panel E, where the osmolality at the loop bend is almost 300 mOsm/kg H_2O higher than the osmolality of the fluid entering the loop, a significant osmolality differential is produced along the flow direction. Thus, the process of countercurrent multiplication has multiplied a 20 mOsm/kg H_2O difference, or the "single effect," axially down the length of the loop.

The countercurrent multiplication process in short Henle loops is comparable to that depicted in Figure 3.2. At roughly 290 mOsm/kg H_2O, the tubular fluid that emerges from the end of the proximal tubule and enters the outer medulla is isotonic to plasma. As the tubular fluid enters the thin descending limb of the loop of Henle and travels through the proximal straight tubule (pars recta), it becomes concentrated. At the bend of the Henle loop, the osmolality of the tubular fluid reaches approximately twice that of blood plasma. After that, the fluid is diluted as it ascends the loop of Henle's medullary thick ascending limb, leaving the tubular fluid that emerges from this nephron segment hypo-osmotic to plasma. There is almost no water permeability in the thick ascending limb, and this nephron segment does not contain any aquaporin proteins. Although the thick ascending limb has a low NaCl permeability, it uses an active transport mechanism to vigorously transport NaCl from the tubular lumen to the medullary interstitium.

3.3.1.2. Countercurrent Exchange

The ascending and descending vasa recta, which supply blood to the medulla, are positioned in a counter-flow configuration and are linked by a capillary plexus. Vasa recta are freely permeable to water, urea, and sodium, which allows them to achieve osmotic equilibration by a combination of water absorption and solute secretion. Ascending vasa recta gain solute and lose water, and descending vasa recta lose solute and gain water. "Countercurrent exchange" refers to the flow of water and solute between the ascending and descending vasa recta and the surrounding interstitium.

Since both hypertonic fluid carried away from the medulla and hypotonic fluid carried into the medulla tend to dissipate the work of countercurrent multiplication, the countercurrent exchange must be extremely efficient to produce a concentrated urine. Therefore, to minimize wasted work, fluid entering the cortex from the ascending vasa recta must have an osmolality close to that of blood plasma, and fluid flowing through the vasa recta must achieve near osmotic equilibrium with the surrounding interstitium at each medullary level. Volume depletion and other conditions that reduce medullary blood flow enhance urine concentrating ability and countercurrent exchange efficiency by giving blood in the ascending vasa recta more time to lose solute and reach osmotic equilibration. On the other hand, disorders like osmotic diuresis that enhance medullary blood flow reduce the capacity to concentrate urine and reduce the effectiveness of countercurrent exchange. (Pallone et al., 2003).

3.3.2. Urine Concentrating Mechanism: History and Theory

The conceptual history of the concentrating mechanism can be separated into three time periods. A study by Kuhn and Ryffel, which suggested that the creation of concentrated urine is the consequence of the countercurrent multiplication of a "single effect," marked the beginning of the first period (1942–1971). Kuhn and Ryffel created a functional device that demonstrated the ideas behind countercurrent multiplication. During this initial phase, the countercurrent multiplication hypothesis was refined and experimental data was gathered to bolster the theory's validity as the explanation for the outer medulla's urine-concentrating mechanism. In particular, the source of the outer medullary single effect was found to be the active transport of NaCl from the thick ascending limbs of the loops of Henle.

The simultaneous publication of two groundbreaking studies, one by Stephenson and one by Kokko and Rector, suggesting that a "passive mechanism" provides the single effect for countercurrent multiplication in the inner medulla, signaled the start of the second period (1972 to 1992). The passive mechanism hypothesis states that favorable transepithelial urea and NaCl gradients—which are caused by the separation of urea and NaCl, which is fueled by the outer medullary concentrating mechanism—lead to a net solute efflux from the thin ascending limbs of the loops of Henle.

The passive mechanism was first supported by a substantial body of experimental evidence, but results from multiple follow-up studies are incongruent with this theory. Furthermore, the models did not predict a significant inner medullary concentrating effect when the measured transepithelial permeabilities were incorporated into the models. For over 30 years, there has been a persistent discrepancy between the very effective inner medullary concentrating effect and the consistently negative results from mathematical modeling studies. Although the discrepancy has prompted the development of numerous extremely complex mathematical models and studies on the transport characteristics of the inner medulla's renal tubules, no model study has been able to satisfactorily address the discrepancy for both modelers and experimentalists.

With the serious consideration of new theories regarding the inner medullary concentrating mechanism starting in 1993, it is possible to date the start of a third phase of conceptual thought. Knepper and associates proposed in 1993 that the papilla's peristalsis plays a crucial role. Jen and Stephenson (1994) examined the concept of "externally driven" countercurrent multiplication, which could arise from the net production of osmotically active particles in the interstitium, for example. The inner medullary urine concentrating mechanism cannot be explained by the passive mechanism, as was first proposed, according to experimental measurements conducted around the same time in chinchilla perfused tubules, which can produce extremely concentrated urine. Current research has aimed to advance theories concerning the papilla's peristalsis and the possible production of osmotically active particles, particularly lactate. In 2004, experimental data indicating the lack of significant urea transport proteins in Henle loops extending deep into the inner medulla caused theories regarding the passive mechanism to be re-examined. Recently, Pannabecker and colleagues proposed that a solute-separation, solute-mixing mechanism for the inner medullary urine concentrating mechanism is most consistent with the spatial arrangements of the loop of Henle subsegments and the identification of multiple countercurrent systems in the inner medulla, along with their initial mathematical model.

3.3.2.1. Urine Concentrating Mechanism in the Outer Medulla

In the outer medulla, the mechanism responsible for concentrating urine is thought to function as follows. The active transport of NaCl from the tubular fluid of the thick ascending limbs of the loops of Henle into the surrounding interstitium is carried out by Na-K-ATPase in the basolateral plasma membrane and the Na-K-2Cl cotransporter NKCC2/BSC1 in the apical plasma membrane. The osmotic reabsorption of water from the tubular fluid of descending limbs and collecting ducts is facilitated by this active NaCl reabsorption, which also increases the osmolality of interstitial fluid. The fluid that is supplied to the ascending limbs has a high NaCl concentration that promotes transepithelial NaCl transport from ascending limb fluid due to the reabsorption of fluid from the descending limbs of the loops of Henle. NaCl diffusion into the fluid of the descending limb is also possible. The thick ascending limb tubular fluid is diluted by NaCl reabsorption, resulting in a fluid osmolality that is lower in the cortex than in the other tubules and vessels at each medullary level. Additionally, the fluid delivered to the cortex is diluted in comparison to blood plasma. Active NaCl reabsorption from cortical thick ascending limbs further dilutes the ascending limb fluid that enters the cortex, causing its osmolality to be lower than that of blood plasma. Vasopressin, an antidiuretic hormone, causes cortical collecting ducts to become extremely permeable to water, and enough water is reabsorbed to bring the fluid back to isotonicity with blood plasma. The fluid that re-enters the medulla through the collecting ducts puts a significant load on the urine concentrating mechanism, which is lessened by this cortical water reabsorption. The collecting ducts transport diluted plasma to the outer and inner medulla borders when vasopressin is not present. This means that the entire system is only partially permeable to water. Despite this, some water is reabsorbed because of the extreme osmotic pressure gradient.

Recent mathematical modeling studies using parameters compatible with perfused tubule and micropuncture experiments support this modern conceptual formulation of the outer medullary urine concentrating mechanism (which is very similar to the proposal of Hargitay and Kuhn as modified by Kuhn and Ramel). Specifically, the osmolality increases by a factor of 2–3 in tissue slice experiments are consistent with the outer medullary osmotic gradients predicted by mathematical simulations (Pallone et al, 2003; Sands & Layton, 2008).

3.3.2.2. The Passive Mechanism Hypothesis for the Inner Medulla

Isolated perfused tubule experiments in rabbit thin ascending limbs showed no significant active NaCl transport, in contrast to the outer medulla where the single effect was generated by active NaCl transport from thick ascending limbs. Rather, the thin ascending limb was impermeable to water but possessed relatively high permeabilities to sodium and urea. The inner medullary thin descending limb, on the other hand, has low urea and sodium permeabilities but a high water permeability. Furthermore, evidence from certain species indicated that urea tended to accumulate in the inner medulla, with concentrations comparable to those of NaCl. It was also well known that urea administration increases maximum urine concentration in protein-deprived rats and humans. Numerous published models of the inner medullary concentrating mechanism were not well received. (Sands JM et al., 2008)

In 1972, Kokko and Rector, along with Stephenson, put forward the theory that the single effect in the inner medulla occurs through a “passive mechanism.” This mechanism involves the active absorption of NaCl from the thick ascending limb, followed by the absorption of water from the cortical and outer medullary collecting ducts, leading to an increase in urea concentration in the collecting duct fluid. Urea then diffuses into the inner medullary interstitium through the highly urea-permeable terminal IMCD, where it is trapped by a countercurrent exchange in the vasa recta. The thin ascending limb, possessing relatively high NaCl permeability compared to urea, causes NaCl to flow down its concentration gradient into the interstitium, resulting in the dilution of fluid within the thin ascending limb and subsequent flow into the thick ascending limb. This process removes dilute fluid from the inner medulla, maintains mass balance, and progressively elevates interstitial osmolality along the tubules of the inner medulla.

The increased osmolality will draw water from the thin descending limbs, increasing the descending limb flow's NaCl concentration as it enters the thin ascending limbs. Furthermore, an accumulation of NaCl in the interstitium will tend to sustain a transepithelial urea concentration gradient that is favorable to urea reabsorption from the terminal IMCD. This is because the elevated osmolality of the inner medullary interstitium will draw water from the water-permeable IMCD, raising the concentration of urea in collecting duct fluid.

3.3.2.3. Several Matters Regarding the Passive Mechanism Merit Discussion

First of all, despite the stepwise description given above, this process should be viewed as continuous and steady-state. Second, despite being labeled as "passive," the mechanism relies on the active reabsorption of NaCl by thick ascending limbs, which maintains the separation of urea and NaCl. A net transport of solute from the thin ascending limbs is affected by the distinct high-concentration flows of urea (in the collecting ducts) and NaCl (in the loops of Henle). These flows provide a source of potential energy. Therefore, the laws of thermodynamics are not broken. Third, while NaCl and urea are described as having equal standing in the description above, NaCl is almost entirely dissociated into Na and Cl ions, meaning that each NaCl molecule has almost twice the osmotic effect of each urea molecule. This distinction needs to be represented in formal mathematical descriptions. Fourth, insofar as it depends on net solute absorption from the thin ascending limb to dilute thin ascending limb fluid and increase the osmolality in the vasa recta and collecting ducts, the passive mechanism hypothesis is very similar to the outer medullary urine concentrating mechanism. As a result, the thin ascending limbs produce a greater volume of slightly diluted urine flow to balance the small amount of highly concentrated urine produced. Equilibration in countercurrent flows is incomplete, despite the fact that the osmolality gradient along the inner medulla depends on countercurrent exchange, particularly exchange between the descending and ascending vasa recta. Therefore, the dissipative effect of ascending flows that are marginally concentrated in comparison to descending flows limits the achievable urine osmolality.

The above-described passive mechanism hypothesis closely resembles the formulation proposed by Kokko and Rector, who drew upon important concepts from a primarily experimental study conducted by Kokko. Niesel and Rosenbleck's theory that IMCD urea reabsorption contributes to the inner medullary osmolality gradient was recognized by Kokko and Rector. The conceptual model of the passive mechanism hypothesis presented by Kokko and Rector did not show that the measured loop of Henle permeabilities were consistent with the hypothesis, nor did their presentation include a mathematical treatment. However, it was supported by a reasonable set of solute fluxes, concentrations, and fluid flow rates that are consistent with the requirements of mass balance. In addition to introducing the highly influential central core assumption and providing more mathematical treatment, Stephenson's formulation of the passive mechanism hypothesis lacked a mathematical reconciliation between the hypothesis and tubular transport properties.

The medullary architecture and tubular transport in mathematical simulations of the urine concentrating mechanism have improved in sophistication and breadth in recent years. This evolution results from the combination of growing experimental knowledge, faster computers with greater computational power, and simulations that consistently fail to show a discernible inner medullary concentration gradient.

Using immunohistochemical labeling and computer-aided reconstruction, Pannabecker, Dantzler, and colleagues' studies have uncovered a wealth of new information regarding the functional architecture of the rat's inner medulla. Their results specifically show that loops of Henle turning within the upper first millimeter of the IM do not have significant aquaporin-1 (AQP-1) in their descending thin limbs (DTLs). On the other hand, loops turning below the first millimeter have three functional subsegments that can be clearly identified: 40% of these DTLs express AQP-1, while 60% do not; additionally, the final ~165 microns express ClC-K1, as does the contiguous thin ascending limb.

Layton and associates. have recently put forth two theories that are strongly connected to the passive mechanism; these theories were inspired by the results of recent research conducted in rats by Pannabecker et al. One theory is based directly on the principles of the passive mechanism: since loops extending deep into the inner medulla did not exhibit significant labeling for urea transport proteins, it was assumed that the thin limbs of Henle loops had low urea permeabilities. In a second, more creative theory, there was zero water permeability and restricted NaCl permeability in thin descending limbs that extended deep into the inner medulla, but extremely high urea loop of Henle urea permeabilities were assumed. Thus, urea secretion would raise the osmolality of the thin descending limb fluid, tubular fluid urea concentration in loops of Henle would nearly equilibrate with the local interstitial urea concentration in the deepest part of the inner medulla, and the prebend segment and early thin ascending limb would experience substantial NaCl reabsorption.

In both theories, the decreasing loop of Henle population plays a key role in facilitating a spatially distributed NaCl reabsorption from prebend segments and early thin ascending limbs along the inner medulla. The focus on NaCl reabsorption from the IMCDs as a crucial active transport process that separates NaCl from tubular fluid urea and indirectly promotes water and urea reabsorption from the collecting ducts is a distinguishing feature of both hypotheses. Urine flow, concentrations, and osmolality consistent with urine from moderately antidiuretic rats were predicted by computer simulations for both hypotheses. It has been argued that urea transport may be paracellular rather than transepithelial, and that the first hypothesis is critically dependent on low loop of Henle urea permeabilities. Further definitive experiments are needed to determine the properties of urea transport in rats. The second hypothesis, in which high loop urea permeabilities have been measured, may help explain the mechanism of chinchilla urine concentration.

3.3.2.4. Alternatives to the Passive Mechanism

There are three categories of alternative hypotheses to the original passive mechanism hypothesis. The first category includes simulation studies that suggest a more accurate representation of medullary anatomy or transepithelial transport is necessary for the passive mechanism to work effectively. The second category involves steady-state mechanisms that focus on a single effect generated in either the collecting ducts or thin descending limbs. The third category of alternatives involves hypotheses that revolve around the peristaltic contractions of the pelvic wall and their effect on the papilla.

Schmidt-Nielsen postulated a theory that is dependent on the pelvic wall's peristaltic contractions: the cycle of contraction and relaxation produces interstitial negative pressures, which act to transfer water—more than solute—from the collecting duct system. This theory states that a water flux into collecting duct cells would be encouraged by the compression wave's increase in hydrostatic pressure in the collecting duct lumen. Without a corresponding solute flux, pressure would induce water flow through aquaporin water channels. Consequently, in comparison to the contents of collecting duct cells and the surrounding interstitium, the remaining luminal fluid would be concentrated. Following the peristaltic wave's passage, the collecting ducts would collapse. The wave's temporary narrowing and lengthening of the papilla would cause it to rebound, creating a negative hydrostatic pressure in the elastic interstitium—a region high in hyaluronic acid and glycosamine glycans. The negative pressure would draw water out of the collecting duct cells (via aquaporins) and into the vasa recta, which would reopen during the contraction's relaxation phase and transport reabsorbate in the direction of the cortex. This theory doesn't seem to explain the significant NaCl gradient created in the papilla, nor does it seem to explain the function of long loops of Henle or the unique function of urea in producing concentrated urine.

Recently, Knepper and associates proposed that hyaluronic acid, which is abundant in the inner medullary interstitium of rats, might function as a mechano-osmotic transducer, i.e., that the mechanical work of papillary peristalsis could be converted into osmotic work that could be used to concentrate urine by using the inherent visco-elastic properties of hyaluronic acid. They put forth three different peristalsis-derived concentrating mechanisms. (1) Cations immobilized by pairing with fixed negative charges on hyaluronic acid would decrease interstitial sodium activity during the contraction phase. As a result, the fluid that can be expressed from the interstitium would have a lower NaCl concentration, and the relatively diluted fluid would enter the ascending vasa recta. In the relaxation phase, water would be absorbed from descending thin limbs (2) due to a drop in interstitial pressure and (3) due to elastic forces generated by the hyaluronic acid-induced expansion of the elastic interstitial matrix. In contrast to other flows, the tubular fluid in the descending limb would be relatively concentrated if water were to be reabsorbed in this way without proportionate solute.

Peristalsis-dependent hypotheses are intricate cycles involving critical combinations of pressure, flow rates, permeabilities, compliances, and peristalsis frequencies. Furthermore, evaluating the viability of these theories would seem to necessitate a thorough understanding of the physical characteristics of the renal inner medulla as well as proof that the energy input from the contractions and any additional energy sources accessed is adequate to explain the osmotic work completed. Therefore, evaluating these theories through experiments or mathematical models poses a formidable technical challenge.

3.3.3. Role of the Collecting Duct

3.3.3.1. Water Transport

The nephron segment that controls water excretion by controlling water reabsorption is the collecting duct, which is influenced by vasopressin. The cortico-medullary osmotic gradient required for water reabsorption is produced by countercurrent multiplication in the loops of Henle, and countercurrent exchange in the vasa recta reduces the dissipative effect of vascular flows. Nevertheless, the collecting duct system, which originates in the cortex and terminates at the papillary tip, is an additional structural element necessary for water excretion. With the exception of the terminal IMCD, which has a moderate water permeability even in the absence of vasopressin, all collecting duct segments are almost impermeable in the absence of the hormone. Since the fluid that leaves the thick ascending limb and enters the cortical collecting duct is diluted relative to plasma, excretion of diluted urine only requires a small amount of water to be absorbed and a small amount of solute to be secreted along the collecting duct.

Vasopressin causes the collecting duct to become extremely water-permeable throughout. This happens in the manner described below. Hypothalamic osmoreceptors, which are sensitive to changes as small as 2 mOsm/kg H_2O in blood plasma osmolality, such as those caused by water deprivation, cause the posterior pituitary gland to secrete more vasopressin when blood plasma osmolality is raised. Vasopressin binds to IMCD and the collecting duct principal cellular basolateral plasma membrane V_2-receptors. Water absorption across the collecting duct is increased when AQP2 water channels are inserted into the apical plasma membrane, phosphorylating aquaporin 2 (AQP2) at serines 256, 261, 264, and 269, and activating protein kinase A. All of these processes are triggered by the binding of AQP2 to cAMP. Vasopressin primarily controls the trafficking of AQP2 between sub-apical vesicles and the apical plasma membrane, which is how it acutely regulates water reabsorption. According to the "membrane shuttle hypothesis," which was first put forth by Wade and associates, water channels are kept in vesicles and are exocytically inserted into the apical plasma membrane in response to vasopressin. The shuttle hypothesis was experimentally verified in the rat inner medulla after AQP2 was cloned. The function of the cytoskeleton, many signal transduction pathways that control AQP2 trafficking (the insertion and retrieval of AQP2), and vesicle targeting proteins (SNAP/SNARE system) have all been clarified by later research.

The ascending vasa recta returns the reabsorbed water to the systemic circulation when vasopressin is present. Water is reabsorbed across the collecting ducts at a high enough rate to achieve near osmotic equilibrium with the hyperosmotic medullary interstitium. The cortex and outer medulla's collecting ducts reabsorb the majority of the water. Even though the inner medulla has a higher osmolality than the outer medulla, it only plays a significant part in water absorption when the greatest amount of water conservation is needed. Because of the significant transepithelial osmolality difference that occurs during diuresis, the IMCD reabsorbs more water during diuresis than during antidiuresis.

3.3.3.2. Urea Transport

A unique function of urea is to aid in the mechanism of urine concentration. Since 1934, when Gamble and associates reported "an economy of water in renal function referable to urea," the significance of urea has been understood. Numerous studies demonstrate that in protein-deficient or malnourished mammals, the maximum capacity to concentrate urine is reduced and that urine concentration can be restored through urea infusion. Recently, it was demonstrated that three knockout mice—UT-A1/UT-A3; UT-A2; and UT-B—all exhibited abnormalities related to urine concentration. Therefore, any explanation for how the inner medulla concentrates urine must include an effect resulting from urea or urea transporters. Vasopressin has no effect on the low urea permeability of the initial IMCD. The terminal IMCD, on the other hand, has a higher basal urea permeability than other areas of the collecting duct; urea permeability can be increased by a factor of 10 when combined with either vasopressin or hypertonicity. Individually, these factors can increase urea permeability by 4–6. Three groups demonstrated in the 1980s that in isolated perfused rat IMCDs, vasopressin could raise passive urea permeability. In rat and rabbit terminal IMCDs, a particular facilitated or carrier-mediated urea transport mechanism was first postulated in 1987.

The apical plasma membrane of the IMCD expresses UT-A1. When stably expressed in UT-A1-MDCK cells, vasopressin stimulates urea transport by UT-A1, and when expressed in Xenopus oocytes, cAMP does the same. In various investigations, UT-A3 has been found in the basolateral and apical plasma membranes and is also expressed in the IMCD. In four studies, but not in the fifth, urea transport by UT-A3 is stimulated by cAMP analogs when expressed in MDCK cells, human embryonic kidney (HEK) 293 cells, or Xenopus oocytes. The first cloned urea transporter, UT-A2, is expressed in thin descending limbs. cAMP analogs do not stimulate urea transport by UT-A2 when it is expressed in HEK-293 cells or Xenopus oocytes.

In humans, UT-B is also known as the Kidd blood group antigen. It was first cloned from a human erythroid cell line, and subsequently from rodents. In the descending vasa recta, UT-B protein and phloretin-inhibitable urea transport are found. Whether UT-B transports water and urea together, or just urea, has been the subject of several recent studies. A UT-B/AQP1 double knock-out mouse's red blood cells demonstrate that UT-B can act as a water channel. However, compared to AQP1, the volume of water carried by UT-B under physiological conditions is negligible, and it is most likely not physiologically significant to the urine concentrating mechanism.

3.3.3.3. Rapid Regulation of Facilitated Urea Transport in the IMCD

The perfused rat inner medullary collecting duct (IMCD) has long been used as a method for studying the rapid regulation of urea transport. While this approach offers valuable functional data, it does not distinguish between UT-A1 and UT-A3 isoforms, both of which are present in this nephron segment. Recent research indicates that vasopressin promotes the phosphorylation and accumulation of both UT-A1 and UT-A3 in the apical plasma membrane of rat IMCDs. Vasopressin targets serines 486 and 499 on UT-A1, and mutating these residues abolishes vasopressin-induced increase in UT-A1 levels in the plasma membrane and urea transport. The specific phosphorylation site on UT-A3 by vasopressin remains unknown, although it is determined that it is not one of the consensus PKA sites. In rat IMCD, UT-A1 interacts with the SNARE machinery through snapin, suggesting that this interaction plays a key role in regulating urea transport.

Even in the absence of vasopressin, raising osmolality to high physiological values as those experienced during antidiuresis—either by adding NaCl or mannitol—acutely increases urea permeability in rat terminal IMCDs, indicating that hyperosmolality is a separate activator of urea transport. The presence of vasopressin when osmolality rises stimulates urea permeability in an additive manner. Phloretin and thiourea, a urea analog, both inhibit hyperosmolality-stimulated urea permeability. Kinetic studies show that hyperosmolality, like vasopressin, increases urea permeability by increasing V_{max} rather than K_m. However, hyperosmolality stimulates urea permeability via increases in activation of PKC and intracellular calcium while vasopressin stimulates urea permeability via increases in adenylyl cyclase. Hypersomolality, like vasopressin, increases the phosphorylation and the plasma membrane accumulation of UT-A1 and UT-A3 (Pallone et al, 2003; Sands & Layton, 2008).

3.4. The Importance of Tubular Function in Chronic Kidney Disease

The renal functional parameters that are currently used to assess the severity of chronic kidney disease (CKD) are glomerular filtration rate (GFR) and proteinuria-albuminuria. In addition, the amount of urine protein-albumin excretion also contributes to the prediction of a patient's cardiovascular risk, CKD progression, and death in cases of chronic nephropathy, just as the patient's GFR value helps determine how to adjust the dosage of some medications. However, despite GFR and urinary protein-albumin excretion parameters, tubular secretion is another important renal functional variable to be taken into account for the following reasons:

Primimal tubule (PT) secretion serves as the primary pathway for the urinary excretion of endogenous organic anions and the majority of medications. Furthermore, unlike GFR, PT secretion possesses a variety of transporter machinery that aids in the basolateral absorption and luminal excretion of solutes, including members of the organic cation/anion/zwitterion solute carrier family (SLC) (Suchy-Dicey et al., 2016).

Second, around 24 of the 153 compounds, which have been confirmed as characteristic uremic toxins, interact with organic anion transporters (OATs), and 7 of these substances: acid uric, indoxyl sulfate (IS), p-hydroxyhippuric acid, 3-carboxy-4-methyl-5-propyl-2-furanopropanoic acid (CMPF), xanthine, indoleacetic acid, hippuric acid, have been documented to present elevated serum levels in uremic patients.

Third, the OATs are involved in the metabolism of metabolites from the gut microbiome and handle drugs (antibiotics, antivirals, diuretics, nonsteroidal anti-inflammatory drugs), toxins (mercury, aristolochic acid), and nutrients (vitamins, flavonoids). OATs have a strong selectivity for specific signaling molecules (such as sex steroids, odorants, etc.) and are expressed in a variety of organs.), they might be involved in distant interorgan communication by controlling the concentrations of important metabolites and signaling molecules in bodily fluids and tissues. The remote sensing and signaling hypothesis (RSSH) is the name given to this mechanism.

Fourth, OATs—in particular, OAT1, OAT2, OAT3, OAT4, and URAT1—play a critical role in the pathophysiologic processes involving the toxicity and intracellular build-up of uremic toxins. Renal injury, whether acute or chronic, can significantly lower the expression of the OAT gene and protein. The PT's down-regulation of OAT expression may be an adaptation to high levels of toxin exposure.

Fifth, studies on solute clearance indicate that GFR and PT secretion may decline at varying rates in the elderly and patients with chronic nephropathy. As a result, since tubular secretion plays a role in the excretion of medications, assessing tubular secretion activity may be essential in determining the appropriate dosage of medication for these patients.

3.4.1. Creatinine and Uric Acid Renal Tubular Transport

The creatinine clearance is a commonly used measure to assess a patient's GFR; however, active tubular secretion in the PT accounts for 10–40% of this clearance, and this phenomenon is even more pronounced in renal disease. Although the SLC22A2 gene has been linked to serum creatinine and estimated GFR values in several studies, the SLC22A2 genotype has also been linked to a net tubular creatinine secretion phenotype (OCT2), demonstrating the obvious bias in using creatininemia as a kidney function indicator. Since the administration of para-aminohippuric acid, an OAT inhibitor, markedly decreased creatinine secretion and increased its plasma level, the role of OAT in creatinine excretion has been established in animal models. Furthermore, investigations utilizing OAT1- and OAT3-deficient mice validated the previously mentioned phenomenon, indicating a more significant function for OAT3. About uric acid, the balance between its tubular secretion and reabsorption—two processes that occur in PT—determines how the acid is handled by the renal tubules. Research on humans has shown that urate transporter 1 (URAT1; slc22a12) is primarily responsible for mediating uric acid reabsorption and that uricosuric drugs, such as probenecid, inhibit URAT1's activity. Furthermore, studies have indicated that all four OATs—including URAT1—may mediate urate transport in both renal secretion and reabsorption because they have been localized at the basolateral and luminal areas of the PT. Additionally, PT urate reabsorption may be aided by the renal-specific transporter RST, which is primarily found at the apical surface of the PT. Urate tubular reabsorption is stimulated by increased oxidative stress and hypovolemia, and angiotensin II, epinephrine, and insulin hormones may function as mediators. Hippuric and kynurenic acids have the potential to accelerate the course of chronic kidney disease by increasing solute retention. In an animal model used to study how elevated serum uric acid levels affected uremic toxin levels, kynurenic acid was discovered to be a substrate for the tubular transporters MRP4 and BCRP. It has been shown that the accumulation of the toxin kynurenic acid was linked to high serum uric acid levels, most likely as a result of uric acid-induced carrier dysfunction. Therefore, adequate function of several kidney carriers (BCRP and MRP4) is required to maintain normal serum urate levels. Thus, it has been proposed that uremic toxin retention caused by elevated serum uric acid levels may indirectly cause chronic kidney disease (CKD).

3.4.2. Drugs and Renal Tubular Transport

OCT2 (SLC22A2) is primarily expressed in human kidneys and is essential for eliminating cationic drugs from blood, including metformin, cimetidine, cisplatin, antihistamines, and some antibiotics. Furthermore, the SLC47A gene family encodes the multidrug and toxin extrusion protein 1 (MATE1) and its isoforms (MATE2 and MATE2-K), which frequently interact with OCTs. Further, MATE2-K is exclusively found in PT, whereas MATE1 is primarily expressed in the liver and kidney. Because genetic variations in MATE1 and MATE2-K polymorphisms have been linked to variations in renal drug handling and toxicity, these carriers may significantly impact the pharmacokinetics of medications. Four multidrug carriers (P-gp, MRP2, MRP4, and BCRP) in the kidney work together to pump various substances into the urine. Glucuronide, glutathione, and sulfate conjugates are among the organic anionic substances and their metabolites that are transported by the MRPs. Moreover, MRP4 has been linked to the efflux of prostaglandins and nucleotides.

OATs can transport a wide range of endogenous chemicals and clinically relevant xenobiotics, including adefovir, tetracycline, mercuric conjugates, and ochratoxin A, according to substrate studies. Due to their ability to interact with multiple toxins, OATs are prime targets for toxicity, which renders them vulnerable. Because of substrate competition for extrarenal OATs transport and delayed toxin clearance, mutations in OATs sequences may cause these carriers to malfunction and accumulate toxins at the PT, further exacerbating extrarenal toxicity. Thus, one mechanism of altered urinary excretion of many medications (e.g., digoxin, etc.) may be the OATP4C1 reduction in the PT during uremia and uremic poisons seen in renal impairment. Research has shown that overexpressing human SLCO4C1 in the kidney reduces renal insufficiency and inflammation in addition to hypertension. Therefore, medications that increase the kidney's SLCO4C1 expression may aid in the excretion of uremic toxins, thereby decreasing renal damage progression, kidney inflammation, and the time at which dialysis is initiated. It is important to note that pravastatin and fluvastatin significantly increased the expression of SLCO4C1 mRNA in human PT cells. Additionally, studies conducted in vitro have shown that pravastatin and fluvastatin facilitated the uptake of thyroid hormone (T3), a substrate of SLCO4C1, indicating an increase in PT's SLCO4C1 function. Studies conducted in vivo have also shown that animals treated with pravastatin exhibited a significant increase in tubular excretion. Thus, it appears from all these studies that statins may enhance the transcription of SLCO4C1 to aid in the excretion of uremic toxins. It has been suggested that medications that upregulate SLCO4C1, like pravastatin, may have therapeutic effects in patients with chronic kidney disease (CKD). Toyohara et al. discovered that different statins upregulate SLCO4C1 transcription.

Lastly, it's important to note that these transporters might also contribute to the RSSH as a component of a network of molecules that communicates with the body in both healthy and unhealthy conditions, like acute or chronic kidney injury.

3.4.3. Uremic Toxins in Chronic Kidney Disease

Uremic syndrome is identified by the buildup of uremic toxins in the body, which is not just caused by a decrease in glomerular filtration rate (GFR), but also by the loss of proximal tubule (PT) function. The PT is responsible for secreting active metabolites, and studies have shown that around 54% of indoxyl sulfate (IS) is excreted by the kidneys alongside urea, highlighting the importance of tubular secretion in IS excretion. Additionally, uremia appears to hinder the function of efflux carriers to a significant degree, leading to further accumulation of uremic toxins and various complications associated with chronic kidney disease. It is well-established that many uremic toxins have the potential to cause cell death in smooth muscles, neutrophils, and PT cells, as well as disrupt cell metabolism, especially in the mitochondria. The buildup of these toxins can also interfere with drug transportation mechanisms in the kidneys, leading to changes in how drugs are processed by the body. Additionally, retained uremic metabolites have been linked to the progression of chronic kidney disease and an increased risk of cardiovascular issues. Polyamines, which are produced during the breakdown of amino acids like lysine, arginine, and ornithine, are known to be toxic to cells by causing damage to proteins and DNA. As a result, lowering the accumulation of uremic toxins can help protect against hypertension and the progression of kidney damage in patients with chronic kidney disease. Recent studies have shown that increasing the expression of the OAT transporter SLCO4C1 in the kidneys of rats can reduce levels of uremic toxins in the blood, as well as lower blood pressure, prevent heart enlargement, and decrease inflammation in cases of kidney failure.

Many biological pathways, including those regulated by drug-metabolizing enzymes and ATP-binding cassette (ABC) and solute carrier (SLC) transporters—many of which are also involved in pharmacokinetics—are impacted in uremic syndrome. The RSSH identifies communication between the gut microbiota and/or the host, mediated by SLC and ABC transporters, as being essential to the homeostasis of metabolites, antioxidants, signaling molecules, products derived from the microbiota, and dietary components within the organism. According to Wu et al., OAT1 and/or

OAT3 play a crucial role in the metabolism of more than 35 uremic toxins, including those that come from the gut microbiome (such as CMPF, phenylsulfate, and indole-3-acetic acid). Numerous of these molecules are involved in interorgan and interorganismal communication, as described in the RSSH, indicating that uremia may be caused by a malfunction of this remote communication system, at least partially. In rats fed a high-fat diet, Wanchai et al. observed a marked rise in serum lipopolysaccharide, serum lipids, and insulin resistance in addition to renal dysfunction and a decrease in renal Oat 3 function. Treatment with *Lactobacillus paracasei* HII01 improved these changes. Thus, it appears that in this animal model, probiotic supplementation reduced renal inflammation and enhanced renal Oat3 function. According to this study, probiotics may help the kidneys handle products of the gut microbiota by improving Oat3 function, which in turn may help the RSSH between the kidneys and the intestines.

3.4.4. Kidney Disease and Renal Tubular Transporters

Since preserved residual diuresis in dialysis patients maintains active PT transport processes, it is currently known that this condition is associated with better clinical outcomes than anuria. Highly protein-bound toxins (e.g., IS, p-cresyl sulfate, and CMPF) that are not sufficiently eliminated by traditional dialysis can be effectively removed by these transport processes. According to available data, active PT secretion rather than GFR is the primary mechanism for renal excretion of uremic toxins. Toxin clearance increased by artificial OAT up-regulation, however, may be accompanied by increased PT cell death from toxic exposure and residual renal function diminution if OAT down-regulation seen in kidney insufficiency patients and animal models indicates PT cells adaptation to reduce the intracellular retention of, and cellular damage from, uremic toxins. Since polyamine uremic toxins, including putrescine, spermine, cadaverine, spermidine, and the polyamine breakdown product (acrolein), as well as guanidino compounds (guanidine and methylguanidine), caused inhibition of OCT2-mediated transport, the uptake transporter is down-regulated in animal models of acute and chronic kidney injury. It is important to note, though, that not all tubular transporters are affected in the same way by renal failure patients, as P-glycoprotein (P-gp) is unaffected, multidrug resistance-associated protein 2 (MRP2) is elevated, and basolateral OATP4C1 expression is reduced. The structural and physiological changes of these carriers during acute renal injury have a direct impact on systemic clearance of their substrate drugs, leading to drug accumulation and adverse events. by-products, and SLC22A organic carriers mediate the urinary excretion of these substances. When ischemia or toxic agents like cisplatin induce dysregulation in SLC22A carriers during acute renal failure, it can lead to uremic syndrome and/or negative drug effects. Furthermore, the progression of acute renal damage brought on by renal ischemia or toxicity may be mediated by an OAT1/3 substrate (such as IS) and a uremic toxin.

3.4.4.1. Uremic Toxins and Renal Tubular Transporters

Tubular secretion is the mechanism by which the kidneys eliminate many organic anionic uremic toxins (e.g., IS, CMPF, indoleacetate, hippurate), which bind to serum albumin. OATs are essential to this process. On the other hand, phenylacetic acid and indoleacetic acid only lower MRP4 uptake, whereas hippuric acid, IS, and kynurenic acid inhibited MRP4 or BCRP uptake. On the other hand, putrescine, oxalate, and quinolinic acid had no effect on MRP4 or BCRP-mediated transport. Furthermore, many cationic endogenous metabolites or xenobiotics are secreted by the kidneys through OCT2-mediated uptake, and when this process fails, cationic metabolites accumulate—a phenomenon that has been linked to cardiovascular consequences. Furthermore, it has been reported that guanidino cationic uremic toxins and polyamines inhibited OCT2-mediated uptake. Wikoff et al discovered that many chemicals, including IS, interact with the renal Oat1 transporter (Slc22A6) and accumulate in chronic nephropathy. IS is one of these substances that is derived from hepatic Phase II metabolism of enteric gut precursors. This discovery validates the intricate and distant communication that occurs between the gut microbiome, liver metabolism, and elimination through renal Oats. It also highlights the significance of Oat1 in the management of endogenous toxins in uremia. Takada et al. found that ATP-binding cassette transporter subfamily G member 2 (ABCG2) is a significant transporter of the uremic toxin IS and that ABCG2 plays a significant role in the advancement of chronic kidney disease. OATs are believed to play a key role in the tubular secretion of the toxin p-cresyl sulfate (PCS), which is a substrate for OAT1 and OAT3. Most low-molecular-weight uremic toxins are eliminated through urine, with protein-bound uremic toxins playing a minor role in tubular secretion. Protein-bound uremic toxins like IS, CMPF, indoleacetate, and hippurate are excreted from the kidneys via OATs, particularly rat OAT1/OAT3 and human OAT1/OAT3. Since OATs are present in the kidneys, blood vessels, and osteoblasts, it has been suggested that these toxins may be transported by OATs and accumulate in various tissues. The main uremic toxins of intestinal origin that are primarily eliminated through proximal tubule (PT) secretion are PCS, IS, cinnamoylglycine (CMG), and hippurate. Higher excretion of CMG has been linked to lower fractional excretion of potassium and phosphate, while increased net clearances of PCS and IS have been associated with lower fractional excretion of sodium, calcium, and uric acid, as well as higher levels of bicarbonate. Conversely, lower excretion of hippurate has been linked to higher mortality rates after adjusting for factors like race, sex, age, and glomerular filtration rate (GFR), whereas lower CMG excretion has been associated with an increased risk of needing dialysis. Studies have shown that serum levels of PCS increase significantly as kidney disease progresses, and elevated levels of PCS and IS are linked to higher mortality rates, cardiac issues, and progression of chronic kidney disease.

3.4.5. Renal Tubular Structural Evaluation

The most prevalent urine protein, Tamm-Horsfall protein (uromodulin), is only produced in the early distal tubule and thick ascending limb of the Henle's loop (TAHL). The majority of uromodulin is released into the lumen, where it forms a layer on the surface of the tubules. This layer is likely there to shield tubular cells from urolithiasis and ascending urinary tract infections. As renal function declines, uromodulin concentration progressively drops; as a result, there is a positive correlation between it and GFR. Serum uromodulin therefore aids in the differentiation of patients with and without chronic nephropathy. Uromodulin is a reliable indicator of the number of TAHL cells that are intact and, thus, of their functionality rather than an indirect GFR marker. Moreover, uromodulin may function as a predictor of the advancement of chronic kidney disease (CKD) given its strong correlation with proteinuria. Furthermore, since the abundance of OAT1, OAT3, and OAT4 protein from membrane fraction samples (exosomes) has been shown in the urine of patients with acute kidney injury, OATs themselves can be used as biomarkers for renal tubular injury. Urine OAT1 and OAT3 levels were high in patients with early PT damage and low in those with acute renal failure; all three carriers were present in high concentrations in patients with acute renal failure (Pallone et al, 2003; Sands & Layton, 2008).

A Closer Look

Urine Composition

Urine is a liquid waste product that the body produces and eliminates. It is excreted through the urethra after being secreted by the renal tubules and building up in the bladder. Although water makes up 91–96% of its composition, it also contains a variety of other liquid and solid substances.

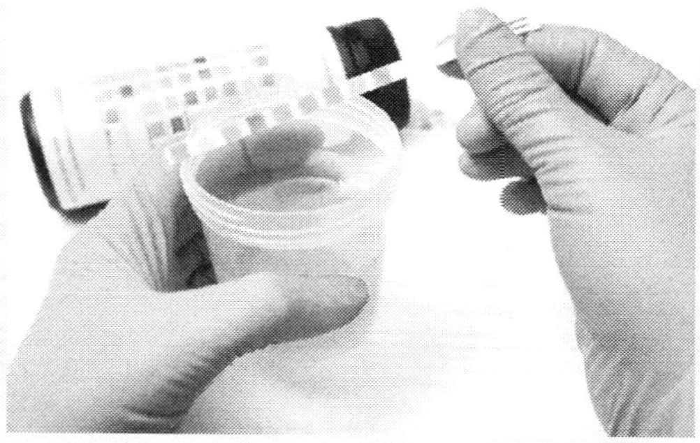

Source: *https://www.news-medical.net/health/Urine-Composition-Whats-Normal.aspx*

- **Urine Osmolarity:** An indicator of urine concentration, urine osmolarity can range from 50 to 12,00 mOsmol/kg on average. Urinary solute levels are approximately 1,000 mOsmol/day, and 1–4 liters of urine are secreted daily. The degree of exertion, the surroundings, the degree of hydration, and the consumption of salt and protein all affect the quantity and concentration of urine produced. Because meat contains a significant amount of urea, people who eat meat have higher solute concentrations; in contrast, vegetarians, who primarily obtain their energy from carbohydrates, have lower solute concentrations.
- **Urinary Physical Characteristics:**
    - o The pH of urine is normally around 6.2 with a range of 5.5–7.0. A high dietary protein and alcohol intake leads to lower pH, while vegetables and fruit bring about a more alkaline pH.
    - o The specific gravity of urine may range from 1.002 to 1.037.
    - o The mean calorific content of urine may be approximately 100 kcal/day.
- **Urine Composition:** Just 68 compounds make up more than 99% of urinary solutes and have concentrations of at least 10 mg/L. In actuality, 42 compounds are involved.

They may be classified as follows:

- o Electrolytes such as sodium, potassium, calcium, magnesium and chloride
- o Nitrogenous chemicals such as urea and creatinine
- o Vitamins

- Hormones
- Organic acids such as uric acid
- Other organic compounds

- **Total Dissolved Solids:** The total dissolved solids range from 24.88 to 37.01 g/kg in urine. The majority of organic matter in urinary solids is volatile solids. There is a lot of potassium, phosphorus, and nitrogen in urine. Urine has a high nitrogen content, primarily in the form of urea, which accounts for over half of the total organic acids. This includes sodium and potassium from food, as well as urea from protein metabolism. Thus, 14–18% of dry solids are nitrogen, 13% are carbon, and 3.7% are each of potassium and phosphorus. Urine is how the body excretes these substances in the greatest amount.
- **Nitrogen Excretion:** The majority of nitrogen excreted in urine is urea, with an average daily excretion of 11 g. Dietary protein intake has the greatest impact on it; urine nitrogenous components and protein in the diet have a correlation of 0.91. The excretion of nitrogenous compounds in the urine balances about 80% of the nitrogen that is consumed through diet. The concentration of urine urea varies from 9 to 23 g/L.

Another significant nitrogenous substance found in urine is creatinine, the amount of which varies with age, body mass, and muscle mass. These could have a correlation with gender differences. The average daily production of creatinine in the body is approximately 1.6 grams.

The third nitrogenous compound in urine is nitrate, which is present in higher concentrations in those who consume a high-protein diet.

Dietary protein influences not only the concentrations of urine nitrogen but also the levels of other minerals like potassium and phosphorus. Furthermore, a very low protein diet may have an impact on calcium levels.

- **Calcium in Urine:** As mentioned above, protein intake has an impact on calcium excretion, which is also significantly influenced by sodium excretion. Therefore, a diet low in sodium will also reduce the excretion of calcium and vice versa.

  A normal adult urine sample taken over the course of 24 hours should have a calcium level of 100–250 mg.
- **Other Ions:** Depending on the levels of parathyroid hormone, urine may also contain less common ionic groups such as phosphates, sulfates from amino acids and ammonium.
- **Overall Solute Concentrations:** The concentration of the following constituents in urine may be regarded as a careful approximation:
  - Urea: 9.3 g/dL
  - Creatinine: 0.670 g/ L
  - Sodium: 1.17 g/L
  - Potassium: 0.750 g/L
  - Chloride: 1.87 g/L

Summary

- Urine is a liquid or semi-solid solution of waste produced by humans and animals due to physiological activities and also contains harmful compounds produced by excretory organs during fluid circulation.
- Urine formation is a very complex process including glomerular ultrafiltration, tubular resorption and excretion.
- The kidney has many functions, which a well-functioning kidney realizes by filtering blood in a process known as glomerular filtration.
- The glomerular filter is permeable for substances in a manner as if it were provided by pores with a diameter measuring 10 nm.
- Tubular secretion participates substantially in the regulation of acid-base balance and in the maintenance of isotonia.
- The countercurrent mechanism in the kidney is a process of concentrating urine. It involves the flow of filtrate in opposite directions in the two limbs of the loop of Henle, which creates an osmotic gradient.
- Countercurrent multiplication primarily occurs in the nephrons of the kidney, specifically in the loop of Henle, a hairpin-shaped structure.
- The mammalian kidney maintains nearly constant blood plasma osmolality and nearly constant blood plasma sodium concentration utilizing mechanisms that independently regulate water and sodium excretion.
- The collecting duct, under the influence of vasopressin, is the nephron segment that, by regulating water reabsorption, is responsible for the control of water excretion.
- Glomerular filtration rate (GFR) and proteinuria-albuminuria are the renal functional parameters currently used to evaluate chronic kidney disease (CKD) severity.
- The kidneys in human beings mainly express OCT2 (SLC22A2), which is crucial for removing cationic substances from the blood, such as metformin, cimetidine, cisplatin, antihistamines and some antibiotics.
- In uremic syndrome, multiple biological pathways are affected, including those controlled by solute carrier (SLC) and ATP-binding cassette (ABC) transporters and drug-metabolizing enzymes, many of which are also involved in pharmacokinetics.
- Tamm-Horsfall protein (uromodulin), the most abundant urinary protein, is exclusively produced in the thick ascending limb of the Henle's loop (TAHL) and early distal tubule.

References

1. Emami Riedmaier, A., Nies, A. T., Schaeffeler, E., & Schwab, M. (2012). Organic anion transporters and their implications in pharmacotherapy. *Pharmacological Reviews, 64*(3), 421–449.
2. Henriksen, U. L., & Henriksen, J. H. (2015). The clearance concept with special reference to determination of glomerular filtration rate in patients with fluid retention. *Clinical Physiology and Functional Imaging, 35*(1), 7–16.

3. Knepper, M. A., Saidel, G. M., Hascall, V. C., & Dwyer, T. M. (2003). Concentration of solutes in the renal inner medulla: Interstitial hyaluronan as a mechano-osmotic transducer. *American Journal of Physiology-Renal Physiology, 284*, F433–F446.

4. Kuhn, W., & Ryffel, K. (1942). Herstellung konzentrierter Lösungen aus verdünnten durch blosse Membranwirkung: Ein Modellversuch zur Funktion der Niere. *Hoppe-Seylers Zeitschrift für Physiologische Chemie, 276*, 145–178.

5. Musso, C. G., Juarez, R., Vilas, M., Navarro, M., Rivera, H., & Jauregui, R. (2012). Renal calcium, phosphorus, magnesium and uric acid handling: Comparison between stage III chronic kidney disease patients and healthy oldest old. *International Urology and Nephrology, 44*(5), 1559–1562.

6. Pallone, T. L., Turner, M. R., Edwards, A., & Jamison, R. L. (2003). Countercurrent exchange in the renal medulla. *American Journal of Physiology-Regulatory, Integrative and Comparative Physiology, 284*, R1153–R1175.

7. Rocha, A. S., & Kokko, J. P. (1973). Sodium chloride and water transport in the medullary thick ascending limb of Henle. Evidence for active chloride transport. *Journal of Clinical Investigation, 52*, 612–623.

8. Sands, J. M., & Layton, H. E. (2008). The urine concentrating mechanism and urea transporters. In R. J. Alpern & S. C. Hebert (Eds.), *The Kidney: Physiology and Pathophysiology* (Vol. 1, pp. 1143–1178). Academic Press.

9. Shen, H., Liu, T., Morse, B. L., et al. (2015). Characterization of organic anion transporter 2 (SLC22A7): A highly efficient transporter for creatinine and species-dependent renal tubular expression. *Drug Metabolism and Disposition, 43*(7), 984–993.

10. Suchy-Dicey, A. M., Laha, T., Hoofnagle, A., et al. (2016). Tubular secretion in CKD. *Journal of the American Society of Nephrology, 27*(7), 2148–2155.

11. Wanchai, K., Yasom, S., Tunapong, W., et al. (2018). Probiotic Lactobacillus paracasei HII01 protects rats against obese-insulin resistance induced kidney injury and impaired renal organic anion transporter 3 function. *Clinical Science (London), 132*(14), 1545–1563.

Chapter 4

RENAL ENDOCRINE FUNCTIONS

Contents

Introduction

Erythropoietin, calcitriol (1,25-dihydroxycholecalciferol), and renin are the three major hormones that the kidneys produce. Prostaglandins, which are produced by them as well, have an impact on several kidney functions. The kidneys are involved in the breakdown of some hormones as well as their synthesis, including parathyroid hormone and insulin (which is broken down by the enzyme insulinase).

Orientation and Directional Terms

Term	Definition	Illustration
Autocrine	Chemical signal that elicits a response in the same cell that secreted it.	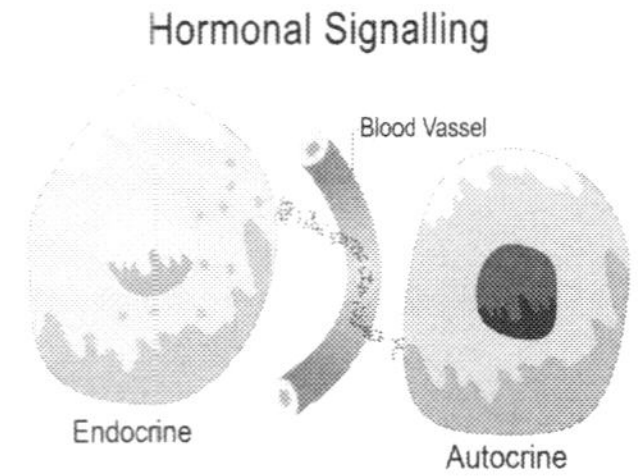
Epinephrine	Also known as adrenaline, is a hormone and neurotransmitter and produced by the adrenal glands.	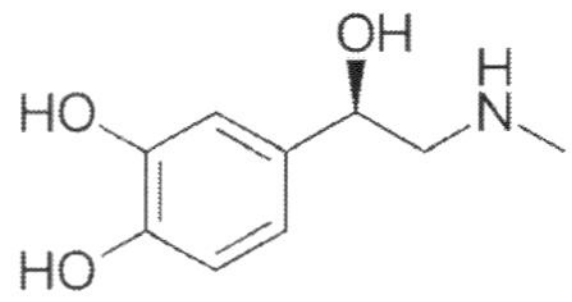
Hormone	Secretion of an endocrine organ that travels via the bloodstream or lymphatics to induce a response in target cells or tissues in another part of the body.	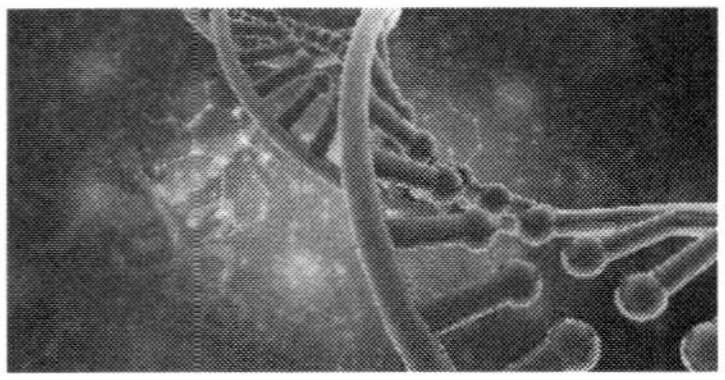
Paracrine	Chemical signal that elicits a response in neighboring cells; also called paracrine factor.	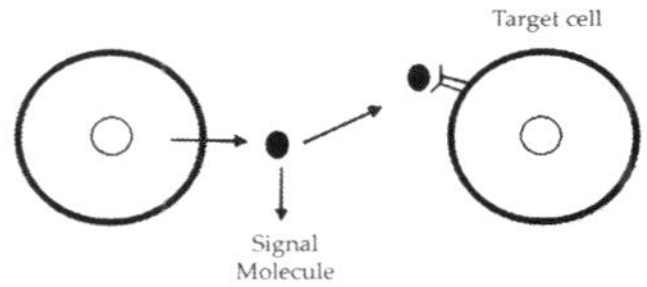
Proliferation	A rapid increase in numbers.	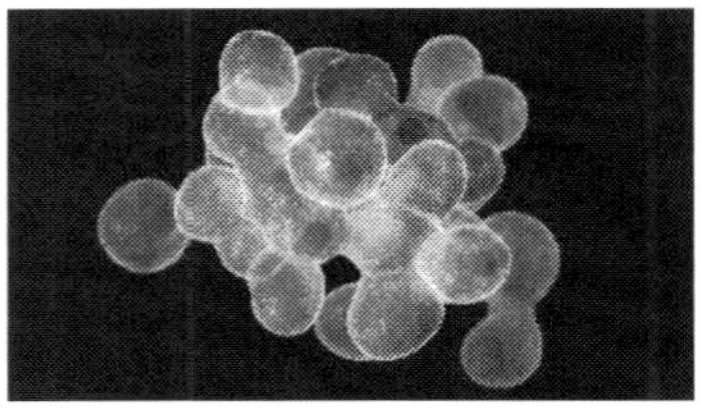
Synthesis	The production of chemical compounds by reaction from simpler materials.	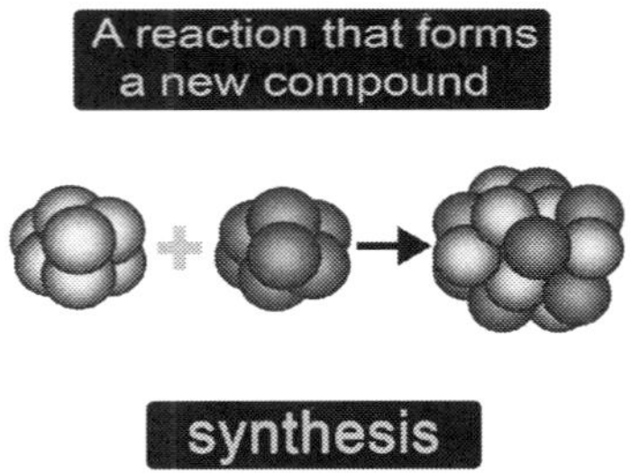

4.1. Erythropoietin Production and Its Role in Erythropoiesis

Human erythropoietin (EPO) is a peptide hormone that is made in the kidneys of adult humans and the liver of fetuses during the early stages of development. Major hematopoietic growth factor (HGF), it promotes the daily massive production (200 billion) of red blood cells (RBCs) containing hemoglobin A ($\alpha_2\beta_2$), which carries oxygen and transfers it from the lungs to tissues (Bunn, 2013) (Figure 4.1). Structure-wise, EPO is a glycoprotein with a starting mass of 193 aa, which includes a signaling peptide at the N-terminus that is 27 aa long. The mature form of EPO (UniProt P01588) is produced through post-translational cleavage of this premature polypeptide.

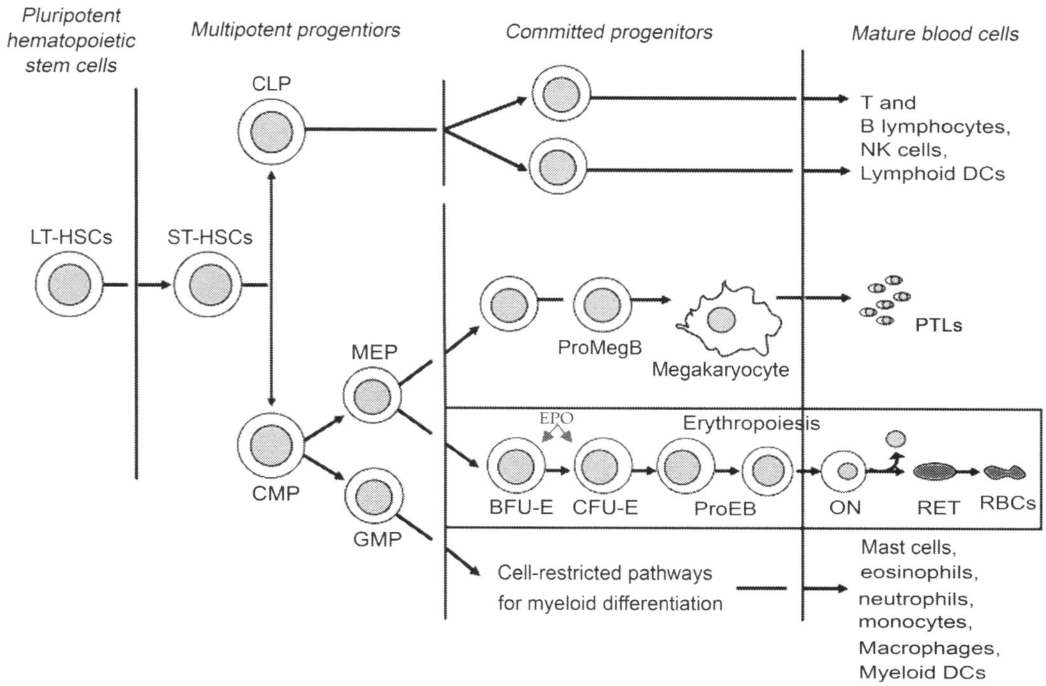

Figure 4.1. *Illustration of the human bone marrow cell restricted pathways of the differentiation of hematopoietic stem cells into mature blood cells.*

Source: Tsiftsoglou AS. (2021). Erythropoietin (EPO) as a key regulator of erythropoiesis, bone remodeling and endothelial transdifferentiation of multipotent mesenchymal stem cells (MSCs): implications in regenerative medicine. Cells, 10(8), 2140. doi: 10.3390/cells10082140. PMID: 34440909; PMCID: PMC8391952.

The restricted lineage differentiation by erythroid cells is depicted in Figure 4.1, lower right box. Common myeloid progenitors (CMP) and common megakaryocyte erythroid progenitors (MEP) are derived from HSCs. The latter are distinguished into BFU-E and CFU-E clones that respond to erythropoietin, as indicated by the arrows where human EPO acts on them. Hemoglobin biosynthesis is increased through cell signaling pathways activated by interactions between EPO and its homodimeric EPO-R. As erythropoiesis proceeds in proerythroblasts, orthochomatic normoblasts (ON), reticulocytes, and mature red blood cells (RBCs) after the nucleus is extruded, the amounts of hemoglobins rise. Homeostatic regulation of erythropoiesis is achieved by low oxygen conditions (hypoxia) and the final end product through a feedback action loop. With an estimated molecular weight of 30.4 kDa, the full-length human erythropoietin's primary structure consists of 166 amino acids. Two disulfide (-S-S-) bonds are present in this acidic glycoprotein, which supports the overall molecular structure between Cys29 and Cyst33 and Cys7 and Cys161. Asparagine residues 24, 38, and 83 contain three N-linked carbohydrates, while Serine residue 126 contains one O-linked carbohydrate. EPO's three-dimensional structure is made up of four alpha helices. While Helices A and B are connected by Cys29 and Cys33, Helix A is connected to Helix D via Cys7 and Cys171. Recombinant human erythropoietins (rhEPOetins) have been produced using a variety of gene-cloning-expression platforms over time. These include insect cell systems infected with yeast and baculovirus, as well as genetically altered mammalian CHO (McDonald J. et al., 1986) and HEK293 cells. Some of the differences between the biosimilar epoetins can be attributed to variations in their glycosylation patterns. Since 1989, rhEPO has been offered for sale after receiving FDA authorization (EPOGENR) to be used as a valuable biologic medication in replacement protein therapy (RPT) for chronic renal failure (CRF), which is typified by insufficient synthesis of EPO.

The history of the hunt for EPO dates back to 1875 when patients with low blood oxygen levels and anemia-like symptoms were identified. Furthermore, as previously mentioned, it required extensive research for the previous 50 years to determine that EPO is the primary driver of BM erythropoiesis, purify it from urine obtained from patients suffering from aplastic anemia, clone the EPO gene, and create recombinant EPO (Lin et al., 1985). The EPO-receptor (EPO-R) was discovered in 1989 (D'Andrea, Lodish, & Wong, 1989) thanks to the skillful work of the Lodish group at MIT. This finding sparked additional research on the EPO–EPO–R interactions and downstream signaling processes.

4.1.1. Homeostatic Regulation of EPO Production Via an Oxygen-Sensitive Feedback Loop

Early in the 1990s, a complex molecular mechanism for oxygen sensing was identified (Kietzmann, 2020) to account for the control of EPO production in hypoxic environments. The adult kidneys produce more EPO in response to ischemia stress, anemia, hypoxia at high altitude, and other conditions (tissue injuries, degeneration). EPO is secreted into plasma, where it activates the EPO-R on the BM erythroid progenitors, causing them to mature into RBCs (Tsiftsoglou et al., 2009). However, the biological effects of EPO on other tissues make this hormone, also known as hematopoietic growth factor, an extremely intriguing pleiotropic macromolecule. This is because the EPO-R is not only expressed on erythroid cells but also on many other tissues, including the heart, bone, brain neurons, adipose tissue, endothelial cells, and immune cells.

EPO has been discovered to be produced and secreted by the kidney's interstitial peritubular cells (IPCs) throughout adulthood. A growing number of IPCs generate and release EPO into the plasma when there is hypoxia. Even though other tissues produce far less EPO than the kidney, this does not replace what the kidney secretes. The HIF transcription factor, which is made up of the heterodimer HIF1α/HIF1β, binds to a hypoxia response element in the EPO gene promoter to control the production of the hypoxia-inducible hormone EPO. When there is normal oxygen availability or normoxia, the hydroxylases that are dependent on proline phosphates reduce the stability and activity of HIF1α. This is because the pVHL complex ubiquitinates the hydroxylated HIF1α, which is then broken down by the 26S proteasome (Sasaki, 2003). In contrast, HIF1α is structurally stabilized and upregulated in the renal EPO-producing cells under hypoxia (lower oxygen availability), where it binds to the EPO gene's promoter region and transactivates it. A rise in the end product of EPO then causes a feedback loop that inhibits the transactivation of HIF1α by preventing interactions with co-activator proteins. In short, the proteins involved in the hypoxia pathway are master regulators of erythropoiesis (Watts et al., 2020). The regulation of EPO synthesis was explained mechanistically by the identification of the hypoxia-inducing factor (HIF) as the primary transactivator of EPO gene expression. This finding also laid the foundation for William to be awarded the Nobel Prize in Physiology or Medicine (Kaelin Jr. Gregg L. & Sir Peter John Ratcliffe, 2019's Semenza).

4.1.2. EPO Binds to EPO-R in BM Hematopoietic Progenitors and Promotes Erythroid Differentiation

The EPOR gene encodes the protein cell surface receptor chain known as ERO-R (Goldwasser & Kung, 1971). It has one N-linked carbohydrate chain, which adds to its approximate 56–57 kDa molecular weight overall. ERO-R belongs to the superfamily of type I cytokine receptors. Three structural domains make up this single transmembrane protein: (i) an extracellular domain spanning 226 aa that binds EPO; (ii) a transmembrane helical domain spanning 23 aa that enables the crucial intracellular transfer of any extracellular EPO-induced conformational changes; and (iii) a C-terminal intracellular domain spanning 235 aa that contains 8-tyrosine phosphorylation sites and JAK2 binding sites that function as binding sites for transcription factors like STAT5, which in turn activates downstream processes (Bhoopalan, Jun-Huang, & Weiss, 2020).

It typically exists as a homodimer and experiences the conformational changes described, which are caused by the receptor-associated JAK2 kinase autophosphorylating (Figure 4.2). In addition to being expressed to varying degrees in other tissues, EPO-R is highly expressed in EPO-responsive BM erythroid progenitors (BFU-E and CFU-E) that are descended from the common precursor of myeloid-erythroid and megakaryocyte (MEK) (Palis & Koniski, 2018). At the proerythroid cell level, EPO and EPO-R interact to stimulate proliferation, improve survival, and encourage cell-restricted lineage erythroid differentiation.

Through a series of intra-conversions to pro-erythroblasts (ProE, BasoE, and PolyE), the EPO-induced cells irreversibly commit to the erythroid pathway before fully differentiating into orthochromatic erythroblasts (normoblasts). The latter then emerge from their nucleus to change into reticulocytes, which develop into red blood cells (RBCs) at a later stage (Figure 4.1). In numerous model systems, this pathway of hematopoietic cell differentiation has been thoroughly investigated (Tsiftsoglou, Vizirianakis, & Strouboulis, 2009). The major erythroid transcription factors GATA-1 and TAL-1 are activated when EPO binds to EPO-R, stimulating the cell signaling pathway and transactivating the expression of the EPOR gene. Additionally, EPO stimulates the mitochondria to produce heme, and in erythroid progenitors, it activates the transferrin-mediated transport of iron through the cell surface transferrin receptor cycling complex. The BM erythropoiesis program is activated when EPO binds to the homodimeric EPOR to form a complex (Tsiftsoglou, Vizirianakis, & Strouboulis, 2009). The expression of the EPOR gene is transcriptionally downregulated as erythroid differentiation completes. As previously reviewed (Bhoopalan, Jun-Huang, & Weiss, 2020), comprehensive studies of the EPO–EPO-R-induced signaling pathways in disease states have recently started to identify many inherited and acquired disorders linked to either excessive or insufficient RBC production. Novel "designer" biopharmaceuticals are therefore required to regulate such erythropoiesis abnormalities.

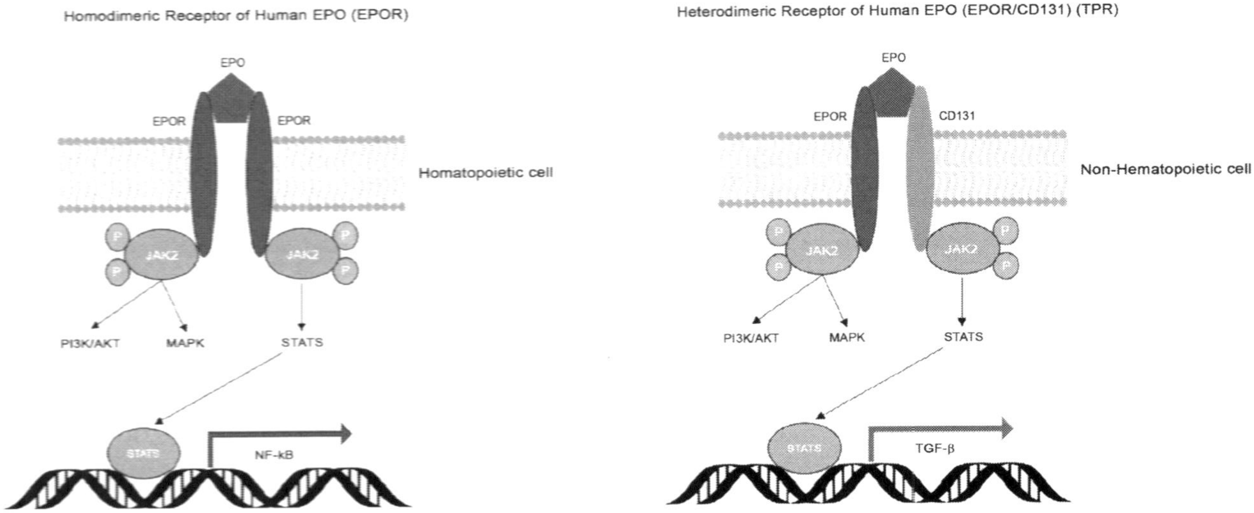

Figure 4.2. *Illustration of the interactions of human EPO with its homodimeric (EPO-R) and heterodimeric receptor (EPO-R/CD131, or tissue protection receptor (TPR)). These receptors are activated in hematopoietic (erythroid progenitors) and non-hematopoietic cells (brain, heart, skeletal muscle cells, etc.), respectively. Activation of the homodimeric EPO-R receptor leads to cell signaling in BM proerythroid cells, while activation of the heterodimeric EPO-R/CD131 leads to the increase of cell renewal, survival and protection of non-hematopoietic cells. For both cases of EPO-R signaling, the activation pathways shown above are mediated by the phosphorylated JAK2 kinases, which then interact with the intracellular regions of the receptor and activate the PI3K/AKT, MAPK and STAT5 molecules by a phosphorylation cascade. The transcription regulator STAT5 interacts with consensus DNA sequences that facilitate the activation of the NF-kB transcription factor (Suresh. et al., 2019). In the case of the activation of the EPO-R/CD131 receptor by EPO in non-hematopoietic tissues, the induced cell signaling promotes the phosphorylation of similar molecules, the activation of STAT5 and eventually the expression of TGF-β (Cantarelli, Angelleti, &Cravedi, 2019).*

Source: Tsiftsoglou AS. (2021). Erythropoietin (EPO) as a key regulator of erythropoiesis, bone remodeling and endothelial transdifferentiation of multipotent mesenchymal stem cells (MSCs): Implications in regenerative medicine. Cells, 10(8), 2140. doi: 10.3390/cells10082140. PMID: 34440909; PMCID: PMC8391952.

4.1.3. EPO Promotes Bone Remodeling

In addition to the BM erythroid progenitors, EPO-R receptors have been found on many different cell types and tissues (Wang et al., 2014). These comprise, among other things, bone marrow mesenchymal stromal cells (BMMSCs), skeletal muscle cells (Park et al., 2012), heart and neuron cells (Van Der Meer et al., 2005), and other cells like dental MSCs (Bianco et al., 2001). According to the stimuli and conditions in their microenvironment, MSCs are multipotent stem cells that can differentiate into osteoblasts, osteoclasts, chondrocytes, odontoblasts, adipocytes, and endothelial cells (Bianco, 2015). It is crucial for maintaining bone homeostasis that EPOR is expressed in osteoblasts, which form new bone, and osteoclasts, which resorb existing bone. According to a recent review by Suresh et al., many in vitro and in vivo biological model systems have been used thus far to examine whether EPO promotes bone remodeling (Suresh et al., 2019). Studies using BM MSCs cultured in vitro have shown that EPO increases osteoblastic activity but not osteoclastic activity (Li, Wang, & Niyibizi, 2010). Fascinatingly, research utilizing adherent and primary osteogenic BMMSCs has demonstrated that the capacity of EPO to enhance osteoblastic differentiation is dose-dependent (low: 5 IU/mL vs. high: 250 IU/mL and above. Moreover, the effect of EPO was age-dependent in patients with myelodysplastic syndromes (MDS). A high dose of EPO induced bone mineralization and endochondral ossification in a fracture repair model. Furthermore, studies have demonstrated that EPO facilitated endosteal vascularization and bone remodeling. In research intended to use EPO to attract BMMSCs to rat bone defect sites, i.e., BMMSCs activated by EPO injection are used for modeling and repair (Li, Wang, & Niyibizi, 2010). Additionally, in patients with tibiofibular fractures, two weeks following surgery, a high-dose (4,000 IU/dose) injection of EPO sped up bone repair by speeding up bone healing. The synopsis of the reviewed studies indicates that more research is required to pharmacologically optimize the dosage of EPO required to support bone remodeling and preserve regenerative bone homeostasis (Suresh, Lee, & Noguchi, 2020).

4.1.4. EPO Induces Angiogenic Differentiation of Human Endothelial Cells (ECs) and Mesenchymal Stem Cells (MSCs)

In vitro angiogenesis of endothelial cells (ECs) has been demonstrated to be facilitated by the expression of EPOR in human umbilical vein endothelial cells (HUVEC cells). Previous research has demonstrated that EPO induces signaling that increases STAT5 phosphorylation and the downstream transcriptional activation of several genes involved in proliferation, migration, and capillary vessel formation (Kimakova et al., 2017). Innovative work by Anagnostou and associates. established in the 1990s that ECs express EPOR mRNA and that EPO has a mitogenic and chemotactic effect on cultured HUVEC cells in vitro. Subsequent research revealed that EPO stimulates the mobilization of endothelial progenitor cells and causes a pro-angiogenic phenotype in ECs that are cultured, ultimately leading to the promotion of new vascularization in vivo (Ribatti et al., 1999).

It has been demonstrated that ECs produce more nitric oxide (NO) and promote EPOR-mediated vascularization in response to EPO and hypoxia. This was instead brought about by the EPO–EPOR interactions activating the signaling pathway AKT-e-Nos-MMP2, not by the endothelin 1 that ECs produce. The vascular tone of the vascular bed is impacted by NO production. A review has previously been conducted on the angiogenic effects of human EPO in ECs with regard to ischemic heart and retinal neovascularization, tumor angiogenesis, and other pathologies (Carlini, Reyes, & Rothstein, 1995). Further research by Wan et al., as well as Holstein et al. As previously mentioned, (Holstein et al., 2011) showed that EPO stimulates chondrogenesis and angiogenesis during bone remodeling and repair, offering an alternate strategy for skeletal cell regeneration. MSCs are widely distributed in tissues and are comparatively simple to separate, describe, and cultivate as adherent cells in culture.

In addition to expressing distinct cell surface markers that allow for identification (Bakopoulou et al., 2015), human MSCs have the unusual capacity to be guided into differentiating into a variety of cell types, including adipocytes, osteoblasts and osteoclasts, chondrocytes (which produce cartilage), endothelial cells, and potentially neuron-like cells. They also express the EPO-R, have anti-inflammatory properties, inhibit immune responses, and respond to EPO. It's interesting to note that MSCs can create and secrete exosomes, or secretomes, which contain a variety of growth factors and cytokines, including VEGF and angiopoietin, among others. These exosomes may one day be used as cutting-edge treatments for in situ tissue regeneration, which is a symptom of many degenerative and metabolic disorders. As a result, without producing significant immunogenicity, MSCs can be an appropriate model system to develop autologous and even allogeneic cell therapy products.

MSCs are fibroblast-shaped adherent cells that can develop into colony-forming units-F (CFU-F). They also have the previously mentioned multipotency, immunomodulatory, and anti-inflammatory properties, as well as a remarkable secretome that can synthesize and secrete a wide range of molecules, including cytokines, chemokines, and growth factors (Bakopoulou et al., 2015).

Numerous studies involving stromal BMMSCs have demonstrated that, after angiogenesis was upregulated, exposure to EPO before transplantation infarcted heart tissue increased the expression of proangiogenic and survival factors, such as HIF1α, angiopoietin, VEGF, VEGFR2, EPO, Bcl-2, and Bcl-xL. Under hypoxic conditions, MSC-mediated cell therapy for heart infarction was more advantageous because it promoted the formation of CD31+ micro-vessel cells and improved transplanted cellular survival (Kobayashi et al., 2008).

The role of endogenous and exogenous EPO on non-erythroid cells, like osteoblasts and adipocytes, was shown in a more recent study by Noguchi's group using transgenic mice with chronic overexpression of EPO and hematocrit, as well as other mice with genetically deficient EPOR in BM stromal cells. The latter showed a decreased capacity to form BM osteoblasts and adipocytes, and they were devoid of EPO–EPO-R-induced signaling. Overall, this elegant work concluded that loss of EPO signaling promotes fat accumulation in the BM at the expense of osteogenesis and facilitates the production of adipocytes. Additionally, the same study showed that aberrant EPO levels contribute to the impaired differentiation of bone marrow stromal cells and that endogenous EPO signals regulate their fate.

We used human dental pulp MSCs (DPSC) and apical papilla mesenchymal stem cells (SCAP) as suitable model systems to: (i) investigate the angiogenic potential of such cells growing under microenvironmental stress conditions (serum, glucose, and/or oxygen deprivation, separately or in combinations); and (ii) explore whether the exposure of SCAP cells to EPO activates the EPO/EPOR signaling pathway, leading to angiogenesis in vitro. Researchers were quite interested in learning more about the angiogenic potential of human MSCs, as discussed earlier. A group of highly intriguing multipotent MSCs known as human SCAP cells express a variety of cell surface markers related to epithelium, endothelium, neurons, hematopoietic cells, and embryonic development. Researchers demonstrated endothelial transdifferentiation of SCAP cells growing under various stress conditions (Bakopoulou et al., 2015) or treated with EPO in culture by employing a variety of methodologies (RT-PCR, flow cytometry, antibody protein microarrays, Western blotting, growth on Matrigel-coated plates to confirm the capillary vessel formation).

Additionally, we evaluated the SCAP cellular secretome, or their ability to secrete a variety of growth factors (VEGF, VEGFR2, angiopoietin-1, and others) that may be useful treatments for tissue regeneration. When conditioned medium from stress-grown SCAP cell cultures was added to human HUVEC cell cultures, it stimulated the formation of capillary vessels *in vitro* (Bakopoulou et al., 2015). In addition, SCAP cells treated with human EPO in culture showed changes in cell morphology, longer cell survival, and endothelial transdifferentiation, as evidenced by the development of microvascular structures on surfaces coated with Matrigel. Ultimately, these cells expressed the maturation marker for endothelial cells, CD31. Ultimately, the research verified the capacity of dental SCAP cells for angiogenesis and stimulated vascularization brought about by stress hypoxia (Bakopoulou et al., 2015) or endodontic pressure (Koutsoumparis et al., 2018). The development of tissue-engineered medicinal products (TEPs) for cell therapies that aim to repair damaged or degenerated dental tissue or non-erythroid tissues like brain tissue can greatly benefit from these findings.

4.1.5. EPO: From Tissue Protection to Modulation of the Innate and Adaptive Immune Responses

Recent data suggests that EPO not only stimulates erythroid progenitor-derived BM erythropoiesis by binding to the homodimeric receptor EPO-R, but also binds to the heterodimeric complex EPO-R on non-erythroid tissues such as the kidney, heart, cornea, and brain. This heterodimeric complex is made up of one EPO-R chain and a widely distributed CD131 (colony-stimulating factor 2) receptor β-chain. (Figure 4.2). It has been suggested that this heterodimeric receptor is the tissue protective receptor (TPR) of EPO. Although the interaction between EPO and TPR does not start erythropoiesis, it does signal biochemical cascades that protect cells from apoptosis, degeneration, and cytotoxicity in general by activating PI3K, MARK, STAT5, and other pathways. Although at comparatively higher concentrations than those that promote erythropoiesis, the binding of EPO with TPR cytoprotects a variety of cell types.

Research on both in vitro and in vivo has shown that EPO via TPR shields the heart from myocardial infarction-related ischemia reperfusion injury (RPI). Clinical research hasn't, however, been able to conclusively show that EPO improves left ventricular function or the infarct site in the weeks following myocardial infraction. Under hypoxic stress, brain (CNS) cells also release EPO. By improving oxygen delivery through the revascularization of the ischemic zone and stimulating TPR signaling, EPO safeguards astrocytes, oligodendrocytes, and neurons. By shielding cells from harm (apoptosis, inflammation, neurotoxicity), EPO also enhances the long-term neurologic result by promoting neuronal regeneration, injury healing, and general survival. Major neurodegenerative disorders and stroke are being studied in relation to the protective effects of EPO on neurons.

Through the activation of TPR signaling, EPO also seems to protect against retinopathy in the retina. Additionally, the survival of stress- and injury-stricken kidney proximal and distal renal tubular cells has been shown to benefit from the protective effects of EPO. Furthermore, in models of chronic kidney transplant rejection, EPO has been found to potentially protect renal transplants. Monocytes, T- and B-lymphocytes are immune cells that express EPO-R functionally, which suggests that EPO may have positive and modulating effects on both the innate and adaptive immune systems. It was discovered that monocytes produce EPO, and that immune self-tolerance is maintained by their autocrine EPO–EPO-R signaling. EPO appears to promote the development and growth of regulatory T-cells (Tregs), but it also has a rather direct inhibitory effect on memory T-cells, according to studies conducted on humans. Furthermore, it was discovered that EPO directly activates immune cellular TPR and inhibits their proinflammatory cytokines, preventing apoptosis. Additionally, it was discovered that EPO directly influences immune cell activation, differentiation, and function (Peng et al., 2020).

4.1.6. EPO Biosimilars

Amgen (Epogen®) was the first company to use recombinant DNA technology to develop human erythropoietin alpha as a valuable biopharmaceutical (biologic) medicine in the late 1980s. This innovation marked a significant advancement in the treatment of anemia in patients receiving chemotherapy for cancer or chronic renal failure. Epoetin alpha (rhEPO) has also been effectively i.v. given to patients to lower the frequency of blood transfusions for adults with moderate anemia or myelodysplastic syndromes (MDS), raise hemoglobin levels and RBC content. Barcoding tracing analysis has provided evidence that EPO influences single-cell hematopoietic stem cell differentiation following transplantation (Eisele et al., 2020). Over the past 10 years, a second generation of biologics with remarkably similar primary structures has been developed in response to the growing global demand for epoetins and other first-generation biologics (peptide hormones, growth factors, antibodies, and others).

Biosimilars are biologics that are subject to regulations in the USA and Europe regarding their manufacture, assessment, and approval for market use. Tight industrial conditions are used to manufacture biosimilars that share the same primary structures, indications, and biological properties. A full-scale comparability study based on quality, preclinical, and clinical evaluation is used to assess the biosimilars' biological similarities in vitro and in vivo, and the biosimilar is then authorized and approved for use on the market. Biosimilars function similarly to the original agent in terms of pharmacokinetics and pharmacodynamics, but they frequently differ in terms of immunogenicity. The original Epogen® and several other epoetin-alpha biosimilars have been used in the clinic because EPO primarily acts in the bone marrow to stimulate erythropoiesis and hemoglobin synthesis in several disorders, including anemias associated with chronic kidney failure, Zidovudine treatment of HIV, and cancer chemotherapy (Peng et al., 2020). These consist of the currently being developed Procrit, Abseamed, epoetin-alpha Hexal, Binocrit, Retacrit, and several others. As previously mentioned, EPO-alpha biosimilars differ slightly in immunogenicity, but otherwise share comparable physicochemical and pharmacological characteristics. The fact that EPO acts through the heterodimeric receptor EPO-R/CD131 (TPR) on non-hematopoietic tissues (brain, heart, skeletal muscle, mast cells, and others) has also "triggered" the development of a new class of EPO-alpha derivatives, which include the carbamylated EPO, the B-surface peptide (HBSP), and the Cyclic Helix B-peptide, all of which are being evaluated clinically for their potential to treat a range of degenerative disorders, as was previously discussed (Peng et al., 2020).

4.1.7. Implications of EPO-Induced Differentiation of HSCs and Multipotent MSCs in Regenerative Medicine

Long-term research using MSCs and multipotent hematopoietic cells has suggested that severe disorders may be cured as well as damaged tissues may be able to regenerate (Hofer & Tuan, 2016). BMMSCs and MSCs from various sources, such as dental, have garnered a lot of interest because of their special qualities. Together with the creation of induced pluripotent stem cells (iPSCs) and cloning techniques, these advancements provided a favorable environment for the emergence of regenerative medicine (RM) as a novel field of applied biomedical science. Through stem cell research, cell phenotype interconversion, and the general development of novel gene- and cell-based therapies for the possible treatment/cure of degenerative disorders are among the main goals of RM. Growth factors, like erythropoiesis in the bone marrow and the ability to induce bone remodeling, prevent tissue degeneration, and promote angiogenic differentiation of MSCs, can be useful agents in the development and production of Advanced Therapy Medicinal Products (ATMPs), which aim to treat/cure severe pathologies and/or promote tissue regeneration.

Pathologies that are classified as severe unmet medical needs include genetic/metabolic disorders, erythroid tissue homeostatic disorders like sickle cell anemia (SCA), thalassemia, and other anemias, degenerative disorders of bones, skeletal muscles, cartilage-forming tissue, and the vascular bed, and certain types of cancer. To replace, repair, and regenerate the damaged tissues, autologous or even allogeneic MSCs derived from various tissues can be transplanted. The Regulation of the European Community (Reg. dated September 13, 2007, regarding ATMPs, has already authorized and approved cell-based ATMPs derived from human MSCs for use in treating bone lesions and cartilage defects caused by chondrocyte and bone osteoblast degeneration. The potential for treating "red foot" type diseases in diabetic patients as well as other disorders may arise from the development of more ATMPs based on EPO's capacity to stimulate endothelial transdifferentiation (angiogenesis) of MSCs (Tsiftsoglou, 2021).

4.2. Renal Regulation of Calcium and Phosphate Metabolism

In general, texts on elementary physiology and biochemistry do not include sections on inorganic elements or metals. This is not to suggest that bioinorganic chemistry is uninteresting. To put it simply, in-depth discussions about other metals and trace elements are typically limited to specialized texts that deal with bioinorganic chemistry. There is no shortage of candidates for focused discussion, aside from the halogen anions chlorine and iodine and the alkaline earth cations sodium and potassium. These include iron, copper, zinc and magnesium, cobalt and nickel, manganese, vanadium and chromium, and the increasingly common selenium. Interestingly, despite their significant abundance, two of the most significant inorganic elements—calcium (Ca^{2+}) and phosphorus—rarely receive their own section. Phosphorus makes up roughly half of the total body weight at 1% (~0.5 Kg), while calcium makes up the remaining 1–2% (or 1.0–1.2 Kg) (based on a 73 Kg human). While phosphorus (85%) and Ca^{2+} (99%) are found in bone as a complex, each ion has a variety of important, frequently unrelated, nonstructural roles connected to cell homeostasis. The complex hormonal regulation linked to each element reflects the significance of both Ca^{2+} and phosphorus in the body. The regulation of these two elements has been the subject of a plethora of exciting recent advances.

4.2.1. Intestinal Absorption

During intestinal uptake, phosphorus (as "phosphate," or Pi/HPO_4^{-2}) and Ca^{2+} both use passive diffusion and saturable/facilitated absorption. P_i uptake is saturable (between cells or transcellular), whereas Ca^{2+} uptake is typically passive (or paracellular). Reduced Ca^{2+} intake will increase facilitated (active/transcellular) Ca^{2+} absorption, but in the P_i system, facilitated uptake will always seem to predominate. It should be highlighted, though, that opinions regarding the amount of passive diffusion that takes place during intestinal Pi uptake are incongruent.

4.2.2. Calcium

Regarding Ca^{2+}, an average daily intake will comprise 1,000 mg of elemental Ca^{2+}. There will be an absorption of about 200 mg and an excretion of 800 mg. Although Ca^{2+} is absorbed throughout the intestine, the duodenum and jejunum's low luminal pH (5 to 6) facilitates Ca^{2+} ionization and effective absorption. A transepithelial electrochemical gradient is probably responsible for the Ca^{2+} exit from the intestinal lumen when the paracellular route is used, which is typically in the jejunum/ileum. While the majority of research on Ca^{2+} diffusion has focused on the renal epithelium, it is reasonable to presume that a comparable mechanism takes place in the intestines as well. Therefore, the brush border NKCC2 (Na-K-Cl-2 transporter) and ROMK (ATP-sensitive K+ channel), as well as the basolateral CLCNKB (Cl-channel) and Na/K ATPase, will produce the gradient. Through NKCC2, ions such as Na^+, K^+, and 2 Cl-first exit the intestinal lumen and enter the cell. This is countered by a K^+ flux through ROMK. On the basal side, Cl- leaves the cell through CLCNKB channels, Na^+ leaves the cell, and K+ enters the cell through Na/K ATPase.

All things considered, this produces an electrochemical gradient that forces Ca^{2+} through a paracellular pathway and out of the lumen and into the extracellular fluid. Even though paracellular diffusion can be conceptualized as straightforward cell-to-cell diffusion, this is probably not the case. Tight junctions connect cells physically and act as a barrier to free intercellular diffusion, as would be expected for the epithelium. It has been discovered that a special type of junctional complex molecule in the kidney controls the transit of both Mg^{2+} and Ca^{2+} through tight junctions. It belongs to the claudin superfamily of junctional molecules and is known as paracellin-1. Together with occludin and JAM (junctional adhesion molecule), it forms a trimeric complex. Other claudins, including claudin-2, -15, and -20, are present in the small intestine and probably function as regulators of divalent cation transit, even though this particular claudin is only found in the kidney.

In reality, a distinct set of ion transporters and channels are used in the duodenum and jejunum for assisted, or transcellular, Ca^{2+} transport. As previously mentioned, there are both luminal and basolateral transporters/channels, primarily based on research on renal epithelial cells. Transcellular transport is characterized by its sensitivity to active $1,25(OH)_2$ vitamin D3 (abbreviated as VitD) levels. Transient receptor potential-vanilloid 6 channel (TRPV6) is present on the luminal side. This channel protein has six transmembrane domains and can be found as either a homotetramer or heterotetramer with TRPV5. Its levels rise in response to vitamin D. It is inactivated by both phosphorylation and a Ca^{2+}-calmodulin complex, and it is upregulated by low cytosolic Ca^{2+}. It also opens in the presence of low luminal Ca^{2+}. Because of an electrochemical gradient, Ca^{2+} enters the cell. Once inside, Ca^{2+}-binding proteins (calbindins), whose synthesis is stimulated by vitamin D, mediate its passage through the cell.

The two Ca^{2+}-binding sites of calbindin-D9K are used in the intestine. Ca^{2+} is delivered by calbindin-D9K to one of two basolateral transporters/pumps: 138 kDa PMCA1b (plasma membrane Ca^{2+}-dependent ATPase) or 120 kDa NCX1 (a Ca^{2+}-Na^{+} exchanger). While PMCA1b pumps Ca^{2+} out at the expense of ATP, the NCX1 exchanger internalizes three Na^{+} for one Ca^{2+}. The predominant route for Ca^{2+} extrusion in the intestine is represented by PMCA1b. VitD positively regulates PMCA1b gene expression, just like it does for TRPV6. Estrogen also positively regulates PMCA1b, which may be very significant during pregnancy and lactation.

Regarding the TRPV system, three points need to be made. First, TRPV6 and TRPV5 are both present in the intestine. However, it is proposed that TRPV6 predominates in the intestine and TRPV5 predominates in the kidney. Second, klotho, a transmembrane multifunctional protein with beta-glucuronidase activity, controls the expression of TRPV5 in the kidney. Glycosylated and constitutively active renal TRPV5. TRPV5 turnover is prevented by membrane-associated klotho deglycosylation, which keeps TRPV5 within the membrane and increases its duration of activity. Although it is unknown, it would seem possible that the intestine experiences the same phenomenon. The last molecule involved in cellular Ca^{2+} transport is known to be positively regulated by parathyroid hormone (PTH) in the kidney. Although the precise effects of PTH on intestinal molecules are unknown, they most likely resemble those in the kidney.

4.2.3. Phosphorus

Phosphorus comes from both natural and artificial sources, including carbonated drinks and dairy products, cereals, and meat. It is a remarkably abundant mineral. Depending on the study, the total daily intake can vary, but for women, it can range from 1,000 mg to 1,500 mg (in men). About 70% of the phosphorus in food is absorbed, mostly in the jejunum. Once more, there are two possible ways for this to happen: an intracellular route for facilitated transport or a passive intercellular route. It is said that phosphorus absorption is little regulated. The question is whether the majority of absorption is facilitated or passive.

Because the extracellular fluid beneath the epithelium is electropositive in comparison to the intestinal lumen and the intestinal lumen has a higher phosphorus concentration than the extracellular fluid, paracellular/intercellular transport is electrochemically favored. The main point to note, however, is that intercellular junctions are extremely impermeable to phosphate ions. Therefore, paracellular transport seems to have a negligible overall impact on phosphate absorption.

At least three factors contribute to transcellular/facilitated diffusion: a basolateral Na^{+}/K^{+} ATPase, a luminal Na^{+}/P_i co-transporter, and an as-yet-unidentified but putative basolateral Pi transporter. One Na^{+} and one P_i ion are simultaneously transported into the cell by the 80 kDa, eight-transmembrane domain protein known as the Na^{+}/Pi transporter, or NPT2b. P_i leaves the cell via the basolateral side after internalization. According to reports, VitD positively regulates NPT2b, and NPT2b probably reacts to variations in intracellular Na^{+} concentration. It's unclear exactly what part VitD plays. Although it appears to boost NPT2b expression or "activity," since the NPT2b gene lacks a VitD response element, it must act at the posttranscriptional level. It could have an indirect effect on NPT2b by increasing the activity of the Na^{+}/K^{+} ATPase, decreasing intracellular Na^{+}, and attracting luminal Na^{+} with P_i. It has also been reported that STC-1/stanniocalcin-1 increases P_i uptake. The kidney produces the dimeric phosphoglycoprotein known as STC-1, which is secreted. Uncertainty surrounds the uptake mechanism, but it surely involves the recently identified STC receptor or receptors. Related protein STC-2 has been demonstrated to control kidney NPT2a expression. High luminal levels of both Ca^{2+} and P_i, which produce insoluble CaHPO4 complexes, and the use of antacids containing aluminum, which makes Pi insoluble, are examples of non-hormonal factors that affect both Ca^{2+} and P_i absorption.

4.2.4. Serum Calcium and Phosphorus

Phosphorus and Ca^{2+} are absorbed and then circulate in different forms. About half of the Ca^{2+} in serum is free to ionize, 50% is bound to proteins, and 5% is present in poorly defined complexes. 30% of phosphorus is inorganic, while 70% is organic. 30% of the inorganic phosphorus is ionic and freely filtered by the kidney, with the remaining 10% ionically bound to protein and not filtered by the kidney. About 5% of the "ionic 90%" is made up of free phosphate ions, 30% is Na^+ salt, and the remaining 65% is divalent phosphate salt (Mg or Ca). Since HPO_{4-}^{2} makes up about 80% of free phosphate ions and $H_2PO_{4-}^{1}$makes up 20%, the term "P_i" is typically understood to refer to HPO_{4-}^{2}. Organic phosphorus can be found in a variety of forms, such as phospholipids, phosphonucleotides, phosphoproteins, and phosphate esters.

4.2.5. Molecules Regulating Calcium and Phosphorus Metabolism

4.2.5.1. Vitamin D

Numerous hormones that affect Pi metabolism and Ca^{2+} levels are in circulation. Vitamin D3 ($1,25(OH)_2$) is the first (Vitamin D). Basal keratinocytes naturally produce 7-dehydrocholesterol, the precursor for vitamin D. It's the last stage of the cholesterol synthesis process. When sterol D7-reductase is present, 7-dehydrocholesterol (7DHC), also referred to as provitamin D, transforms into cholesterol. When 7DHC is exposed to UV-B radiation (290–319 nm), its B ring is broken, and vitamin D3 is created by spontaneous isomerization. Although it is bio-inactive, this will attach to the 53 kDa vitamin D-binding protein (VDBP) that is produced by endothelia. Before moving on to the kidney, where a second -OH is added at position 1, each VDBP-vitamin D3 complex transits first to the liver, where a -OH is added at position 25.

Although 1,25 $(OH)_2$ vitamin D3/VitD is thought to be the active form, 25(OH) vitamin D3 is also thought to have specific bioactivity, especially in terms of encouraging intestinal Ca^{2+} uptake. 1 alpha-hydroxylase, an enzyme that is highly regulated by several factors, carries out the second, or position 1 hydroxylation. Ca^{2+}, Pi, and Klotho decrease 1 alpha-hydroxylase activity, whereas PTH, IFN-gamma, and IGF-I increase it.

The VDBP-25(OH) vitamin D3 complex's detour during the second, or kidney-based, hydroxylation is the most noteworthy feature of this process. It is filtered through the glomerulus before binding to luminal, 550 kDa megalin on proximal tubule cells, as opposed to binding to basolateral VDBP receptor(s) on proximal tubule cells. Internalization and seeming complex dissociation are caused by this. Freshly liberated 25(OH) vitamin D3 now attaches to a novel intracellular VDBP called IDBP-1, which guides it to the alpha-hydroxylase of mitochondrial CYP1/1. Following formation, vitamin D ($1,25(OH)_2$ vitamin D3) diffuses freely out of the cell to interact with either the incompletely characterized 60 kDa membrane receptor that triggers fast, non-transcriptional responses in cells, or the 48 kDa vitamin D receptor/VDR. Vitamin D probably has the noteworthy effect of downregulating its own activity in addition to its significant effects on bone and renal metabolism. To inactivate the vitamin, it accomplishes this by increasing the activity of 24-hydroxylase, an enzyme that swaps out the hydroxide at position 1 for one at position 24.

The take-home message for vitamin D is, in essence, that it keeps serum Ca^{2+} concentrations within normal limits. The process involves upregulating certain elements like TRPV6 and calbindin-D9K that are linked to the intestinal Ca^{2+} absorption process. It is involved in immunity, reproduction, and the metabolism of phosphate. It also has intricate interactions with other important hormones related to the metabolism of bone. In summary, however, it targets the intestines.

It is stated that sufficient vitamin D3 levels can be produced by four hours of intense sun exposure per week on the face or upper extremities. To get the necessary amount of vitamin D3 during the winter or in other gloomy conditions, one must either consume fatty fish, fortified milk, or nutritional supplements. Dietary vitamin D3 is absorbed by the stomach, then chylomicrons carry it to the liver where it is either converted to 25(OH) vitamin D3 or stored as fat. Vitamin D2 or vitamin D3 may be found in nutritional supplements. The source (D2/ergocalciferol from plants versus D3/calciferol from animals) is the only distinction. Both can be converted to $1,25(OH)_2$ vitamin D that is active.

While vitamin D supplementation is frequently advised for "healthy bones," other research strongly suggests taking a dual supplement that combines vitamin K and vitamin D2/3. Adequate Ca^{2+} absorption is only one aspect of the story, as will be demonstrated later. Additionally, it needs to be properly integrated into bone mineral, a process that is significantly influenced by vitamin K.

4.2.5.2. Parathyroid Hormone (PTH)

The parathyroid gland's Chief cells produce the 9.4 kDa polypeptide known as parathyroid hormone (PTH). PTH controls the distribution of total body Ca^{2+}, whereas VitD ensures sufficient stores of the mineral. The quick mobilization of Ca^{2+} from bone follows its release. Its secretion is highly sensitive to the current Ca^{2+} concentration, making it the primary regulator of minute-to-minute circulating Ca^{2+} levels. The 140 kDa, 7-transmembrane domain receptor (CaSR), which is the receptor for circulating Ca^{2+}, inhibits the release of PTH from Chief cells when it is activated. It is recommended that the CaSR be able to quickly identify a 200 μM variation in extracellular Ca^{2+}. Reduced CaSR signaling and the release of PTH occur when circulating levels drop below a threshold.

PTH would appear to exist in a confusing variety of isoforms upon release. It starts off as a 115 amino acid (aa) prepropeptide that has an N-terminal pro-segment of six aa and a signal sequence of 25 aa. The mature, circulating form of PTH is composed of 84 amino acids (aa). PTH pharmacological analogs are based on the fact that bioactivity requires only the first 34 amino acids of the mature polypeptide. Typically, 20% of circulating PTH (aa # 1–84) is full-length, and 80% exhibits some N-terminal truncation (C-PTH; note that different authors use different abbreviations; C-PTH here refers to any form that is not full-length). Fragments that differ at the C-terminus may be found starting at aa position # 4, 7, 8, 10, 15, 34, 35, 37, 41, and 43. All appear to be targets of cathepsins and other proteases. Hepatocytes produce some of these, while Chief cells produce others. The molecules appear to become inactive toward the PTH receptor (PTH1R) upon cleavage of the first six aa. Surprisingly, PTH molecules with N-terminal truncations appear to have their own receptor, known as C-PTHR. It hasn't been described yet. C-PTHs frequently exhibit anticalcemic, antagonistic activity in comparison to PTH. The amount of Ca^{2+} in the surrounding air affects the ratio of full-length to truncated forms. At low Ca^{2+} concentrations, full-length PTH makes up 30–40% of total PTH (~18 pM), and more Ca^{2+} must be taken from mineral stores. On the other hand, total PTH drops to 5 pM in high Ca^{2+} environments, and full-length PTH accounts for only 5% of this value. Apart from the variability induced by Ca^{2+}, PTH exhibits a circadian rhythm. The baseline difference between the peak (10 PM-3 AM) and trough (10 AM-Noon) releases is 30%. Notably, individuals with osteoporosis appear to lose this cadence.

PTH receptor PTH1R/PTHR1 is a G protein-coupled receptor (GPCR) with a 7-transmembrane domain that is present on a variety of cell types, such as osteoblasts, osteoclasts, hematopoietic stem cells, and renal tubule cells (proximal and distal epithelium). As mentioned previously, a C-PTH receptor has also been proposed. Osteocytes and osteoblasts appear to express this receptor highly, and when it is ligated, intracellular Ca^{2+} is increased but not cAMP. A decrease in circulating Ca^{2+} and P_i, the stimulation of bone formation, and an increase in osteoclast activity and formation are among the functional outcomes linked to C-PTHR.

PTH is a normo-calcemic hormone by definition. In other words, its purpose is to keep the Ca^{2+} levels in blood and extracellular fluid within a certain range. It accomplishes this by raising renal 1a-hydroxylase expression, causing Ca^{2+} release from bone, and decreasing Ca^{2+} loss through urine. It affects phosphorus in an important but indirect way. PTH carries out its primary role, which is to facilitate Ca^{2+} release from bone, by encouraging phosphorus excretion and consequently lowering the total phosphorus load.

4.2.5.3. FGF-23

Fibroblast growth factor-23 (FGF-23) represents the latest addition to the extensive and varied FGF protein family. FGF-23 exhibits a typical beta-trefoil structure, just like the other members. However, FGF-23 differs from the majority of members in that it has an extended C-terminus/pro-segment, an atypical intrachain disulfide bond, and a signal sequence. It belongs to the small FGF-19 subfamily as a result. The glycoprotein FGF-23, with a molecular weight of 30 kDa, is secreted and subsequently processed. Mature FGF-23, which has a length of 155 aa, is produced after the signal sequence and pro-segment between Arg179 and Ser180 are removed. The C-terminal pro-segment appears to be necessary for bioactivity, as this mature form is bio-inactive. It is thought that osteoblasts produce it in reaction to vitamin D. Its receptor was long unknown, but it now appears to bind to FGF R1c, FGF R2, FGF R3, and FGF R4. Klotho, along with its corresponding carbohydrate moiety, is said to be the most likely physiological co-receptor for FGF-23.

FGF-23 in its full length is regarded as a phosphatonin. Phosphotonins promote phosphate excretion, which is one way they lower plasma phosphate levels. They are thought to function similarly to calcitonin, which lowers serum Ca^{2+} levels. FGF-23 primarily stimulates the excretion of phosphate in the urine and inhibits the synthesis of vitamin D. Its capacity to downregulate phosphorus transporters on the luminal side of the renal epithelium mediates its effect on phosphate resorption. It works on VitD synthesis by inhibiting kidney 1a-hydroxylase activity.

The connections among VitD, PTH, and FGF-23 are intricate and possibly counterintuitive. One could argue that FGF-23 regulates the Pi-VitD axis and PTH regulates the Ca^{2+}-VitD axis. According to one model, PTH is released from Chief cells when there is insufficient Ca^{2+} in the extracellular fluid or circulating blood (a simple Ca^{2+} deficiency). In the short term, this has the effect of removing Ca^{2+} from the bone. To produce active VitD, it also stimulates kidney 1 alpha-hydroxylase activity. VitD accomplishes two crucial tasks. It does this by first encouraging the absorption of Ca^{2+}, which raises total body stores. Second, it raises intestinal phosphorus absorption, most likely to supply hydroxyapatite/ $Ca^{2+}{}_{10}(PO_4)_6(OH)_2$, the mineral equivalent of Ca^{2+} required for mineralization. There is no concurrent phosphorus deficit when there is only a simple Ca^{2+} deficiency. But phosphorus is now excess due to increased VitD activity. PTH can promote excretion rather than reabsorption in the short term, which has the same effect as FGF-23 on P_i excretion. Overall, this should remove excess phosphorus; however, we know that PTH release is inhibited by the Ca^{2+}-CaSR interactions on Chief cells, which cause an increase in circulating Ca^{2+} as a result of VitD-mediated absorption. Longer-term phosphatonin supplementation is required to restore normal phosphorus levels. FGF-23 is that molecule (and maybe MEPE and/or sFRP-4). FGF-23 will downregulate 1a-hydroxylase activity and upregulate 24-hydroxylase activity to "catch up" with continuous Ca^{2+} and P_i absorption, thereby eliminating the stimulus for excess phosphorus uptake.

It appears that osteoblasts produce FGF-23, but what causes its expression to be induced? Apparently, VitD does. Additionally, it has been proposed that FGF-23 is released in response to circulating phosphorus, which makes sense given that FGF-23 is meant to guard against too much phosphorus. e. -reaction to a stimulus. In fact, extracellular Pi alone can independently upregulate several genes, such as osteopontin, STAT5, and beta5 integrin; this finding would be consistent with an upregulation of the FGF-23 gene. However, phosphorus intake has no effect on FGF-23 levels in healthy subjects. In people with intact kidneys, high-phosphorus diets do cause increased excretion, but they do not alter FGF-23 levels. Surprisingly, a high-phosphorus diet does raise serum phosphorus in rats, which in turn raises FGF-23.

4.2.5.4. Calcitonin

A member of the calcitonin gene-related peptide family, calcitonin is a 3 kDa, 32 aa peptide. It is allegedly produced by the thyroid gland's C cells in reaction to high blood Ca^{2+} levels. It begins life as a 141 aa preproprecursor and matures into a 32 aa peptide through processing. The calcitonin GPCR, also known as the calcitonin R., has a strong inhibitory effect on osteoclasts. It might function as a stress-related molecule in mature humans.

4.2.5.5. Soluble Frizzled-related Protein-4 (sFRP-4)

A small family of secreted proteins called sFRP-4 shares structural similarities with the extracellular domain of the frizzled family of receptors. The mature sFRP-4 molecule has a length of 328 aa and is composed of two regions: a 100 aa netrin-like region and a 120 aa frizzled/cysteine-rich domain. The molecule is extensively spliced in rats, and variations can be found at the C-terminus. In humans, similar variations might exist. Similar to other sFRPs, sFRP-4 binds to frizzled receptors-1 and -4 as well as Wnt ligands. The family is widely known to inhibit Wnt signaling. Other things might be going on. For example, it has been reported that sFRP1 binds to RANK L, which induces the formation of osteoclasts.

Similar to FGF-23, kidney osteoblasts and unidentified cells have been reported to express sFRP-4. It is also believed that sFRP-4 is a phosphatonin. Renal phosphate transporters internalize in response to FGF-23, most likely via FGF R signaling. sFRP-4, on the other hand, appears to sabotage rather than activate Wnt signaling. There are at least three potential mechanisms of action, albeit very speculative. Firstly, FGF-23 exhibits phosphatonin activity when it is present in its entirety. It becomes inactive upon cleavage into mature N- and C-termini. According to certain theories, cleavage is caused by a molecule resembling matrix metalloproteinase (MMP), and FGF-23 activity would persist if MMP was inhibited by a tissue inhibitor of metalloproteinase (TIMP). Because sFRP-4 possesses a TIMP-like domain, it may be able to neutralize MMPs, protecting FGF-23's integrity and enhancing its phosphatonin activity. It should be mentioned that cleaving FGF-23 has also been reported to occur with Furin-type convertases. Additionally, a lack of Wnt signaling in osteoblasts can result in cell death. Osteoblasts play a key role in the formation of bones, so a decrease in their numbers could lead to a slower mineralization rate and a decreased requirement for phosphate. As a result, there would be a decrease in kidney phosphate resorption due to lower demand. Furthermore, sFRP-4 hinders the production of Vitamin D through 1a-hydroxylase. Vitamin D is known to enhance phosphate absorption, so blocking its effects would lead to an increase in phosphate excretion.

4.2.5.6. MEPE (Matrix Extracellular Phosphoglycoprotein)

A third phosphatonin is called MEPE. It is a secreted glycoprotein with a molecular weight of 45–65 kDa that is a member of the SIBLING (short integrin-binding ligand interacting glycoprotein) family. The mature molecule has a length of 508 amino acids, is serine-rich, and has a C-terminal Ser-Asp-Gly-Asp motif linked to glycosaminoglycans in addition to an RGD motif for cell attachment. Osteocytes and osteoblasts synthesize MEPE, especially during mineralization. It is connected to PHEX, a type II transmembrane metalloproteinase found on the surface of osteoblasts, and the extracellular matrix (ECM). PHEX shields MEPE from being broken down by cysteine-proteases like cathepsin B, rather than having any proteolytic action on MEPE. This is probably because PHEX functions as a cathepsin pseudosubstrate (s). Upon gaining functional access to MEPE, cathepsins cleave the molecule between Arg507 and Asp508, producing ASARM, an 18 aa C-terminal peptide. This particular peptide appears to have two distinct functions: it inhibits mineralization and promotes the loss of phosphate in the urine. MEPE (or its cleavage product) may have its primary role in controlling mineralization. Even though it is material, the phosphatonin effect can be complementary—that is, unless uncontrolled conditions exist.

4.2.6. Renal Resorption of Calcium and Phosphorus

4.2.6.1. Calcium

Urinary Ca^{2+} reabsorption works similarly to intestinal enterocyte reabsorption. Specifically, it is discovered that there are both paracellular and transcellular processes. 40% of the Ca^{2+} in blood is bound to albumin, 10% is linked to organic ions, and 50% is free ions and can attach to CaSR. Since the glomerulus does not filter albumin, this Ca^{2+} fraction cannot be reabsorbed. With the exception of about 200 mg, the remaining fractions supply about 9,000 mg of Ca^{2+} per day, all of which is reabsorbed. 30% of the glomerular filtrate is resorbed in the distal convoluted tubule and collecting duct, 20% in the thick ascending loop of Henle, and 70% in the proximal tubule.

Nearly all paracellular resorption takes place in the thick ascending limb and proximal tubule. In the distal segments, transcellular (hormone-sensitive) resorption takes place.

The same ion transport pathways found in enterocytes and paracellin-1 are likely involved in passive uptake in the proximal and straight tubules. These comprise basolateral Na/K ATPases and CLCNKB (Cl- channels), as well as luminal NKCC2 transporters and ROMK channels. CaSR is also involved in paracellular transport in the ascending loop of Henle. This membrane's basolateral region contains this receptor. When the Ca^{2+} levels in extracellular fluid are high enough, the receptor is activated and ROMK is inhibited. As a result, the lumen's K+ content decreases, the typical electrochemical gradient is distorted, and the paracellular Ca^{2+} flow is disrupted.

Hormone-sensitive transcellular absorption is predominant in the distal tubule. There is a PMCA1 Ca^{2+} pump, a basolateral NCX1 Na/Ca exchanger, and a TRPV Ca^{2+} channel (TRPV5), just like in the intestine. Calbindin-D28K is utilized for intracellular Ca^{2+} transport instead of calbindin-D9K. Several molecules influence the uptake of Ca^{2+}. PTH is released and the Chief cell CaSR is inactivated when blood Ca^{2+} levels fall. Three things are increased when PTH binds to PTH1R on the basolateral surface of distal tubule cells: the levels of NCX1 and calbindin-D28K, as well as PMCA1's affinity for Ca^{2+}. Regarding whether TRPV5 is a target of PTH, opinions vary.

Nevertheless, Klotho is aiming for TRPV5. In addition to having two glycosyl hydrolase type-1 regions devoid of a crucial Glu in the "active" site, Klotho also has both soluble and membrane forms. However, it appears that the transmembrane form interacts with TRPV5 in the cell membrane and eliminates some of its glycosylation. As a result, it becomes trapped in the luminal membrane and is compelled to keep moving Ca^{2+}. It's unclear what part VitD plays. It is hypothesized that the ion transporters/channels involved in Ca^{2+} flow and calbindin D are not especially sensitive to VitD action. Further research is required on this topic.

CaSRs in the collecting duct keep a close eye on the urine's Ca^{2+} content. Ca^{2+} activates collecting duct CaSRs when there is a decrease in resorption, resulting in high levels. This prevents the collecting duct epithelium from being affected by ADH/vasopressin-mediated water absorption through native aquaporin channels. Kidney stone formation is prevented, the mM concentration of Ca^{2+} drops, and the urine becomes diluted.

4.2.6.2. Phosphorus

Renal resorption essentially controls the levels of extracellular and circulatory phosphate. The glomerulus freely filters circulating P_i, with 85–90% of it being resorbed. The figures are astounding. About 7,000 mg of P_i are added to the glomerular filtrate daily, whereas 6,300–6,000 mg are removed. The mechanism of intestinal P_i absorption and renal P_i resorption is similar, as is the case with Ca^{2+}.

Within the nephron, the proximal tubule accounts for 60–75% of Pi resorption, the loop of Henle accounts for 15–20%, and the distal tubule accounts for 5–10%. The main factor influencing resorption is the activity of the luminal Na/P transporters NPT2a. P_i must actively enter the cell in the proximal tubule from the urine despite a strong electrochemical gradient. There is an inhibitory electronegative gradient and the concentration of P_i in the cell is at least equal to that of P_i in the urine or lumen. Therefore, luminal Na^+ is needed as a "co-transportee" for P_i transport. The Na/P co-transporter gene family is composed of three members. NPT1, 3, and 4 are members of the Type 1 family. Their physiological role is unknown, and their transport function is not restricted to Na^+ and P_i. Pit1 and Pit2 are the two members of the type 3 family.

Their role includes keeping the necessary intracellular phosphate levels. They are found on the basolateral side of the kidney and carry Na^+ and Pi into the tubule cell. There are three members of the type 2 family, and each one is the result of a different gene. They are located in the tubular epithelium's luminal border. NPT2b is confined to the intestine, NPT2a to the kidney, and NPT2c to the fetal transporter. It is only in proximal tubule cells that NPT2a is present. It is a protein with eight transmembrane domains that shows intricate regulation. Resorbed Pi leaves the cytosol through passive but aided transport after passing through it without becoming complex. It is unknown who the basolateral transporter is.

The significance of NPT2a is reflected in the quantity of extracellular regulators. VitD is known to upregulate the expression of molecules that support NPT2a activity, most likely via a transcriptional mechanism. The NPT2a promoter has elements related to vitamin D response. Stanniocalcin-1, or STC-1, is another molecule that facilitates the uptake of P_i. It is a phosphoprotein that is secreted and is created by gathering duct epithelium. Through the upregulation of Pit-1 (type 3 family) transporters, STC-1 mediates osteoblast P_i uptake in bone. It is proposed that STC-1 regulates NTP2a expression in the kidney. This still needs to be proven.

Furthermore, NPT2a is down-regulated by phosphatonins and phosphatonin-like compounds. Phosphateuria (high urine phosphate) results from this decreased phosphate absorption. There are several molecules at play, including FGF-23, sFRP-4, MEPE, and PTH. It has been reported that FGF-23, PTH, and sFRP-4 influence NPT2a activity. Although the effects of sFRP-4 are not fully understood, it has been proposed that NPT2a is removed from the luminal membrane. PTH and FGF-23 both lower the quantity of luminal transporters. In one scenario, PTH actually causes transporter internalization, but FGF-23 decreases NPT2a protein levels and mRNA synthesis. Existing NPT2a keeps working until its lifespan is reached in the absence of PTH. Notably, megalin co-expresses with NPT2a and may be a major target for PTH-mediated NPT2a internalization. Megalin is the vitamin D binding protein that internalizes 25(OH) vitamin D3 from urine. According to alternative theories, FGF-23 mediates NPT2a internalization. On this matter, nothing is set in stone. MEPE is phosphatonin that may be the least understood. It has been discovered that the C-terminal ASARM motif is phosphaturic, though the exact mechanism is unknown. Interestingly, MEPE and FGF-23 are linked to PHEX, pointing to an underappreciated dynamic amongst these three molecules.

4.3. Other Hormones Produced by the Kidneys and Their Functions

Numerous hormones play distinct yet significant roles in controlling kidney function. They function to either promote or prevent blood flow. While some of these operate locally and are paracrine, others are endocrine and act remotely.

4.3.1. Renin–Angiotensin–Aldosterone

The granular cells of the afferent arteriole at the JGA produce the enzyme renin. It does this by enzymatically converting the freely circulating angiotensinogen produced by the liver into angiotensin I. When the volume of extracellular fluid decreases, prostaglandins and NO from the

JGA trigger its release. Although ACE is not a hormone, it plays a crucial role in controlling kidney and systemic blood pressure. Although it is made in the lungs, it attaches itself to the glomerulus' and afferent arterioles' endothelial cellular surfaces. It changes inactive angiotensin I into active angiotensin II through an enzymatic process. A crucial factor in increasing blood pressure is ACE. ACE inhibitors are occasionally prescribed to people with high blood pressure to lower their blood pressure.

Strong vasoconstrictor angiotensin II directly contributes to blood pressure regulation. Its systemic effects include constriction of the afferent and efferent arterioles of the glomerulus in addition to vasoconstriction. It limits fluid loss and maintains blood volume in cases of blood loss or dehydration by lowering both GFR and renal blood flow. Its main function is to maintain appropriate blood pressure because drops in blood pressure typically trigger its release.

The adrenal cortex releases aldosterone, sometimes known as the "salt-retaining hormone," in reaction to either angiotensin II or elevated plasma K^+ levels. It facilitates the nephron's Na^+ absorption, which helps the body hold onto water. It plays a crucial role in controlling and encouraging the excretion of K^+. Its origin in the adrenal cortex and its dual action on two minerals account for its classification as a mineralocorticoid. Renin therefore affects blood pressure in two ways: first, through angiotensin II-stimulated vasoconstriction, which happens immediately; second, through aldosterone-induced Na^+ recovery, which takes time to happen. Aldosterone causes a greater loss of K^+ in addition to an increased recovery of Na^+.

Aldosterone and progesterone share a structural resemblance. It increases water recovery and weakly stimulates Na^+ reabsorption by binding to the aldosterone receptor. In men, this process is insignificant because progesterone levels are low. When progesterone levels rise in women during specific stages of the menstrual cycle, it may result in increased water retention.

4.3.2. Antidiuretic Hormone (ADH)

Diuretics are medications that can cause an increase in water loss by preventing solutes and water from being recaptured from the urine that is being formed. They are frequently administered to reduce blood pressure. Diuretics like coffee, tea, and alcohol are well-known. The posterior pituitary secretes the 9-amino acid peptide known as ADH, which has the exact opposite effect. It lowers urine volume, encourages water recovery, and keeps blood pressure and plasma osmolarity constant. By inducing the movement of aquaporin proteins into the principal cellular apical cell membrane in the collecting ducts, it creates water channels that facilitate the transcellular osmosis process that moves water from the collecting duct lumen into the kidney's interstitial space. It then re-enters the circulation by entering the vasa recta capillaries. The deep kidney medulla's high osmotic environment draws water.

4.3.3. Endothelin

Vasoconstrictors of great potency are 21-amino acid peptides called endothelins. These are generated by mesangial cells, DCT cells, and endothelial cells of the renal blood vessels. Endothelin release is triggered by the hormones bradykinin, epinephrine, and angiotensin II. For most healthy individuals, they have no effect on blood pressure. Conversely, sodium retention occurs when endothelin levels are persistently raised in individuals with diabetic kidney disease. Furthermore, by injuring podocytes and strongly constricting both afferent and efferent arterioles, they lower GFR.

4.3.4. Natriuretic Hormones

Peptides known as natriuretic hormones cause the kidneys to excrete sodium, the opposite of what aldosterone does. Natriuretic hormones work by preventing the release of aldosterone, which prevents the collecting ducts from recovering Na^+. Water will be lost concurrently with the formation of urine if Na^+ is still present because of its osmotic force. Additionally, natriuretic hormones block the release of ADH, which naturally reduces the amount of water recovered. Natriuretic peptides therefore prevent the recovery of both Na^+ and water. Atrial natriuretic hormone (ANH), a 28-amino acid peptide produced by the heart atria in response to the atrial wall being overstretched, is one example of a hormone from this family. People who have heart failure or high blood pressure tend to overstretch. By simultaneously vasodilating the afferent arteriole and constricting the efferent arteriole, it raises GFR. The resulting urine loses more water and salt as a result of these occurrences. Additionally, it lessens the DCT's reabsorption of sodium. The heart's ventricles also produce 32 amino acids that make up the B-type natriuretic peptide (BNP). It has fewer effects than ANH because of its 10-fold lower affinity for its receptor. Its function might be to "fine-tune" blood pressure regulation. Because of its extended biologic half-life, BNP is a useful diagnostic tool for congestive heart failure.

4.3.5. Parathyroid Hormone

The parathyroid glands release the 84-amino acid peptide known as parathyroid hormone (PTH) in reaction to a drop in the blood levels of Ca^{++}. One of its targets is the PCT, where it induces calcidiol to hydroxylate into calcitriol, the active form of vitamin D (1,25-hydroxycholecalciferol). Furthermore, it inhibits the reabsorption of phosphate (PO_3^-), leading to its excretion in urine. Phosphate retention would cause calcium phosphate to form in the plasma, which would lower the amount of Ca^{++} in circulation. Higher levels of Ca^{++} are allowed to circulate by eliminating phosphate from the blood.

Whereas paracrine hormones function locally, endocrine hormones function remotely. Angiotensinogen is changed into angiotensin I by the renal enzyme renin. Angiotensin I is changed into active angiotensin II by the lung enzyme ACE. Blood pressure is raised by the active vasoconstrictor angiotensin II. Additionally, angiotensin II increases the adrenal cortex's release of aldosterone, which causes the collecting duct to hold onto Na^+. This promotes water retention and a prolonged rise in blood pressure. By encouraging the insertion of aquaporin water channels into cell membranes, ADH facilitates water recovery via the collecting ducts. When diabetic kidney disease is present, endothelin levels are raised, which lowers GFR and increases Na^+ retention. When the heart's atria contract, it releases hormones called natriuretic hormones, which promote the excretion of Na^+ and lower blood pressure. PTH decreases phosphate reabsorption and increases the last stage of the production of active vitamin D3, which raises the levels of Ca^{++} in the blood (Tsiftsoglou, 2021).

A Closer Look

Hematopoiesis

- **Erythropoiesis:** The process of making blood-circulating cells is known as hemopoiesis. Erythropoiesis, in particular, is the process that results in the production of erythrocytes, or red blood cells. The body produces an amazing 2.5 billion red blood cells per kilogram per day on average. A complex line of cells gives rise to erythrocytes, and their rate of production is carefully controlled to guarantee that the right amount of red blood cells—not too many, not too few—are produced.
- **Sites of Erythropoiesis:** Throughout life, the location of erythropoiesis shifts. It takes place in the yolk sac of an extremely young fetus. It starts in the liver and spleen between two and five months of pregnancy and eventually settles in the bone marrow around five months. Erythropoiesis can happen in the bone marrow of most bones in children. But in adults, it only develops in the bone marrow of the proximal femur, sacrum, ribs, sternum, and vertebrae. Extramedullary hemopoiesis, or i.e., can occur when bone marrow erythropoiesis is insufficient. e. hemopoiesis taking place outside of the bone marrow. This is frequently observed in hemoglobinopathies like myelofibrosis and thalassemias.
- **Stages of Erythropoiesis:** The hemocytoblast, a multipotent hematopoietic stem cell, is the starting point for the synthesis of all blood cells. Of all adult cells, hemocytoblasts are the most capable of self-renewal. When necessary, they can be released from the bone marrow and added to the bloodstream.

Certain hemocytoblasts differentiate into common myeloid progenitor cells, which generate mast cells, megakaryocytes, myeloblasts, and erythrocytes. There are various steps involved in the transformation of common myeloid progenitor cells into fully developed red blood cells. Initially, they develop into normoblasts, also known as erythroblasts, which are exclusively found in the bone marrow.

Then, as they develop into reticulocytes—essentially, immature red blood cells—they lose their nucleus. A portion of these are discharged into the peripheral bloodstream. Ultimately, as reticulocytes develop into erythrocytes—fully developed red blood cells—they lose the last of their organelles. A red blood cell has an average life span of 120 days.

In this maturation process, nuclear extrusion occurs, i.e., Nuclei are absent from mature erythrocytes. The release of immature cells can be indicated by nucleated red blood cells found in a bone marrow sample. This may transpire in pathologies like thalassemia, severe anemia, or hematological cancer.

- **Regulation of Erythropoiesis:** The glycoprotein cytokine hormone erythropoietin (EPO) is the primary inducer of erythropoiesis. It is the kidney that secretes EPO. It is continuously secreted in small enough amounts to maintain normal erythropoiesis regulation. On the other hand, the blood becomes relatively hypoxic if the erythrocyte level falls. Renal interstitial peritubular cells sense when the partial pressure of oxygen (pO_2) in the kidney is decreased.

The marrow is stimulated to produce more red blood cells as a result of the spike in EPO production that follows. As a result, there is an increase in hemoglobin levels, which raises pO_2 and lowers EPO levels. The feedback system is finished.

Summary

- Human erythropoietin (EPO) is a peptide hormone produced in the fetal liver during early development and the kidneys in the human adult body.
- Under ischemic stress, anemia, hypoxia at high altitude as well as other factors (tissue injuries, degeneration), the production of EPO is activated in the adult kidneys.
- ERO-R is a protein cell surface receptor chain encoded by the EPOR gene. It carries a single N-linked carbohydrate chain that contributes to an overall approximate molecular weight of 56–57 kDa. ERO-R is a member of the type I cytokine receptor superfamily.
- EPO-R receptors have been detected on several other cell types and tissues in addition to the BM erythroid progenitors. These include, among others, heart and neuron cells, BMMSCs (bone marrow mesenchymal stromal cells), skeletal muscle cells as well as others such as dental MSCs.
- EPO and hypoxia have been shown to stimulate EPOR-mediated vascularization and increase production of nitric oxide (NO) in ECs. This was not induced by the endothelin 1 produced by ECs, but rather through the activation of the signaling pathway AKT-e-Nos-MMP2 by the EPO–EPOR interactions.
- EPO, in addition to stimulating BM erythropoiesis by binding to the EPO-R homodimeric receptor on erythroid progenitors, also binds to the heterodimeric complex EPO-R on non-erythroid tissues (brain, heart, retina, kidney, etc.).
- The development of human erythropoietin alpha via recombinant DNA technology as a valuable biopharmaceutical (biologic) medicine, first by Amgen (Epogen®) in the late 1980s, was a breakthrough in the treatment of anemia in patients suffering from chronic renal failure (kidney disease) or undergoing cancer chemotherapy.
- Both Ca^{2+} and phosphorus (as "phosphate" or P_i/HPO_{4-}^{2}) utilize passive diffusion and saturable/facilitated absorption during intestinal uptake. In general, Ca^{2+} uptake is passive (or paracellular) while P_i uptake is saturable (between cells or transcellular).
- In the case of Ca^{2+}, a typical daily diet will contain 1,000 mg of elemental Ca^{2+}. Approximately 200 mg will be absorbed and 800 mg excreted. Ca^{2+} is absorbed throughout the intestine, but the low luminal pH (5 to 6) associated with the duodenum and jejunum promotes the ionization of Ca^{2+} and its efficient absorption.
- Phosphorus is remarkably abundant and derived from natural sources such as dairy products, cereals and meat, and unnatural sources such as carbonated beverages.
- Several hormones have specific, important roles in regulating kidney function. They act to stimulate or inhibit blood flow. Some of these are endocrine, acting from a distance, whereas others are paracrine, acting locally.

References

1. Anagnostou, A., Liu, Z., Steiner, M., Chin, K., Lee, E. S., Kessimian, N., & Noguchi, C. T. (1994). Erythropoietin receptor mRNA expression in human endothelial cells. *Proceedings of the National Academy of Sciences USA, 91*, 3974–3978. https://doi.org/10.1073/pnas.91.9.3974.

2. Bakopoulou, A., Kritis, A., Andreadis, D., Papachistou, E., Leyhausen, G., Koidis, P., Geutsen, W., & Tsiftsoglou, A. (2015). Angiogenic potential and secretome of human apical papilla mesenchymal stem cells in various stress microenvironments. *Stem Cells Development, 24*, 2496–2512. https://doi.org/10.1089/scd.2015.0197.

3. Bhoopalan, S. V., Jun-Huang, L., & Weiss, M. J. (2020). Erythropoietin regulation of red blood cell production: From bench to bedside and back. *F1000Research, 9*, F1000 Faculty Rev-1153. https://doi.org/10.12688/f1000research.26648.1.

4. Bianco, P. (2015). Stem cells and bone: A historical perspective. *Bone, 70*, 2–9. https://doi.org/10.1016/j.bone.2014.08.011.

5. Bianco, P., Rimunnicci, M., Gronthos, S., & Robey, P. G. (2001). Bone marrow stromal stem cells: Nature, biology and potential applications. *Stem Cells, 19*, 180–192. https://doi.org/10.1634/stemcells.19-3-180.

6. Brines, M., Grasso, G., Fioraliso, F., Sfacteria, A., Ghezzi, P., Fratelli, M., Latini, R., Xie, O. W., Smart, J., Su-Rick, C. J., et al. (2004). Erythropoietin mediates tissue protection through an erythropoietin and common beta-subunit heteroreceptor. *Proceedings of the National Academy of Sciences USA, 101*, 14907–14912. https://doi.org/10.1073/pnas.0406491101.

7. Broxmeyer, H. E. (2013). Erythropoietin: Multiple targets, actions and modifying influences for biological and clinical considerations. *Journal of Experimental Medicine, 210*, 205–208. https://doi.org/10.1084/jem.20122760.

8. Bunn, H. F. (2013). Erythropoietin. *Cold Spring Harbor Perspectives in Medicine, 3*, a011619. https://doi.org/10.1101/cshperspect.a011619.

9. Calvinio, L., Latini, R., Kajsgera, J., Leri, A., Anversa, P., Ghezzi, P., Salio, M., Cerami, A., & Brines, M. (2003). Recombinant human erythropoietin protects the myocardium from reperfusion injury and promotes beneficial remodeling. *Proceedings of the National Academy of Sciences USA, 100*, 4802–4806. https://doi.org/10.1073/pnas.0630444100.

10. Cantarelli, C., Angelotti, U., Cravedi, P., et al. (2019). Erythropoietin, a multifaceted protein with innate and adaptive modulatory activity. *American Journal of Transplantation, 19*, 2407–2414. https://doi.org/10.1111/ajt.15369.

11. Carlini, R. G., Reyes, A. A., & Rothstein, M. (1995). Recombinant human erythropoietin stimulates angiogenesis in vitro. *Kidney International, 47*, 740–745. https://doi.org/10.1038/ki.1995.113.

12. D'Andrea, A. D., Lodish, H. F., & Wong, G. G. (1989). Expression cloning of the mouse erythropoietin receptor. *Cell, 57*, 277–285. https://doi.org/10.1016/0092-8674(89)90965-3.

13. Eisele, A. S., Cosgrove, J., Magniez, A., Tubenf, E., Beuto, T., Cayrac, E., Tak, T., Lyne, A. M., Urbanus, J., & Perie, L. (2020). Erythropoietin directly affects single hematopoietic stem cell differentiation after transplantation. *BioRxiv*. https://doi.org/10.1101/2020/04.20.0501460.

14. Enlev, A. (1953). Humoral regulation of red cell production. *Blood, 8*, 349–357. https://doi.org/10.1182/blood.V8.4.349.349.

15. Goldwasser, E., & Kung, K. H. (1971). Purification of erythropoietin. *Proceedings of the National Academy of Sciences USA, 68*, 697–698. https://doi.org/10.1073/pnas.68.4.697.

16. Hofer, H. R., & Tuan, R. S. (2016). Secreted trophic factors of mesenchymal stem cells support

neovascular and musculoskeletal therapies. *Stem Cell Research & Therapy, 7*, 131. https://doi.org/10.1186/s13287-016-0394-0.

17. Holstein, J. H., Orth, M., Scheuer, C., Tammi, A., Becker, S. C., Garcia, P., Histing, T., Morsdorf, P., Klein, M., Pohlemann, T., et al. (2011). Erythropoietin stimulates bone formation, cell proliferation and angiogenesis in a femoral segmented defect model in mice. *Bone, 49*, 1037–1045. https://doi.org/10.1016/j.bone.2011.08.004.
18. Jackson, W. M., Nosti, L., & Tuan, R. S. (2012). Mesenchymal stem cell therapy for attenuation of scar formation during wound healing. *Stem Cell Research & Therapy, 3*, 20. https://doi.org/10.1186/scrt111.
19. Jacobson, L. O., Goldwasser, E., & Fried, N. (1957). Role of kidney in erythropoiesis. *Nature, 179*, 633–634. https://doi.org/10.1038/179633a0.
20. Jelkman, W. (2013). Physiology and pharmacology of erythropoietin. *Transfusion Medicine and Hemotherapy, 40*, 302–309. https://doi.org/10.1159/000356193.
21. Jia, Y., Susuki, N., Yamamamoto, M., Gassmann, M., & Noguchi, C. T. (2012). Endogenous erythropoietin signaling facilitates skeletal muscle repair and recovery following pharmacologically induced damage. *FASEB Journal, 23*, 2847–2858. https://doi.org/10.1096/fj.11-196618.
22. Kietzmann, T. (2020). Hypoxia inducible erythropoietin expression: Details matter. *Hematologica, 105*, 2704–2706. https://doi.org/10.3324/haematol.2020.261966.
23. Kimakova, P., Solar, P., Solarova, Z., Komel, R., & Debeljak, N. (2017). Erythropoietin and its angiogenic activity. *International Journal of Molecular Sciences, 18*, 1519. https://doi.org/10.3390/ijms18071519.
24. Kobayashi, H., Miura, T., Ischida, H., Miki, T., Tanno, M., Yano, M., Sato, T., Hotta, H., & Shimamoto, K. (2008). Limitation of infarct size by erythropoietin is associated with translocation of AKT to the mitochondria after reperfusion. *Clinical and Experimental Pharmacology, 135*, 799–808.
25. Koutsoumparis, A., Vassili, A., Bakopoulou, A., Ziouta, A., & Tsiftsoglou, A. S. (2018). Erythropoietin (rhEPOα) promotes endothelial trans differentiation of stem cells of the apical papilla. *Archives of Oral Biology, 96*, 96–103. https://doi.org/10.1016/j.archoralbio.2018.09.001.
26. Li, F., Wang, X., & Niyibizi, C. (2010). Bone marrow stromal cells contribute to bone formation following infusion into femoral cavities of a mouse model of osteogenesis imperfecta. *Bone, 47*, 546–555. https://doi.org/10.1016/j.bone.2010.05.040.
27. Lin, F. K., Suggs, S., Lin, C. H., Browne, J. K., & Smalling, R. (1985). Cloning and expression of the human erythropoietin gene. *Proceedings of the National Academy of Sciences USA, 82*, 7580–7584. https://doi.org/10.1073/pnas.82.22.7580.
28. McDonald, J., Lin, F. K., & Goldweisser, E. (1986). Cloning, sequencing and evolutionary analysis of the mouse erythropoietin gene. *Molecular and Cellular Biology, 6*, 842–848. https://doi.org/10.1128/MCB.6.3.842.
29. Miyake, T., Klug, K., & Goldwasser, E. (1977). Purification of human erythropoietin. *Journal of Biological Chemistry, 252*, 5558–5564. https://doi.org/10.1016/S0021-9258(19)63387-9.
30. Oswald, J., Boxberger, S., Jørgensen, B., Feldmann, S., Ehninger, G., Bornhäuser, M., & Werner, C. (2004). Mesenchymal stem cells can be differentiated into endothelial cells in vitro. *Stem Cells, 22*, 377–384. https://doi.org/10.1634/stemcells.22-3-377.

31. Palis, J., & Koniski, A. (2018). Functional analysis of erythroid progenitors by colony-forming assays. In *Methods in Molecular Biology* (Vol. 1698, pp. 117–132). https://doi.org/10.1007/978-1-4939-7404-7_10.

32. Park, D., Spencer, J. A., Koh, B. I., Kobayashi, T., Fujisaki, I., Lin, C. P., Kroneberg, H. M., & Scadden, D. T. (2012). Endogenous BMMSCs are dynamic, fate-restricted participants in bone maintenance and regeneration. *Cell Stem Cell, 10*, 259–272. https://doi.org/10.1016/j.stem.2012.02.003.

33. Parsa, C. J., Matsumoto, A., Kim, J., Riel, R. U., Pascal, L. S., & Walton, G. B. (2003). A novel protective effect of erythropoietin in the infarcted heart. *Journal of Clinical Investigation, 112*, 999–1007. https://doi.org/10.1172/JCI18200.

34. Peng, B., Kong, G., Yang, C., & Ming, Y. (2020). Erythropoietin and its derivatives: From tissue protection to immune regulation. *Cell Death & Disease, 11*, 79. https://doi.org/10.1038/s41419-020-2276-8.

35. Pledge, U., Belhage, B., Guadalupe-Grau, A., Andersen, P. R., Lundby, C., & Dela, F. (2012). Erythropoietin treatment enhances muscle mitochondrial capacity in humans. *Frontiers in Physiology, 3*, 50. https://doi.org/10.3389/fphys.2012.00050.

36. Regmi, S., Pathak, S., Kim, J. O., Yong, C. S., & Jeong, J. H. (2019). Mesenchymal stem cell therapy for the treatment of inflammatory disease: Challenges, opportunities and future perspectives. *European Journal of Cell Biology, 98*, 151041. https://doi.org/10.1016/j.ejcb.2019.04.002.

37. Rey, F., Balsari, A., Giallongo, T., Ottoherghi, S., De Giulio, A. M., Samaja, M., & Carelli, S. (2019). Erythropoietin as a neuroprotective molecule: An overview of its therapeutic potential in neurodegenerative diseases. *ASBMB Reviews, 11*, 1–18. https://doi.org/10.1177/1759091419871420.

38. Ribatti, D., Presta, M., Vacca, A., Ria, R., Giuliani, R., Dell'Era, P., Nico, B., Roncali, L., & Dammacco, F. (1999). Human erythropoietin induces a proangiogenic phenotype in cultured endothelial cells and stimulates neovascularization in vivo. *Blood, 93*, 2627–2636. https://doi.org/10.1182/blood.V93.8.2627.

39. Rundqvist, H., Rullman, E., Sundberg, C. J., Fischer, H., Eisleitner, K., & Stahlberg, M. (2009). Activation of the erythropoietin receptor in human skeletal muscle. *European Journal of Endocrinology, 161*, 427–434. https://doi.org/10.1530/EJE-09-0342.

40. Sasaki, R. (2003). Pleiotropic functions of erythropoietin. *Internal Medicine, 42*, 142–149. https://doi.org/10.2169/internalmedicine.42.142.

41. Suresh, S., de Castro, L. F., Robey, P. G., & Noguchi, C. T. (2019). Erythropoietin modulates bone marrow stromal cell differentiation. *Bone Research, 7*. https://doi.org/10.1038/s41413-019-0060-0.

42. Suresh, S., Lee, J., & Noguchi, C. T. (2020). Effects of erythropoietin in white adipose tissue and bone microenvironment. *Frontiers in Cell and Developmental Biology, 8*, 584696. https://doi.org/10.3389/fcell.2020.584696.

43. Tsiftsoglou, A. S. (2021). Erythropoietin (EPO) as a key regulator of erythropoiesis, bone remodeling, and endothelial trans differentiation of multipotent mesenchymal stem cells (MSCs): Implications in regenerative medicine. *Cells, 10*(8), 2140. https://doi.org/10.3390/cells10082140.

44. Tsiftsoglou, A. S., Vizirianakis, I. S., & Strouboulis, J. (2009). Erythropoiesis: Model systems, molecular regulation and developmental processes. *IUBMB Life, 61*, 800–830. https://doi.org/10.1002/iub.226.

45. Van Der Meer, P., Lipsic, E., Henning, R. H., Van Der Velden, J., & Voors, A. A. (2005). Erythropoietin induces neovascularization and improves cardiac function in rats with heart failure after myocardial infarction. *Journal of the American College of Cardiology, 46*, 125–133. https://doi.org/10.1016/j.jacc.2005.03.044.

46. Wan, L., Zhang, F., He, Q., Tsang, W. P., & Lu, L. (2014). EPO promotes bone repair through enhanced cartilaginous callus and angiogenesis. *PLoS ONE, 9*, e102010. https://doi.org/10.1371/journal.pone.0102010.

47. Wang, L., Di, L., & Noguchi, C. T. (2014). Erythropoietin: A novel versatile player regulating energy metabolism and beyond the erythroid system. *International Journal of Biological Sciences, 10*, 921–999. https://doi.org/10.7150/ijbs.9518.

48. Watts, D., Gaete, S., Rodriguez, D., Hoojewijs, D., Rauner, M., Sormendi, S., & Wielockx, B. (2020). Hypoxia pathway proteins are master regulators of erythropoiesis. *International Journal of Molecular Sciences, 21*, 8131. https://doi.org/10.3390/ijms21218131.

49. Yuan, R., Maeda, Y., Li, W., Lu, W., Cook, S., & Dowing, P. (2008). Erythropoietin: A potent inducer of peripheral immune/inflammatory modulation in autoimmune EAE. *PLoS ONE, 3*, e1924. https://doi.org/10.1371/journal.pone.0001924.

Chapter

5

ASSESSMENT OF KIDNEY FUNCTION

Contents

Introduction

Evaluating kidney function is essential for both tracking general health and identifying and treating renal diseases. The kidneys' main jobs include keeping acid-base homeostasis, controlling fluid and electrolyte balance, and filtering waste products out of the blood. Many clinical tests and indicators are frequently used to assess kidney function. The three most significant ones are glomerular filtration rate (GFR), blood urea nitrogen (BUN), and serum creatinine. The kidneys eliminate serum creatinine, which is a waste product of muscle metabolism. Because higher levels usually indicate impaired kidney filtration, its concentration in the blood offers a rough indication of kidney function. Serum creatinine, however, is not a perfect marker by itself because it can be affected by age, sex, and muscle mass. As a result, it is frequently combined with other strategies. BUN, or blood urea nitrogen, is an additional measure of kidney function. The breakdown of proteins in the liver produces urea, a waste product that is typically eliminated by the kidneys. Reduced kidney function may be indicated by elevated BUN levels; however, similar to creatinine, BUN can also be impacted by variables unrelated to kidney health, such as dietary protein consumption, liver health, and level of hydration.

The most accurate measure of kidney function overall is thought to be the glomerular filtration rate or GFR. The glomeruli, or microscopic filtering units in the kidneys, filter blood on a minute-by-minute basis; this is measured by GFR. Age, sex, and body size all affect what constitutes a normal GFR, but a GFR of 90 mL/min/1.73 m^2 or above is usually accepted as normal. Renal failure is indicated by a GFR below 15 mL/min/1.73 m^2, whereas chronic kidney disease (CKD) is indicated by a GFR below 60 mL/min/1.73 m^2 for three months or longer. GFR can be calculated using formulas, like the CKD-EPI (Chronic Kidney Disease Epidemiology Collaboration) equation, that account for body size, age, sex, and serum creatinine levels. Urinalysis is another crucial instrument for evaluating kidney function in addition to these primary tests. Urine's physical and chemical characteristics, such as the presence of blood, protein, glucose, and other materials, are examined. Excess protein in the urine, or proteinuria, is a warning indication of kidney damage, especially in cases of diabetic nephropathy. Blood in the urine, or hematuria, is a sign of many illnesses, such as kidney stones, infections, or more serious conditions like glomerulonephritis or cancers. The size, structure, and any anomalies of the kidneys can be seen through imaging tests like MRIs, CT scans, and ultrasounds. These imaging methods are helpful in the detection of tumors, obstructions, and structural abnormalities. A kidney biopsy may be necessary in certain circumstances to remove a small sample of kidney tissue for microscopic analysis. Making treatment decisions can be aided by this, which can offer conclusive information regarding the kind and severity of kidney disease.

Orientation and Directional Terms

Term	Definition	Illustration
Hematuria	Hematuria is the presence of blood in the urine. Hematuria can be gross or microscopic.	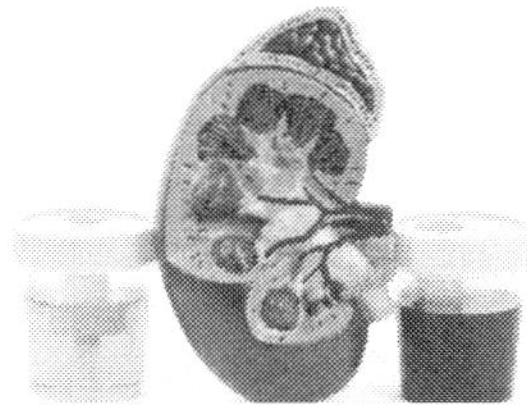
Bladder	A hollow organ in humans and other vertebrates that stores urine from the kidneys before disposal by urination.	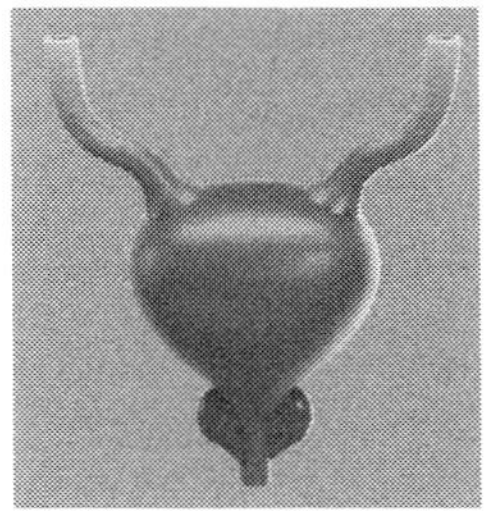
Renal pelvis	Enlarged upper end of the ureter, the tube through which urine flows from the kidney to the urinary bladder.	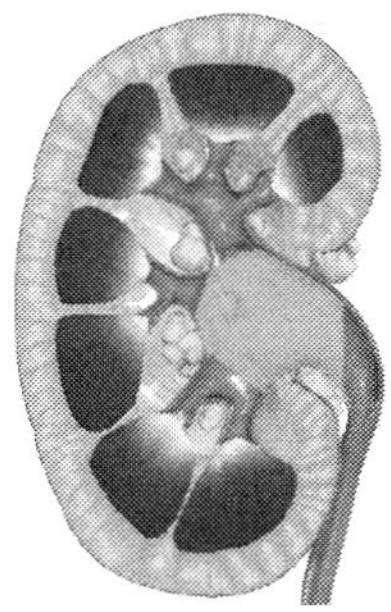
Renal sinus	A compartment inside your kidney that uses fat to cushion important parts like the renal pelvis, lymphatic channels, calyces and renal artery.	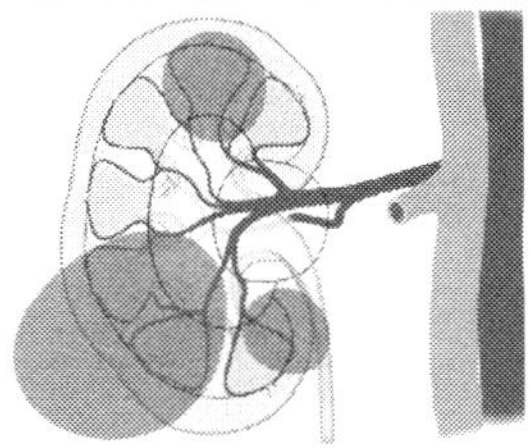
Renal cortex	The outer layer of the kidney, is just deep to the fibrous capsule and surrounding the inner medullary layer.	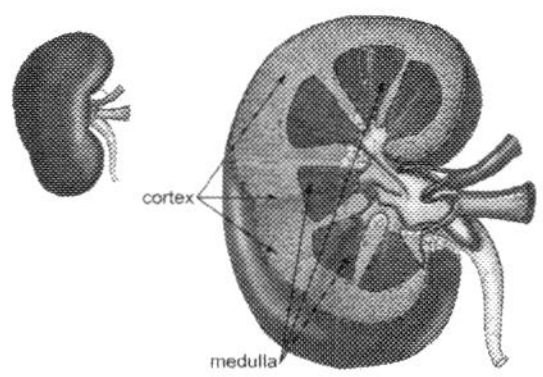

5.1. Kidney and Its Function

The kidneys are two reddish-brown, bean-shaped organs that filter blood. They are a multilobar, multipapillary form of the kidney found in mammals, and they typically lack outward lobulation symptoms. They are roughly 12 centimeters (41/2 inches) long in adult humans and are situated on the left and right in the retroperitoneal space. Blood enters them through the paired renal arteries and leaves through the paired renal veins. The ureters, which are tubes that convey excreted urine to the bladder, are connected to each kidney. The kidney is involved in the regulation of different body fluid volumes, fluid osmolality, acid-base balance, different electrolyte concentrations, and toxin elimination. One-fifth of the blood volume that enters the kidneys is filtered at the glomerulus. Amino acids, sodium, bicarbonate, glucose, and solute-free water are a few examples of materials that are reabsorbed. A few examples of substances secreted are uric acid, hydrogen, ammonium, and potassium. The kidney's anatomical and functional unit is the nephron. A mouse kidney has only about 12,500 nephrons, compared to approximately 1 million nephrons in an adult human kidney. In addition, the kidneys perform tasks without the assistance of the nephrons. For instance, they synthesize the hormones erythropoietin and renin and transform a precursor of vitamin D into its active form, calcitriol.

Chronic kidney disease (CKD) has been recognized as a leading public health problem worldwide. The global estimated prevalence of CKD is 13.4%, and patients with kidney failure needing renal replacement therapy are estimated between 5 and 7 million (Gai Z et al., 2019). A kidney biopsy and CT scan to check for abnormal anatomy are among the procedures used in the management of kidney disease. Other procedures include measuring kidney function by calculating the estimated glomerular filtration rate (eGFR) using the serum creatinine level and chemical and microscopic examination of the urine (urinalysis). Kidney failure is treated with dialysis and kidney transplantation; when renal function falls below 15%, one of these treatments (or both sequentially) is almost always utilized (Lote, 2012). The standard treatment for renal cell carcinoma is nephrectomy. Kidney function is the subject of renal physiology. The medical specialty of nephrology deals with disorders of the kidneys, such as pyelonephritis, acute kidney injury, nephrotic and nephritic syndromes, and chronic kidney disease (CKD). Diseases affecting the anatomy of the kidneys and urinary tract are the focus of urology. These include renal cysts, kidney and ureteral stones, cancer, and obstructions of the urinary tract. The adjective renal has French or late Latin origins and means "pertaining to the kidneys." While some experts believe that the term "renal" should always be replaced with "kidney" in scientific publications, such as kidney arteries, other experts have argued that the term "renal" should still be used when appropriate, such as in renal arteries.

5.1.1. Structure

In humans, the kidneys are situated at a slightly oblique angle in the retroperitoneum, high in the abdominal cavity, one on each side of the spine. Because of the asymmetry in the abdominal cavity brought about by the liver's location, the right kidney usually has a slightly smaller and lower profile than the left, as well as a slightly more central placement. Approximately, the left kidney is located at vertebral level T12 to L3, while the right kidney is located slightly lower.

The right kidney is located posterior to the liver and immediately below the diaphragm. The left kidney is located behind the spleen and beneath the diaphragm. Adrenal glands are located above each kidney. The 11th and 12th ribs provide some partial protection for the upper portions of the kidneys. Every kidney has two layers of fat surrounding it, one layer being superior to the renal fascia and the other between the renal fascia and the renal capsule. This is where the adrenal gland is located. With convex and concave borders, the human kidney is a bean-shaped organ. The renal hilum, a recessed region on the concave border, is where the renal vein and ureter exit the kidney and the renal artery enters. Tough fibrous tissue known as the renal capsule envelops the kidney. Renal fascia, pararenal fat, and perirenal fat encircle the renal capsule. These tissues have the transversalis fascia on the posterior (rear) surface and the peritoneum on the anterior (front) surface. Adjacent to the liver is the superior pole of the right kidney. Next to the spleen is where the left kidney is located. Thus, upon inhaling, both move downward (Table 5.1).

Table 5.1. Standard Reference Range of Kidney

Sex	Weight, Standard Reference Range	
	Right Kidney	**Left Kidney**
Male	80–160 g (2+$^3/_4$–5+$^3/_4$ oz)	80–175 g (2+$^3/_4$–6+$^1/_4$ oz)
Female	40–175 g (1+$^1/_2$–6+$^1/_4$ oz)	35–190 g (1+$^1/_4$–6+$^3/_4$ oz)

Source: https://en.wikipedia.org/wiki/Kidney.

A Danish study measured the median renal length to be 11.2 cm (4+$^7/_{16}$ in) on the left side and 10.9 cm (4+$^5/_{16}$ in) on the right side in adults. Median renal volumes were 146 cm^3 (8+$^{15}/_{16}$ cu in) on the left and 134 cm^3 (8+$^3/_{16}$ cu in) on the right.

5.1.1.1. Gross Anatomy

The human kidney's parenchyma, or functional substance, is composed of two primary structures, namely the inner renal medulla and the outer renal cortex (Thomas, 2005). In general, these structures resemble 8 to 18 cone-shaped renal lobes, with a renal pyramid-shaped section of the medulla encircling each renal cortex. Renal columns are cortical projections that lie between the renal pyramids. Urine is emptied into a minor calyx by the tip of each pyramid, known as the papilla; major calyces empty into the renal pelvis, and minor calyces empty into major calyces. This turns into the ureter. The renal artery enters the kidney at the hilum, where the ureter and renal vein leave. These structures are surrounded by hilar fat and lymphatic tissue that contains lymph nodes. The renal sinus, a cavity filled with fat, is adjacent to the hilar fat. The renal pelvis and calyces are located within the renal sinus, which also divides them from the renal medullary tissue (Figure 5.1).

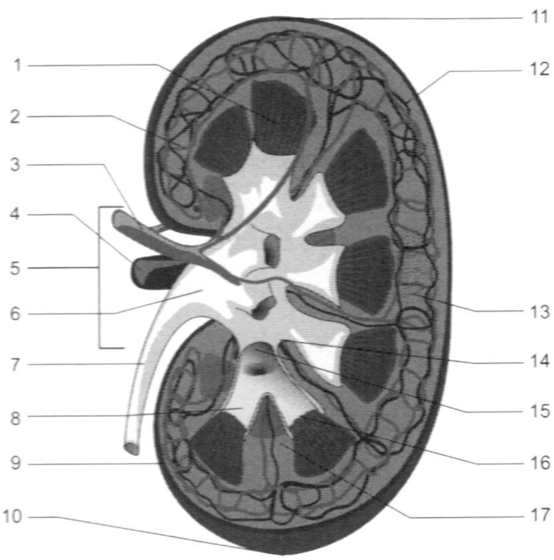

Figure 5.1. *The kidneys possess no overtly moving structures.*

Note: 1. Renal pyramid, 2. Interlobular artery, 3. Renal artery, 4. Renal vein 5. Renal hilum, 6. Renal pelvis, 7. Ureter, 8. Minor calyx, 9. Renal capsule, 10. Inferior renal capsule, 11. Superior renal capsule, 12. Interlobular vein, 13. Nephron, 14. Renal sinus, 15. Major calyx, 16. Renal papilla, 17. Renal column.

Source: https://upload.wikimedia.org/wikipedia/commons/thumb/a/ab/KidneyStructures_PioM.svg/300px-KidneyStructures_PioM.svg.png.

5.1.1.2. Blood Supply

The left and right renal arteries, which emerge straight from the abdominal aorta, supply blood to the kidneys. In an adult human, the kidneys receive about 20–25% of cardiac output. Every renal artery divides into segmental arteries, which then split into interlobar arteries. These arteries then pass through the renal columns and between the renal pyramids, penetrating the renal capsule. The arcuate arteries, which pass through the cortex and medulla's border, subsequently receive blood from the interlobar arteries. Many interlobular arteries that feed into the afferent arterioles that supply the glomeruli are supplied by each arcuate artery. Eventually, blood exits the kidneys through the inferior vena cava. Following filtration, blood passes via a tiny network of venules, which eventually join to form interlobular veins. The veins follow the same pattern as the arteriole distribution: blood is supplied by the interlobular veins to the arcuate veins, which in turn return to the interlobar veins to form the renal veins that leave the kidney.

5.1.1.3. Nerve Supply

The renal plexus, whose fibers travel via the renal arteries to each kidney, serves as a conduit for communication between the kidney and the nervous system. Vasoconstriction in the kidney is caused by input from the sympathetic nervous system, which lowers renal blood flow. The renal branches of the vagus nerve carry information from the parasympathetic nervous system to the kidney; the purpose of these branches is unknown. The corresponding dermatome receives sensory information from the kidney that travels to the T10–11 levels of the spinal cord. Therefore, the related kidney may be the source of flank pain.

5.1.1.4. Microanatomy

Nephrons are the kidney's functional structures that produce urine, and they are found in both the cortex and medulla. Located in the cortex, the renal corpuscle is the first filtering portion of a nephron. A renal tubule that travels deep into the medullary pyramids from the cortex comes next. A medullary ray, which is a group of renal tubules draining into a single collecting duct, is a portion of the renal cortex. The microscopic structure of the kidney is studied in renal histology. At least 26 different cell types can be found in an adult human kidney.

Distinct cell types include:

- Kidney glomerulus parietal cell
- Kidney glomerulus podocyte

- Kidney proximal tubule brush border cell
- Loop of Henle thin segment cell
- Thick ascending limb cell
- Kidney distal tubule cell
- Collecting duct principal cell
- Collecting duct intercalated cell
- Interstitial kidney cells

5.1.2. Function

Numerous waste products from metabolism are eliminated by the kidneys and end up in the urine. The nephron is the kidney's microscopic structural and functional unit. Urine is produced as a result of the filtration, reabsorption, secretion, and excretion processes it uses to process the blood that is supplied to it.

These comprise the nitrogenous wastes uric acid from nucleic acid metabolism and urea from protein catabolism. An intricate countercurrent multiplication mechanism is required for mammals and certain birds to concentrate wastes into a volume of urine significantly smaller than the volume of blood from which the wastes were extracted.

A tight hairpin arrangement of the tubules, water and ion permeability in the loop's descending limb, water impermeability in the ascending limb, and active ion transport out of the majority of the ascending limb are all necessary for this to function. Furthermore, this function cannot be performed without passive countercurrent exchange by the blood vessels supplying the nephron (Figure 5.2).

The kidney plays a role in maintaining homeostasis throughout the body by controlling blood pressure, extracellular fluid volume, electrolyte concentrations, and acid-base balance. These homeostatic tasks are carried out by the kidney both on its own and in coordination with other organs, especially those belonging to the endocrine system.

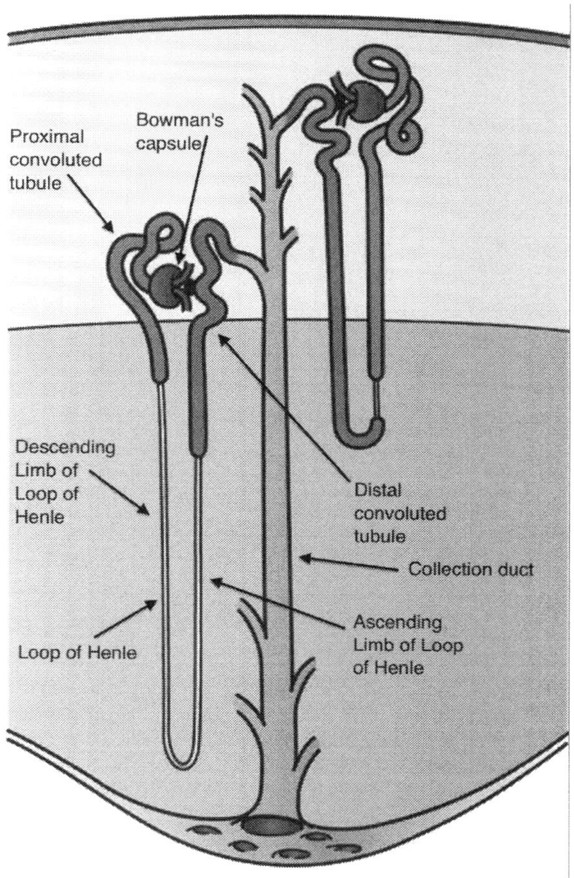

Figure 5.2. *The functional unit of the kidneys. Its parts are labeled except the (gray) connecting tubule located after the (dark red) distal convoluted tubule and before the large (gray) collecting duct (mislabeled collection duct).*

Source: *https://upload.wikimedia.org/wikipedia/commons/9/98/Kidney_Nephron.png.*

These endocrine processes are regulated by many endocrine hormones, which include atrial natriuretic peptide, renin, angiotensin II, aldosterone, and antidiuretic hormone. Located at the lowest point of the rib cage on either side of the spine, the two kidneys are roughly the size of a fist. Up to a million nephrons, or functional units, can be found in each kidney. A glomerulus, a filtering unit made up of microscopic blood vessels, is joined to a tubule to form a nephron. Blood is filtered as it enters the glomerulus, and the residual fluid then travels through the tubule. Urine is the end product that is expelled from the body after chemicals and water are added to or removed from this filtered fluid in the tubule based on the body's needs. Every 24 hours, the kidneys carry out their vital function of filtering and replenishing the bloodstream with approximately 200 quarts of fluid. The body excretes approximately two quarts in the form of urine, and approximately 198 quarts are recovered. Our bladders hold onto the pee we excrete for a maximum of one to eight hours.

5.1.2.1. Formation of Urine

- **Filtration:** The process of filtering, which occurs at the renal corpuscle, keeps cells and large proteins in the blood while removing materials with smaller molecular weights to create an ultrafiltrate that eventually turns into urine. The majority of the 180 liters of filtrate that an adult human kidney produces each day is reabsorbed. 800 to 2,000 milliliters per day is the typical range for a 24-hour urine volume collection. Because the capillary walls are subjected to hydrostatic pressure, the process is also known as hydrostatic filtration (Figure 5.3).

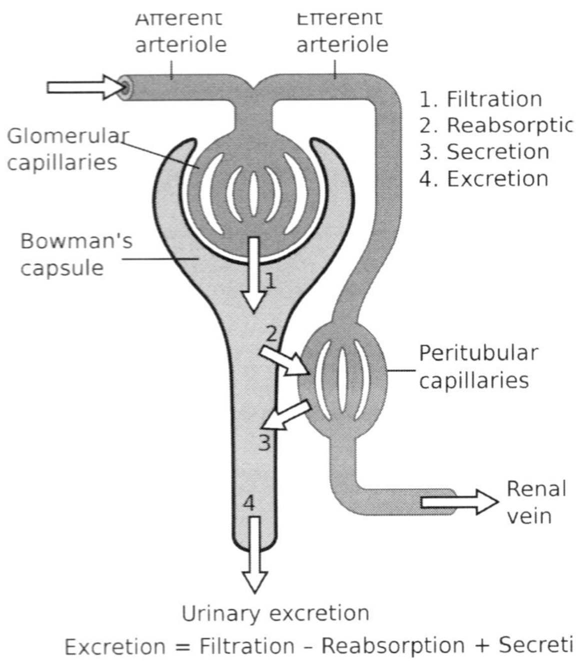

Figure 5.3. *Four main processes are involved in the creation of urine.*

Source: *https://upload.wikimedia.org/wikipedia/commons/thumb/2/2b/Physiology_of_Nephron.png/800px-Physiology_of_Nephron.png.*

- **Reabsorption:** Molecules are transported from this ultrafiltrate into the peritubular capillary through reabsorption. Selective receptors on the luminal cell membrane enable it. In the proximal tubule, water is reabsorbed to the extent of 55%. In the proximal tubule, glucose is fully reabsorbed at normal plasma levels. The Na^+/glucose cotransporter is the mechanism underlying this. The transporters will be fully saturated at 350 mg/dL of plasma, at which point glucose will be lost in the urine. A plasma glucose level of about 160 is needed to cause glucosuria, a crucial clinical indicator of diabetes mellitus. In the proximal tubule, sodium-dependent transporters reabsorb amino acids. Pelagra is the result of a tryptophan amino acid transporter deficiency in Hartnup disease (Table 5.2).

Table 5.2. Examples of Substances that are Reabsorbed in the Kidneys, and the Hormones that Influence Those Processes

Location of Reabsorption	Reabsorbed Nutrient	Notes
Early proximal tubule	Glucose (100%), amino acids (100%), bicarbonate (90%), Na^+ (65%), Cl^- (65%), phosphate (65%) and H_2O (65%)	• PTH will inhibit phosphate reabsorption. • AT II stimulates Na^+, H_2O and HCO_3^- reabsorption.
Thin descending loop of Henle	H_2O	• Reabsorbs via medullary hypertonicity and makes urine hypertonic.
Thick ascending loop of Henle	Na^+ (10–20%), K^+, Cl^-; indirectly induces para cellular reabsorption of Mg^{2+}, Ca^{2+}	• This region is impermeable to H_2O and the urine becomes less concentrated as it ascends.
Early distal convoluted tubule	Na^+, Cl^-	• PTH causes Ca^{2+} reabsorption.
Collecting tubules	Na^+(3–5%), H_2O	• Na^+ is reabsorbed in exchange for K^+, and H^+, which is regulated by aldosterone. • ADH acts on the V2 receptor and inserts aquaporins on the luminal side

Source: https://en.wikipedia.org/wiki/Kidney.

- **Secretion:** Secretion is the reverse of reabsorption: molecules are transported from the peritubular capillary through the interstitial fluid, then through the renal tubular cell and into the ultrafiltrate.
- **Excretion:** Excretion is the final stage of the ultrafiltrate processing system. After leaving the nephron, the ultrafiltrate travels through the collecting duct, a tube that is a part of the collecting duct system, and into the ureters, where it is referred to as urine. Apart from its role in ultrafiltrate transportation, the collecting duct also participates in reabsorption (Figure 5.4).

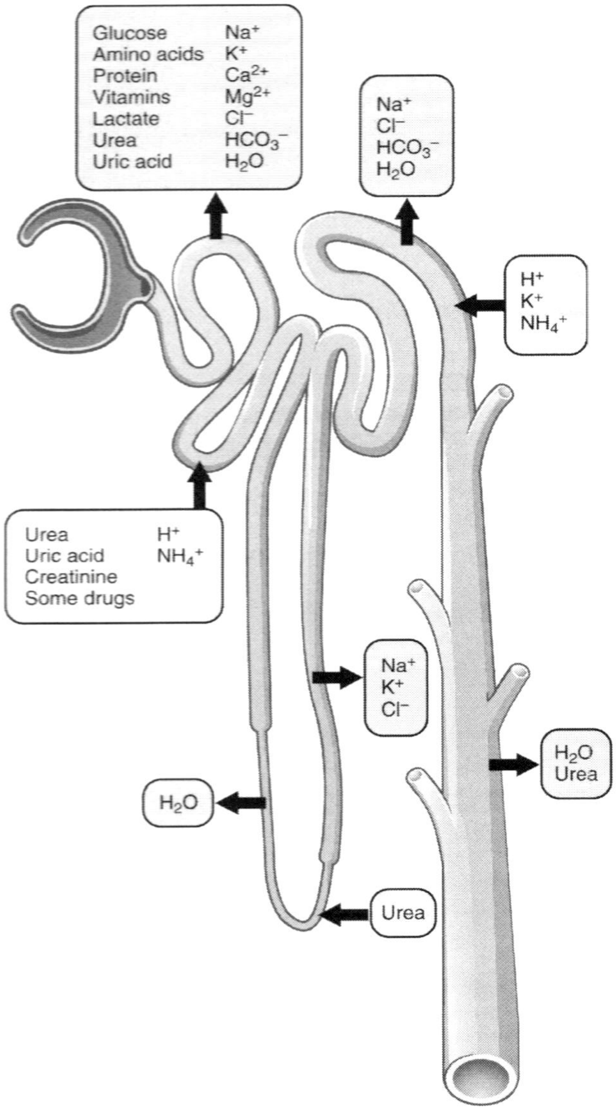

Figure 5.4. *Secretion and reabsorption of various substances throughout the nephron.*

Source: https://upload.wikimedia.org/wikipedia/commons/thumb/2/26/2618_Nephron_Secretion_Reabsorption.jpg/220px-2618_Nephron_Secretion_Reabsorption.jpg.

5.1.2.2. Hormone Secretion

Hormones secreted by the kidneys include calcitriol, renin, and erythropoietin. When there is hypoxia (low oxygen levels at the tissue level) in the renal circulation, erythropoietin is released. It causes the bone marrow to produce more red blood cells or erythropoiesis. The activated form of vitamin D, calcitriol, facilitates the reabsorption of phosphate by the kidneys and the intestinal absorption of calcium. Renin is an enzyme that controls aldosterone and angiotensin levels.

5.1.2.3. Blood Pressure Regulation

Despite the kidney's inability to sense blood directly, it is primarily responsible for long-term blood pressure regulation. The extracellular fluid compartment's maintenance, which is largely responsible for this, is influenced by the concentration of plasma sodium. The renin–angiotensin system consists of several key chemical messengers, the first of which is renin. In the end, variations in renin affect this system's output, primarily the hormones aldosterone and angiotensin II. Both hormones increase the kidney's absorption of sodium chloride, which increases the extracellular fluid compartment and blood pressure. However, their respective mechanisms of action are different. The concentrations of angiotensin II and aldosterone rise in response to elevated renin levels, which causes an increase in blood pressure, an expansion of the extracellular fluid compartment, and an increase in sodium chloride reabsorption. On the other hand, low renin levels cause a drop in angiotensin II and aldosterone, which constricts the extracellular fluid compartment and lowers blood pressure.

5.1.2.4. Acid–Base Balance

The kidneys and lungs are the two organ systems that assist in controlling the body's acid-base balance. Acid-base homeostasis refers to keeping pH levels between 7 and 6.4. As part of the respiratory system, the lungs control blood carbon dioxide (CO_2) concentration, which aids in the maintenance of acid-base homeostasis. The body's first line of defense in the event of an acid-base imbalance is the respiratory system. It regulates the respiratory rate to bring the body's pH back to 7 points. When an acidic environment is present in the body, the respiratory rate increases, which eliminates CO_2 and lowers the H+ concentration, raising the pH. Under normal circumstances, the respiratory rate will slow down to allow the body to retain more CO_2, raise the concentration of H+, and lower the pH.

Intercalated A and B cells are two types of cells found in the kidneys that aid in preserving acid-base homeostasis. Conditions that are acidic to the body stimulate the intercalated A cells. The high blood CO_2 concentration in an acidic environment produces a gradient that allows CO_2 to enter the cell and shifts the reaction $HCO_3 + H \leftarrow H_2CO_3 \leftarrow CO_2 + H_2O$ to the left. There is an H/K exchanger and an H+ pump on the cell's luminal side. These pumps need ATP because they move H+ against their gradient. The blood's pH will rise as a result of these cellular removal of H+ and transfer of it to the filtrate. A Cl/K co-transporter (facilitated diffusion) and an HCO_3/Cl exchanger are located on the basal side of the cell. The HCO_3 concentration in the cell rises when the reaction is pushed to the left, and when HCO_3 is free to enter the blood, the pH rises even more. The response of the intercalated B cell is very similar to that of the intercalated A cells; however, the membrane proteins are reversed, with the proton pumps located on the basal side and the K/Cl co-transporter and HCO_3/Cl exchanger on the luminal side. They still do the same thing, but they now lower the blood's pH by releasing protons.

5.1.2.5. Regulation of Osmolality

The kidneys assist in regulating the body's salt and water balance. Through direct communication with the posterior pituitary gland, the hypothalamus detects any appreciable increase in plasma osmolality. Urine concentration rises as a result of the kidneys reabsorbing more water due to an increase in osmolality, which triggers the gland to release antidiuretic hormone (ADH). Together, the two elements help to bring the plasma osmolality back to normal.

5.1.2.6. Measuring Function

Kidney function is attempted to be measured using a variety of computations and techniques. The amount of plasma from which a drug is entirely removed from the blood in a given amount of time is known as renal clearance. The amount of plasma that really passes through the kidney's filter is known as the filtration fraction. The equation can be used to define this. Due to its complexity, the kidney has been better understood on many levels, including fluid uptake and secretion, through mathematical modeling.

5.1.3. Clinical Significance

The subspecialty of Internal Medicine known as nephrology focuses on kidney function, disease states associated with renal malfunction, and treatment options for these conditions, such as kidney transplantation and dialysis. Urology is a subspecialty of surgery that treats abnormalities of the kidney's structure, including kidney cancer, cysts, and urinary tract issues. Although both are frequently referred to as kidney doctors, urologists are surgeons and nephrologists are internists. Nephrologists and urologists can treat kidney stones and infections related to the kidneys, among other overlapping conditions. Kidney disease has a wide range of causes. Certain causes, like diabetic nephropathy, develop over time, while other causes, like polycystic kidney disease, are inherited. Terms like *renal* and the prefix *nephro* are frequently used in medical terminology pertaining to the kidneys. The prefix nephro- comes from the Ancient Greek word for kidney, nephros (νεφρός), and the adjective renal, meaning related to the kidney, comes from the Latin rēnēs, meaning kidneys. For instance, a nephrectomy is the surgical removal of a kidney, whereas renal dysfunction is the term used to describe a decrease in kidney function.

5.1.3.1. Acquired Diseases

- Diabetic nephropathy
- Glomerulonephritis
- Hydronephrosis is the enlargement of one or both of the kidneys caused by obstruction of the flow of urine.
- Interstitial nephritis
- Nephrolithiasis, or kidney stones, is a rather common and extremely painful condition. Kidney scarring can be the consequence of a long-term illness. Kidney stones are removed by breaking them up into smaller pieces with ultrasound therapy, which allows the stones to pass through the urinary tract. A sharp to incapacitating pain in the middle and sides of the lower back or groin is a common symptom of kidney stones.
- Kidney tumor
    - Wilms tumor
    - Renal cell carcinoma
- Lupus nephritis
- Minimal change disease
- In nephrotic syndrome, the glomerulus has been damaged so that a large amount of protein in the blood enters the urine. Other

frequent features of the nephrotic syndrome include swelling, low serum albumin, and high cholesterol.

- Pyelonephritis is an infection of the kidneys and is frequently caused by complications of a urinary tract infection.
- Kidney failure
  - o Acute kidney failure
  - o Stage 5 Chronic Kidney Disease
- Renal artery stenosis
- Renovascular hypertension

5.1.3.2. Kidney Injury and Failure

Humans can typically survive with just one kidney because they have more functioning renal tissue in one kidney than they need for survival. Chronic kidney disease only appears when there is a significant reduction in the amount of functioning kidney tissue. Dialysis or kidney transplantation, two forms of renal replacement therapy, are recommended when the glomerular filtration rate has dropped significantly or when the renal dysfunction is causing severe symptoms.

5.1.3.3. Dialysis

The treatment known as dialysis takes the place of the kidneys' natural function. A glomerular filtration rate (GFR) of less than 15 indicates that 85–90% of kidney function has been lost, at which point dialysis may be started. Dialysis maintains numerous chemical levels in the body and eliminates metabolic waste products, excess water, and sodium, which helps to control blood pressure. Those receiving dialysis can expect to live for 5 to 10 years; some can live up to 30. Dialysis is usually given three times a week for several hours at free-standing dialysis centers. Recipients are allowed to lead essentially normal lives in between treatments. Dialysis can be performed via the blood (through a catheter or arteriovenous fistula) or through the peritoneum (peritoneal dialysis) (Figure 5.5).

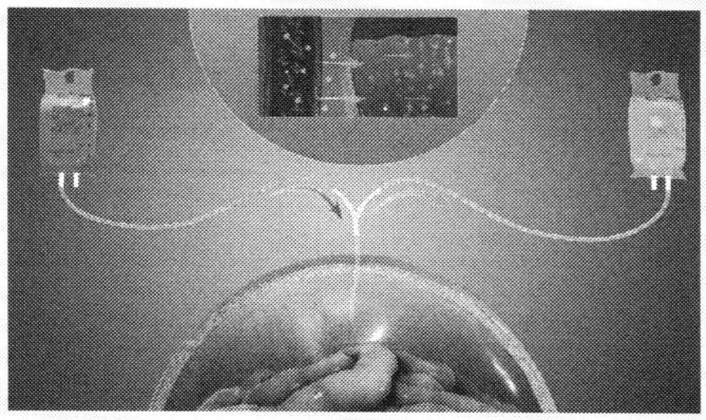

Figure 5.5. *A depiction of peritoneal dialysis.*

Source: *https://upload.wikimedia.org/wikipedia/commons/thumb/b/b6/Peritoneal_dialysis.jpg/1280px-Peritoneal_dialysis.jpg.*

5.1.3.4. Congenital Disease

- Congenital hydronephrosis
- Congenital obstruction of the urinary tract
- Duplex kidneys, or double kidneys, occur in approximately 1% of the population. This occurrence normally causes no complications, but can occasionally cause urinary tract infections.
- Duplicated ureter occurs in approximately one in 100 live births
- Horseshoe kidney occurs in approximately one in 400 live births
- Nephroblastoma (Syndromic Wilm's tumor)
- Nutcracker syndrome
- Polycystic kidney disease
  - o Autosomal dominant polycystic kidney disease affects patients later in life. Approximately one in 1,000 people will develop this condition

  - o Autosomal recessive polycystic kidney disease is far less common, but more severe than the dominant condition. It is apparent *in utero* or at birth.

- Renal agenesis. Failure of one kidney to form occurs in approximately one in 750 live births. Failure of both kidneys to form used to be fatal; however, medical advances such as amnioinfusion therapy during pregnancy and peritoneal dialysis have made it possible to stay alive until a transplant can occur.
- Renal dysplasia
- Unilateral small kidney
- Multicystic dysplastic kidney occurs in approximately one in every 2,400 live births
- Ureteropelvic Junction Obstruction or UPJO; although most cases are congenital, some are acquired.

5.1.4. Diagnosis

An extensive medical history and physical examination are used to diagnose many renal diseases. The medical history considers recent infections, exposure to kidney-toxic substances, family history of kidney disease, and past and present symptoms, particularly those of kidney disease. Urine and blood tests are used to assess kidney function. The most popular blood tests are those for electrolytes, urea, and creatinine. Tests for urine, like urinalysis, can assess pH, protein, glucose, and blood presence. Urinary casts and crystals can also be detected by microscopic analysis. Although it is rarely done in routine practice, the glomerular filtration rate (GFR) can be directly measured (measured GFR, or mGFR). Instead, the GFR (estimated GFR, or eGFR) is computed using unique equations.

- **Imaging:** Renal ultrasonography is essential in the diagnosis and management of kidney-related diseases. Other modalities, such as CT and MRI, should always be considered supplementary imaging modalities in the assessment of renal disease.
- **Biopsy:** The purpose of the renal biopsy is to use noninvasive methods (clinical history, past medical history, medication history, physical examination, laboratory studies, and imaging studies) to diagnose renal disease for which the etiology is unknown. To arrive at a pathological diagnosis, a renal pathologist will typically conduct a thorough morphological evaluation and combine the results with the patient's medical history and laboratory results. A doctor who has completed both general training in anatomic pathology and additional specialized training in the interpretation of renal biopsy specimens is known as a renal pathologist. Optimally, several core sections are extracted and assessed intraoperatively for sufficiency (glomeruli present). The specimen(s) for light, electron, and immunofluorescence microscopy are divided by a pathologist or pathology assistant. Using light microscopy and various staining methods (hematoxylin and eosin/HandE, PAS, trichrome, and silver stain) on several level sections, the pathologist will examine the specimen. Several immunofluorescence stains are used to check for the deposition of complement, proteins, and antibodies. Lastly, electron microscopy is used to perform an ultra-structural examination. This may reveal the presence of electron-

dense deposits or other distinctive abnormalities that could point to the cause of the patient's renal disease.

5.1.5. Other Animals

The mesonephros is only found in the embryo in amniotes; in most other vertebrates, it continues into adulthood, albeit usually fused with the more developed metanephros. In fish and amphibians, the kidneys are usually long, narrow organs that take up a large amount of the trunk. Every cluster of nephrons typically has collecting ducts that empty into an archinephric duct, which is similar to the amniotic vas deferens. The situation is not always straightforward, though, as the posterior (metanephric) portions of the kidney are drained by a shorter duct that resembles the amniote ureter and connects to the archinephric duct at the bladder or cloaca in cartilaginous fish and some amphibians. In fact, the anterior part of the kidney in many cartilaginous fish may degenerate or stop functioning entirely in adulthood. The kidney is remarkably simple in the simplest vertebrates, such as hagfish and lampreys, consisting of a row of nephrons that empty into the archinephric duct. Even in Amphioxus, the excretory organs that invertebrates have that are sometimes called kidneys are never homologous with the kidneys of vertebrates; instead, they are more correctly called nephridia. Monogeneans of the family Polystomatidae are specialized parasites found in the kidneys and urinary bladder of amphibians.

Reptile kidneys are made up of several lobules arranged in a generally linear pattern. The collecting ducts empty into a single ureter branch located in the center of each lobule. In comparison to other amniotes of comparable size, reptiles have comparatively fewer nephrons, perhaps as a result of a slower metabolic rate. The kidneys of birds are elongated and relatively large, with multiple distinct lobes within each kidney. The lobes are made up of multiple tiny, erratically arranged lobules, each of which is centered on a ureteric branch. Compared to mammals of comparable size, birds have roughly twice as many nephrons but smaller glomeruli. The kidney in humans is quite similar to that in mammals. When compared to the kidneys of other vertebrates, the kidney of mammals differs in that it has a distinct cortex and medulla, as well as the presence of renal pyramids and pelvis. The latter characteristic results from elongated Henle loops, which are absent in other vertebrates but considerably shorter in birds (though the nephron frequently has a brief intermediate segment between the convoluted tubules). With a few notable exceptions, such as the multilobed reniculate kidneys of pinnipeds and cetaceans, the kidney only assumes its typical shape in mammals.

- **Evolutionary Adaptation:** Kidneys of various animals show evidence of evolutionary adaptation and have long been studied in ecophysiology and comparative physiology. Kidney morphology, often indexed as the relative medullary thickness, is associated with habitat aridity among species of mammals and diet (e.g., carnivores have only long loops of Henle).

5.2. Renal Function Tests

In addition to producing hormones like erythropoietin, 1,25-dihydroxy vitamin D, and renin, the kidneys are essential for the excretion of waste materials and toxins like urea, creatinine, and uric acid, as well as for regulating the volume of extracellular fluid, serum osmolality, and electrolyte concentrations. The glomerulus, proximal and distal tubules, and collecting duct make up the nephron, the functional unit of the kidney. When managing patients with renal disease or other pathologies impacting renal function, assessment of renal function is crucial. Renal function tests are useful for diagnosing renal disease, tracking the kidneys' response to treatment, and figuring out how far along the disease is. The National Institutes of Health estimates that 14% of people worldwide have chronic kidney disease (CKD) (Boga & Sönmez, 2019). Overseas, diabetes and hypertension are the most frequent causes of chronic kidney disease.

5.2.1. Specimen Collection

The procedure or test that is requested will determine the requirements for collecting specimens. Usually, a random blood sample will be used for measuring serum creatinine and blood urea nitrogen (BUN) levels, and no further patient preparation is needed (Wiles et al., 2019). On the other hand, a recent high-protein diet may have significantly raised serum creatinine and urea levels. Furthermore, BUN measurement may be significantly impacted by one's level of hydration. Urine must be precisely collected over the required period for timed urine collections, such as the 24-hour urine creatinine clearance, as under- or over-collection will impact the outcome. Therefore, it is better to schedule a collection for 5 to 8 hours rather than 24. Since midstream urine is less likely to contain commensal bacteria and epithelial cells, it must be collected for urine analysis.

5.2.2. Procedures

5.2.2.1. Assessment of Renal Function

Many clinical laboratory tests are helpful in examining and assessing kidney function. In clinical settings, estimating the glomerular filtration rate (GFR) and looking for proteinuria (albuminuria) are the most practical methods to evaluate renal function.

5.2.2.1.1. Glomerular Filtration Rate

The glomerular filtration rate (GFR) is the most accurate general measure of glomerular function. GFR, or blood substance clearance, is the measurement of the speed in milliliters per minute at which substances in plasma pass through the glomerulus. An adult male's GFR typically ranges from 90 to 120 mL per minute. The perfect GFR marker should have the following qualities.

- It should appear endogenously in the plasma at a constant rate
- It should be freely filtered at the glomerulus
- It can be neither reabsorbed nor secreted by the renal tubule
- It should not undergo extrarenal elimination.

Exogenous GFR markers are utilized since there isn't currently an endogenous marker of this kind. The polysaccharide inulin is used to assess GFR, and this method is regarded as the standard for GFR estimation. To ascertain the rate of inulin clearance, inulin is infused and blood levels are measured after a predetermined amount of time. Radioisotopes like technetium-99-labeled diethylene-triamine-pentaacetate (99 Tc-DTPA) and chromium-51 ethylene-diamine-tetra-acetic acid (51 Cr-EDTA) are examples of other exogenous markers that are used. Iohexol, a non-radioactive contrast agent, is the most promising exogenous marker, particularly when used in pediatric patients.

The use of endogenous markers has been prompted by the drawbacks of using exogenous markers, such as the need for specialized centers for testing and the challenge of assaying these substances.

1. **Creatinine:** The most commonly used endogenous marker for the assessment of glomerular function is creatinine. The calculated clearance of creatinine is used to provide an indicator of GFR. This involves the collection of urine over a 24-hour period or preferably over an accurately timed period of 5 to 8 hours since 24-hour collections are notoriously unreliable. Creatinine clearance is then calculated using the equation:

$$C = (U \times V) / P$$

C = clearance, U = urinary concentration, V = urinary flow rate (volume/time i.e., ml/min), and P = plasma concentration

It is necessary to adjust creatinine clearance for body surface area. Timed collection is beneficial because one of the main problems affecting the accuracy of this test is improper or incomplete urine collection. Moreover, creatinine overestimates GFR by roughly 10% to 20% as a result of tubular secretion. The body continuously produces creatinine, which is a byproduct of creatine phosphate in muscle. The kidneys remove creatinine from the blood completely most of the time. Blood creatinine rises as a result of reduced kidney clearance. Muscle mass affects how much creatinine is produced daily. Males and females have different creatinine ranges, with lower creatinine values in children and those with less muscle mass. Creatinine levels are also influenced by diet. Red meat consumption can cause a 30% shift in creatinine levels. Lower creatinine levels are observed during pregnancy as GFR rises. Furthermore, renal function must decline by 50% before a rise in serum creatinine is seen, making serum creatinine a late indicator of renal impairment. Additionally, GFR-estimating equations like the CKD-EPI (Chronic Kidney Disease Epidemiology Collaboration) equation and the Modified Diet in Renal Disease (MDRD) equation use serum creatinine. Because these eGFR equations take age, gender, and race into account, they are better than serum creatinine alone. Based on kidney disease, the following stages of GFR are assigned.

Kidney Disease Improving Global Outcomes (KDIGO) stages of chronic kidney disease (CKD):

- Stage 1 GFR greater than 90 ml/min/1.73 m^2
- Stage 2 GFR-between 60 to 89 ml/min/1.73 m^2
- Stage 3a GFR 45 to 59 ml/min/1.73 m^2
- Stage 3b GFR 30 to 44 ml/min/1.73 m^2
- Stage 4 GFR of 15 to 29 ml/min/1.73 m^2
- Stage 5-GFR less than 15 ml/min/1.73 m^2 (end-stage renal disease)

This provides an easier estimation of GFR without the collection of urine or the use of exogenous materials. However, as they utilize serum creatinine, they are also affected by the issues around serum creatinine measurement; hence the correction for the race, gender, and age is required.

2. **Blood Urea Nitrogen (BUN):** BUN, also known as urea, is a nitrogen-containing substance that is produced in the liver as a byproduct of the urea cycle and protein metabolism. The kidneys remove about 85% of urea; the gastrointestinal (GI) tract excretes the remaining urea. When renal clearance is reduced, such as in acute and chronic renal failure or impairment, serum urea levels rise. In addition to renal

diseases, other conditions like upper gastrointestinal bleeding, dehydration, catabolic states, and high-protein diets can also cause an increase in urea. Starvation, a low-protein diet, and severe liver disease may cause a decrease in urea. Although urea increases earlier in renal disease, serum creatinine provides a more accurate measure of renal function. When the BUN is elevated, the ratio of BUN to creatinine can be helpful in distinguishing between pre-renal and renal causes. The ratio is closer to 20:1 in pre-renal illness and closer to 10:1 in intrinsic renal disease. A very high BUN to creatinine ratio (sometimes >30:1) has been linked to upper gastrointestinal bleeding.

3. **Cystatin C:** All of the body's nucleated cells produce the low-molecular-weight protein known as cystatin C, which can inhibit proteases. The kidneys freely filter it and form it at a steady rate. The glomerular filtration rate and serum levels of cystatin C have an inverse relationship (GFR). Stated differently, high values correspond to low GFRs and lower values, like creatinine, correspond to higher GFRs. Cystatin C is handled by the kidneys differently than creatinine. While both are freely filtered by glomeruli, unlike creatinine, cystatin C is reabsorbed and metabolized by proximal renal tubules after it has been filtered. Therefore, cystatin C does not significantly enter the final excreted urine under normal circumstances. Serum and urine are used to measure cyclostatin C. The fact that cystatin C is unaffected by age, muscle mass, or diet gives it an advantage over creatinine. Moreover, many studies have shown that cystatin C is a more accurate indicator of GFR than creatinine, especially in cases of early renal impairment. eGFR equations that include cystatin C, like the creatinine-cystatin KDIGO CKD-EPI equation, have also been updated. The concentration of cystatin C may be impacted by smoking, thyroid conditions, and cancer.

5.2.2.1.2. Albuminuria and Proteinuria

The abnormal presence of albumin in the urine is referred to as albuminuria. Urine albumin is the only term used these days to refer to the biochemical molecule known as microalbumin, which is thought to be obsolete. In diabetics, albuminuria serves as a marker for the early identification of nephropathy. Due to its association with elevated endothelial permeability, it serves as a separate marker for both chronic renal impairment and cardiovascular disease. Urine albumin can be measured as an albumin/creatinine ratio in 24-hour urine collections or in early morning/random specimens. When albuminuria is present twice and a urinary tract infection is ruled out, this suggests glomerular dysfunction. A three-month or longer duration of albuminuria is suggestive of chronic kidney disease. More than 300 mg of protein per day is the threshold for Frank proteinuria. A normal amount of urine protein is 150 mg/day (30% albumin, 30% globulins, and 40% Tamm Horsfall protein).

Increased amounts of protein in the urine may be due to:

- Glomerular proteinuria: Caused by defects in permselectivity of the glomerular filtration barrier to plasma proteins (for example, glomerulonephritis or nephrotic syndrome)

- Tubular proteinuria: Caused by incomplete tubular reabsorption of proteins (for example, interstitial nephritis)
- Overflow proteinuria: Caused by increased plasma concentration of proteins (for example, multiple myeloma-Bence Jones protein, myoglobinuria)
- Urinary tract inflammation or tumor

Urine protein may be measured using either a 24-hour urine collection or random urine protein: creatinine ratio (an early morning sample is preferred since it is a near representative of the 24-hour sample).

The KDIGO classification defines three stages of albuminuria:

- A1: Less than 30 mg/g creatinine
- A2: 30 to 300 mg/g creatinine
- A3: Greater than 300 mg/g creatinine

In nephrotic syndrome, urine protein excretion exceeds 3.5 g per day and is associated with edema, hypoalbuminemia, and hypercholesterolemia.

5.2.2.1.3. Tests of Tubular Function

To reabsorb electrolytes, and water, and to maintain the acid-base balance, the renal tubules are essential. Urine can be used to measure electrolytes such as sodium, potassium, chloride, magnesium, and phosphate in addition to glucose. Urine osmolality measurement enables evaluation of urine tubule concentrating capacity (Kamianowska et al., 2019). A urinary osmolality greater than 750 mOsmol/kg H_2O indicates that tubules are capable of concentrating normally. To rule out nephrogenic diabetes insipidus, a water deprivation test can be utilized. Additionally, if the urine cannot be acidified to a pH of less than 5.3, an ammonium chloride test can be used to confirm the diagnosis of distal renal tubular acidosis (RTA). Aminoaciduria, glycosuria, phosphaturia, and bicarbonate wasting (proximal RTA) are all present in Fanconi's syndrome.

5.2.2.1.4. Urine Analysis

Urine analysis is the evaluation of urine properties to support the diagnosis of illness. It entails microscopic inspection, chemical analysis, and physical observation. During the physical examination, color and clarity are evaluated. Normal urine is straw in color; urine that has been dehydrated is darker in color. Red pee may be a sign of porphyria or hematuria, or it may be an indication of eating foods like beets. When a urinary tract infection is the cause of pyuria, cloudy urine may be observed. The renal concentrating ability can be chemically determined with a urine dipstick or refractometry-based. Specific gravity is a measure of this ability. Specific gravity has a physiological range of 1.003 to 1.030. Urine that is concentrated has a higher specific gravity than urine that is diluted. Urine dipsticks use chemical analysis to provide a qualitative analysis of various analytes found in urine. To find out whether there is protein, glucose, blood, ketones, bilirubin, urobilinogen, nitrite, and leukocyte esterase, Dipstick uses dry chemistry techniques. One test that can be used as a point-of-care is the dipstick. To interpret the results, the color changes that occur when the urine interacts with the chemical reagents that are impregnated on the dipstick's paper are compared to the color chart guide. In healthy urine specimens, analytes tested on urine dipstick protein shouldn't be detectable. Normal urine does not contain bilirubin. When the renal threshold of 180 mg/dl is lowered, glucose can be observed in renal glycosuria, diabetes mellitus, and pregnant patients. It is not detected in healthy individuals. Results may be impacted by the use of some antibiotics and ascorbic acid (vitamin C). After renal tract damage or infection, blood may be present; ascorbic acid can lead to a falsely negative result. The difference between myoglobin and hemoglobin in urine cannot be distinguished by a urine dipstick since it only detects the globin component of hemoglobin.

Hemoglobinuria and undamaged red blood cells (RBC) are also found. When rhabdomyolysis is present on a urine dipstick test and the RBC count is normal, it can be distinguished from hematuria, which also shows RBCs on the urine dipstick. White blood cells (WBC) range from 0 to 5 and red blood cells (RBC) from 0 to 3 in normal urine. Diabetic ketoacidosis, severe vomiting, and fasting all contain ketones. A urine dipstick can identify only acetone and acetoacetate; it cannot identify beta-hydroxybutyrate, a ketone. Conjugated hyperbilirubinemia results in the presence of bilirubin. While urobilinogen may normally be present, it is increased in the presence of prehepatic jaundice and hemolysis and absent in conjugated hyperbilirubinemia. Leucocyte esterase and nitrite are markers of urinary tract infections. Certain bacteria, like those in the Enterobacteriaceae family, change nitrates into nitrites. Urine is subjected to a wet-prep analysis as part of the microscopic analysis to determine whether microorganisms and/or cells, casts, and crystals are present. White blood cell casts are consistent with pyelonephritis, whereas red blood cell casts typically indicate glomerulonephritis. Red blood cells indicate renal injury, white blood cells and WBC casts indicate infection, and RBC casts indicate tubular damage or glomerulonephritis. Protein-based hyaline casts can develop in glomerular disease. Nephrotic syndrome is associated with fatty casts.

Crystals may also be identified in urine and are indicative of the following conditions:

- Triple phosphate crystals have the "coffin-lid" appearance and can be seen in alkaline urine and urinary tract infections.
- Uric acid crystals are needle-shaped and are associated with gout.
- Oxalate crystals are envelope-shaped and are present in ethylene glycol poisoning or primary and secondary hyperoxaluria.
- Cystine crystals are hexagonal and are observed in cystinuria.

The best specimen for urine analysis is freshly voided midstream urine. Midstream urine is less likely to be contaminated by commensal bacteria and epithelial cells.

5.2.2.2. Acute Versus Chronic Renal Impairment

Acute renal impairment or acute kidney injury (AKI) refers to the sudden onset of kidney injury within a period of a few hours or days. Chronic kidney disease (CKD) is caused by long-term diseases such as hypertension and diabetes. Causes of acute kidney injury can be divided into the following:

- Causes that result in decreased blood flow to the kidneys (pre-renal causes), for example, hypotensive and cardiogenic shock, dehydration, and blood loss from major trauma
- Causes that result in direct damage to the kidneys (renal /intrinsic causes) such as damage to kidneys by nephrotoxic medications and other toxins, sepsis, cancers such as myeloma, autoimmune diseases or conditions that cause inflammation, or damage to the kidney tubules
- Causes that result in blockage of the urinary tract such as bladder, prostate, or cervical cancer, large kidney stones, and blood clots in the urinary tract

It is important to note that pre-renal kidney injury may progress to acute tubular necrosis (ATN) and cause intrinsic renal injury.

Guidelines for defining AKI use urine output as a useful tool for assessing kidney function. AKI patients exhibit oliguria (less than 400 milliliters per day). Based on serum creatinine, GFR variations, and urine output determinants, the RIFLE classification system categorizes patients according to risk, injury, failure, loss of kidney function, and end-stage kidney disease. Urine output and changes in serum creatinine are also used by the Acute Kidney Injury Network (AKIN) to classify acute kidney injury (AKI); however, GFR changes and a baseline serum creatinine are not required. In addition to serum creatinine, other laboratory tests are essential for diagnosing AKI and helping to distinguish between various forms of acute kidney injury. This is crucial because it will establish the best course of care for the patient, treating patients with fluid replacement for pre-renal causes. On the other hand, fluids would be administered more cautiously to those with renal and post-renal causes. The specific gravity is measured, and it is increased (greater than 1.020) in dehydration and pre-renal causes. This measurement helps determine whether the renal injury is pre-renal, renal, or post-renal. Under light microscopy, the differential diagnosis can be aided by the identification of casts, crystals, tubular epithelial cells, white and red blood cells, or other materials in the urine sediment.

Acute tubular necrosis and pre-renal uremia can be distinguished from one another using fractional excretion of sodium (FeNa). Measurements of creatinine and sodium in serum as well as creatinine and sodium in spot urine specimens are necessary. The formula for calculating fractional excretion is FeNa = 100 x (urine sodium x serum creatinine) / (serum sodium x urine creatinine). Pre-renal causes are indicated by values less than 1% and intrinsic causes by values more than 2%. However, the FeNa is unreliable in patients on diuretic therapy. Less than 20 mmol/l of sodium in spot urine is indicative of pre-renal acute kidney injury. The presence of pre-renal versus intrinsic AKI can also be assessed by fractional excretion of urea, which is calculated similarly to FeNa but uses urine and serum urea instead of sodium. Values less than 35% indicate pre-renal injury. An osmolality in urine that is comparable to serum (roughly 300 mOsm/kg) indicates an intrinsic cause, whereas a value above 500 mOsm/kg is linked to pre-renal causes.

5.2.2.3. Novel Biomarkers

It has been reported that many novel biomarkers can be used to measure AKI and distinguish it from pre-renal and intrinsic AKI, as well as from AKI and stable CKD. The proteins that are produced in response to cellular or tissue injury include beta-trace protein, kidney injury molecule 1 (KIM-1), L-type fatty acid-binding protein (L-FABP), FGF23 (fibroblast growth factor 23), and NGAL (neutrophil gelatinase-associated lipocalin). Low-molecular-weight proteins that are present in the systemic circulation and undergo glomerular filtration include cystatin C, beta2-microglobulin, and retinol-binding protein. Further research will be necessary to realize their maximum clinical utility.

5.2.3. Indications

Renal function assessments can be performed in a variety of contexts, from acute emergency rooms to long-term care facilities. Renal function tests are primarily carried out to diagnose renal disease, choose the best course of treatment for the patient, and stop further decline in renal function. Further indications for patients in whom renal disease has been diagnosed include determining the type or level of renal disease, tracking its progression to guarantee prompt and effective management, and assessing the effectiveness of interventions. In other situations, when a known or potentially nephrotoxic therapeutic agent is started for patient management, renal function tests might be necessary to determine and track renal function (Okoro & Farate, 2019). Renal function tests are also recommended for transplant candidates to determine their initial suitability as donors and, subsequently, to identify any notable decline in renal function following donation. Renal function tests can also be used to determine the specific area of the kidney's functional unit (nephron) that is impacted, such as tubular versus glomerular disease.

5.2.4. Potential Diagnosis

The glomerular filtration rate can be directly measured or estimated through renal function tests, which can then be used to evaluate overall renal function. The GFR is estimated to ascertain whether renal impairment is present. It can detect the existence and stage of chronic kidney disease if reduced over a predetermined amount of time. Renal function tests can also be used to identify whether the renal disease is acute or chronic. Urine albumin can be used to identify patients who are at-risk for developing nephropathy, such as those who have diabetes. Tests of renal function, specifically the measurement of urine amino acids, glucose, phosphate, and pH, can identify disorders of tubular function, including Fanconi syndrome.

5.2.5. Normal and Critical Findings

An adult male's GFR typically ranges from 90 to 120 ml per minute. End-stage renal failure is defined as a GFR of less than 15 ml/min and necessitates renal replacement therapy, e.g., dialysis. The existence of renal disease, which can be demonstrated by imaging or albuminuria/proteinuria, is not ruled out by a normal GFR. Age and gender determine the reference intervals for serum creatinine and urea. In addition to pathological factors, the length of urine collection, the hydration state, and the clinical context all affect the presence of electrolytes in urine. Reference intervals are frequently broad.

5.2.6. Interfering Factors

- **Creatinine:** Elevated creatinine levels can result from preanalytical factors like a high protein diet and increased muscle mass, but they don't accurately reflect a person's actual renal function. Similarly, serum creatinine is not always a reliable indicator of renal function in people with decreased muscle mass, such as the elderly, amputees, and those with muscular dystrophy. Using an enzymatic assay or a colorimetric reaction called the Jaffe reaction, creatinine is typically measured on automated analyzers. The creation of an alkaline picrate is a step in the Jaffe reaction. It is susceptible to both positive (like bilirubin) and negative (like ketones and proteins) interferences. To address some of these problems, the Jaffe reaction has undergone many modifications.
- **BUN:** Serum urea/BUN concentrations may also be raised in the presence of a high-protein diet or with patients using oral corticosteroids.

- **Urine Albumin and Protein:** Urine albumin or protein may be increased in the presence of conditions not related to renal disease, for example, posture, fever, and exercise. Furthermore, in the presence of a urinary tract infection, urine protein levels may be raised without any intrinsic renal pathology present.

5.2.7. Complications

Aside from issues with venepuncture, most renal function tests have few complications. Isotope-based GFR measurements could result in very little radiation exposure. Short bursts of repeated exposure are not recommended, though. Iodine-containing radiocontrast agents have the potential to cause allergic reactions in certain patients.

5.2.8. Patient Safety and Education

Patients should be informed about the small amounts of ionizing radiation they will be exposed to during the GFR measurement using radioactive isotopes. Before this test is performed, any female of childbearing age must rule out pregnancy. Patients should generally be informed about the possibility of pain and bruising when having blood drawn. Urine collection bottles meant for 24 hours might include trace amounts of preservatives like thymol, so it's important to keep them away from skin and mucous membranes. Keep collection bottles out of the reach of small children so they can't inadvertently swallow the preservatives inside. Before these tests, patients ought to be counseled to continue consuming fluids on a regular basis.

5.2.9. Clinical Significance

- **Creatinine:** Serum creatinine is elevated when there is a significant reduction in the glomerular filtration rate or when urine elimination is obstructed. About 50% of kidney function must be lost before a rise in serum creatinine can be detected. Thus, serum creatinine is a late marker of acute kidney injury.
- **BUN:** Serum urea/BUN level increases in acute and chronic renal disease.

  eGFR equations are used to determine the presence of renal disease, and stage of CKD, and to monitor response to treatment.

5.3. Evaluation of Kidney Function

Most people are aware that the kidneys' primary job is to flush the body of waste materials and extra fluid. The urine eliminates these waste materials and extra fluid. Urine is produced by extremely intricate processes of excretion and reabsorption. This procedure is required to keep the chemical balance in the body steady. The kidneys play a crucial role in controlling the body's salt, potassium, and acid content. In addition, the kidneys generate hormones that impact the operation of other organs. For instance, the kidneys produce a hormone that increases the production of red blood cells. The kidneys also produce other hormones that are involved in blood pressure regulation and calcium metabolism control.

The kidneys are powerful chemical factories that perform the following functions:

- remove waste products from the body
- remove drugs from the body
- balance the body's fluids
- release hormones that regulate blood pressure
- produce an active form of vitamin D that promotes strong, healthy bones
- control the production of red blood cells

Functions of a healthy kidney include maintaining a person's fluid balance, maintaining an acid-base balance; regulating electrolytes including sodium, potassium, and other electrolytes; clearing toxins; regulating blood pressure; and regulating hormones, such as erythropoietin; and activation of vitamin D.

5.3.1. Description

The kidney's many tasks include maintaining the proper ratio of acid to base in the body, controlling fluid balance, regulating sodium, potassium, and other electrolytes, eliminating toxins, absorbing glucose, amino acids, and other small molecules, controlling blood pressure, producing different hormones like erythropoietin, and activating vitamin D. The best indicator of the kidney's overall performance is the glomerular filtration rate (GFR). GFR estimates are used in clinical settings to monitor the course of a patient's illness and assess the extent of kidney impairment. However, the kidney disease's etiology is not disclosed by the GFR. The methods used to achieve this include kidney imaging, urine protein excretion measurement, urinalysis, and, if required, kidney biopsy (Levey et al., 2020).

The nephron, the smallest functional unit of the kidney, is the level at which most research on renal physiology is conducted. The filtration component of each nephron starts the process of filtering the blood that enters the kidney. The filtrate then travels the entire length of the nephron, a tubular organ encircled by capillaries and lined with a single layer of specialized cells. These lining cellular primary jobs include secreting waste products from the blood into the urine and reabsorbing water and other tiny molecules from the filtrate back into the blood. The kidney needs enough blood to be received and filtered for proper function. Renal corpuscles, which are made up of a glomerulus and a Bowman's capsule, are hundreds of thousands of filtration units that carry out this function at the microscopic level. Estimating the rate of filtration, also known as the glomerular filtration rate (GFR), is a common method used to determine a comprehensive evaluation of renal function.

5.3.2. Clinical Assessment

Kidney function can be evaluated through clinical assessment. This is due to the possibility of developing symptoms in an individual with kidney disease. For instance, edema may arise in a patient with chronic kidney disease as a result of the kidneys' inability to control the water balance. They might start to exhibit indicators of chronic kidney disease, such as high blood pressure, osteoporosis, or anemia, which can be used to gauge the disease's severity. The inability of the kidneys to eliminate urea can cause disorientation or a generalized itching sensation. Clinical assessment, which includes a variety of techniques for diagnosing, tracking, and managing renal health, is essential to assessing kidney function. This comprehensive approach combines physical examination, history of the patient, and multiple diagnostic tests to provide a thorough understanding of kidney function. A thorough patient history is the first step in the clinical assessment process. During this time, medical professionals ask about any symptoms—such as weariness, swelling, and changes in urine output, and hypertension— that could point to kidney dysfunction. Additionally examined are risk factors for kidney disease such as diabetes, hypertension, exposure to nephrotoxic agents, and family history of kidney disease. This data directs additional diagnostic testing and aids in the identification of people who are more vulnerable. A physical examination is then performed, with an emphasis on looking for symptoms of renal impairment. This includes looking for edema, as it may indicate fluid retention brought on by compromised kidney function. Since hypertension can lead to kidney disease as well as be a cause of it, measuring blood pressure is essential. A thorough cardiovascular examination is also necessary due to the close relationship that exists between kidney and heart health.

Diagnosing kidney function clinically starts with laboratory testing. Since creatinine is a byproduct of muscle metabolism that the kidneys filter out, serum creatinine levels are regularly measured. Increased levels of creatinine in the serum signify a decrease in kidney filtration. Another important indicator is blood urea nitrogen (BUN), which shows how well the kidneys are able to eliminate urea, a waste product of protein metabolism. However, factors other than kidney function can also affect serum creatinine and BUN levels, so these tests should be used in conjunction with other evaluations. The gold standard for assessing kidney function is the glomerular filtration rate (GFR), which gives an estimate of the volume of blood the kidneys filter minutely. Formulas that take into account body size, sex, age, and serum creatinine levels are used to calculate GFR. GFR values below 60 mL/min/1.73 m^2 for longer than three months indicate CKD, while values above 90 mL/min/1.73 m^2 are considered normal. Kidney failure is indicated by a GFR of less than 15 mL/min/1.73 m^2, which calls for dialysis or kidney transplantation.

The examination of urine for anomalies such as proteinuria (excess protein), hematuria (blood), and the presence of glucose is known as urinalysis, and it is another essential step. Whereas hematuria may indicate kidney stones, infections, or glomerular diseases, proteinuria may be an early sign of kidney damage, frequently observed in conditions such as diabetic nephropathy. Urine examination under a microscope can reveal casts, cells, and crystals, offering more information about the condition of the kidneys. Imaging studies provide visual details about kidney anatomy and function, which improve clinical assessment. Ultrasonography is frequently used to measure kidney size and find blockages, tumors, and cysts. For a thorough anatomical assessment or to direct biopsies, more sophisticated imaging methods like CT or MRI scans might be necessary. Kidney biopsies are sometimes carried out, especially in situations where the etiology of renal dysfunction is unknown or when a precise diagnosis is required to direct medical intervention. A kidney biopsy entails removing a tiny sample of tissue, which is then viewed under a microscope to look for pathological alterations.

5.3.3. Urine Tests

Urine and its contents are measured as part of the evaluation of kidney function. Urine output can be abnormally high or low depending on the kidneys. Urine albumin or urine protein levels are commonly used to assess the kidneys' capacity to filter protein. These tests can be performed once or every 24 hours due to daily variations in the results. A key component of nephrology is the evaluation of kidney function by measuring urine and its contents. This method provides important information about renal health and helps diagnose a variety of kidney disorders. The most popular and non-invasive test for analyzing urine is urinalysis. Urine's physical, chemical, and microscopic characteristics are examined as part of a series of tests that give a thorough picture of renal function and general health. Urine is physically examined to determine its color, clarity, and odor. Normal urine color usually varies, from light yellow to deep amber, based on the amount of hydration. Different conditions can be indicated by abnormal colors. For example, red or brown urine may indicate the presence of blood (hematuria), which can be caused by infections, kidney stones, or more serious conditions like cancer or glomerulonephritis. A urinary tract infection or inflammation may be suggested by cloudy urine, which can also indicate the presence of pus (pyuria). Odd smells can also give hints; for example, sweet-smelling urine may be a sign of diabetes mellitus.

Dipstick tests, which entail dipping a reagent strip into the urine sample, are used to analyze urine chemically. When certain substances are present, the color of the strip changes. pH, protein, glucose, ketones, hemoglobin, bilirubin, urobilinogen, nitrites, and leukocyte esterase are among the important elements that are measured. Urine pH can reveal the body's acid-base equilibrium; deviations from this range may indicate metabolic or respiratory problems. One important indicator of kidney damage is the presence of protein (proteinuria), which is frequently observed in disorders like glomerular diseases and diabetic nephropathy. When a diabetic has poor blood sugar control, it is usually indicated by glucose in the urine (glucosuria). Severe starvation or uncontrolled diabetes may have ketones in their bodies. While bilirubin and urobilinogen levels can point to liver dysfunction or hemolytic disorders, hemoglobin in the urine may indicate hematuria or hemolysis. A urinary tract bacterial infection is indicated by the presence of nitrites and leukocyte esterase. Urine sediment can be examined microscopic by centrifuging a urine sample and looking at the sediment under a microscope. Microorganisms, casts, cells, and crystals can all be found with this analysis. White blood cells suggest pyuria, while red blood cells can confirm hematuria. These are both indicators of potential infection or inflammation. If epithelial cells are detected in large quantities, they may indicate genital tract contamination. Different types of renal pathologies can be indicated by different types of urinary casts, which are cylindrical structures formed in the renal tubules. These types of casts include hyaline, granular, red blood cell, and white blood cell casts. Depending on the kind, crystals in the urine can indicate diseases like kidney stones or metabolic issues.

5.3.4. Blood Tests

Renal function is also evaluated through blood tests. These consist of exams designed to measure kidney function directly as well as exams that evaluate kidney function by searching for signs of issues related to abnormal function. The GFR is one way to assess kidney function. Additional tests that can evaluate the kidneys' function include measuring potassium and phosphate levels in the blood, measuring bicarbonate levels in a vein to determine the acid-base status, and checking the whole blood count for anemia.

5.3.4.1. Glomerular Filtration Rate

The amount of fluid filtered into the Bowman's capsule per unit of time from the renal (kidney) glomerular capillaries is known as the glomerular filtration rate, or GFR. An effective way to approximate the GFR is to measure the volume of blood plasma that is cleared of creatinine per unit of time, or creatinine clearance. The differential basal tone of the afferent and efferent arterioles is essential for the physiologic maintenance of GFR. Stated differently, the filtration rate is reliant on the difference between the lower blood pressure produced by less vasoconstriction of the output, or efferent arteriole, and the higher blood pressure created by the input, or afferent arteriole, vasoconstriction.

When any solute is freely filtered and not secreted or reabsorbed by the kidneys, GFR is equal to the renal clearance ratio. Therefore, the amount of the substance in the urine that came from a calculable volume of blood is the rate that is measured. Applying this idea to the following equation, the mass of the substance expelled during the urine collection period is equal to the product of urine flow and concentration for the substance used. Since nothing is added to or taken out of the nephron, this mass is equal to the mass filtered at the glomerulus. This mass's initial plasma volume can be calculated by dividing it by the plasma concentration. This yields the volume of plasma fluid that entered Bowman's capsule during the previously mentioned time frame. Usually, the GFR is expressed in volume per time, or e.g., mL/min, or milliliters per minute. As opposed to the filtration fraction.

$$GFR = \frac{\text{Urine Concentration} \times \text{Urine Flow}}{\text{Plasma Concentration}}$$

The glomerular filtration rate (GFR or eGFR) can be estimated or calculated using a variety of methods. Only when the GFR equals the Clearance Rate does the aforementioned formula apply to the GFR calculation. When body surface area is taken into account, the normal range of GFR is 100–130: average 125 (mL/min)/(1.73 m^2) for men and 90–120 (mL/min)/(1.73 m^2) for women under 40. Until the age of two years old in both genders, the GFR in children as determined by inulin clearance is 110 (mL/min)/(1.73 m^2), after which it gradually drops. GFR gradually drops with age after the age of 40, by 0–1± mL/min annually. Clinical practice guidelines and regulatory agencies now recommend estimated GFR (eGFR) for routine GFR evaluation, while measured GFR (mGFR) is advised as a confirmatory test when a more precise assessment is needed.

5.3.5. Medical Imaging

Medical imaging can also be used to evaluate kidney function. Certain imaging modalities, like kidney ultrasounds or CT scans, can evaluate kidney function by spotting small or shriveled kidneys, which are signs of chronic disease that can affect function. Other tests, like those in nuclear medicine, measure the perfusion and excretion of radioactive materials through the kidneys to evaluate kidney function directly. A crucial aspect of nephrology and urology is the evaluation of kidney function using medical imaging, which offers comprehensive anatomical and functional details about the kidneys. A range of imaging modalities are employed to facilitate the visualization of the kidneys, detect anomalies, and steer clinical interventions. One of the most popular imaging methods for assessing kidney function is ultrasound. It uses high-frequency sound waves to create images of the kidneys so that their size, structure, and form can be evaluated. When it comes to diagnosing diseases like hydronephrosis—a condition in which the flow of urine is obstructed, leading to kidney swelling—and identifying obstructions like kidney stones or tumors, ultrasound is especially helpful. It is a first-line imaging option in many clinical scenarios because it is non-invasive, safe, and reasonably priced.

When compared to ultrasound, computed tomography (CT) scans provide more precise cross-sectional images of the kidneys. When identifying and characterizing complex renal masses, stones, and infections, CT scans are especially helpful. A specific kind of CT scan called a CT urography uses contrast material to make the urinary tract more visible, which facilitates a thorough evaluation of the bladder, ureters, and renal parenchyma. This method works very well for finding tumors, congenital abnormalities, and obstructions in the urinary tract. An additional sophisticated imaging technique used to evaluate kidney function is magnetic resonance imaging (MRI). For certain patients, like those who need repeat imaging or are pregnant, MRI offers high-resolution images and excellent contrast between various soft tissues without the use of ionizing radiation, making it a safer option. When assessing tumors, vascular disorders, and complex renal cysts, MRI is especially helpful. Renal artery stenosis is one condition that can be evaluated with magnetic resonance angiography (MRA), and it can lead to hypertension and kidney dysfunction.

Renal scintigraphy is one type of nuclear medicine scan that can reveal functional information about the kidneys. With this method, a tiny amount of radioactive material is injected, taken up by the kidneys, and then imaged with a gamma camera. Renal scintigraphy provides quantitative information regarding the health of individual kidneys by evaluating renal perfusion, function, and excretion. When assessing diseases such as obstructive uropathy, renal artery stenosis, and differential renal function in cases of asymmetry, it is especially helpful. Intravenous pyelography (IVP) has been less common with the development of more sophisticated imaging methods, but it is still useful in certain situations. A contrast dye is injected into the bloodstream during intravenous hemodialysis (IVD), where it is filtered by the kidneys and visible on X-rays. By emphasizing the kidneys, ureters, and bladder, this technique can aid in the detection of structural irregularities and blockages. An additional imaging modality that offers fine-grained pictures of the renal vasculature is angiography. It entails giving the blood vessels a contrast agent injection, followed by X-ray imaging to see blood flow and spot obstructions or anomalies in the renal arteries and veins. Digital subtraction angiography (DSA) removes background structures from images to improve blood vessel clarity.

5.3.6. Kidney Function in Disease

Numerous forms of kidney disease can result in a reduced ability to function the kidneys. When a patient presents with reduced kidney function, a renal ultrasound, a urinalysis, and a history and physical examination should all be conducted. Medication, edema, nocturia, gross hematuria, family history of kidney disease, diabetes, and polyuria are the most pertinent aspects of the history. Signs of endocarditis, diabetes, lupus erythematosus, vasculitis, and hypertension are the most significant findings in a physical examination. Even in cases where there is no pathology, a urinalysis is still recommended because this result points to an extrarenal etiology. Urinary sedimentation and/or proteinuria are typical signs of glomerular disease. Both glomerular disease and disorders affecting the urinary tract can result in hematuria. In a renal ultrasound, the most important evaluations are renal sizes, echogenicity, and any indications of hydronephrosis. Typically, focal segmental glomerular sclerosis, myeloma, or diabetic nephropathy are indicated by renal enlargement. Chronic renal disease with a long history is suggested by renal atrophy.

5.3.7. Chronic Kidney Disease Stages

Diabetes, high blood pressure, a family history of kidney disease, aging, ethnicity, and smoking are risk factors for kidney disease. In most cases, a GFR of more than 60 (mL/min)/(1.73 m^2) is sufficient. On the other hand, a marked drop in GFR from a prior test result may be a precursor to kidney disease that calls for medical attention. There is a higher chance of conserving the remaining nephrons and avoiding the need for dialysis if kidney disease is identified and treated early (Table 5.3).

Table 5.3. Risk Factors for Kidney Disease

CKD Stage	GFR Level ((mL/min)/(1.73 m^2))
Stage 1	≥ 90
Stage 2	60–89
Stage 3	30–59
Stage 4	15–29
Stage 5	< 15

Source: *https://en.wikipedia.org/wiki/Assessment_of_kidney_function#Description.*

The severity of chronic kidney disease (CKD) is described by six stages; the most severe three are defined by the MDRD-eGFR value, and the first three also depend on whether there is other evidence of kidney disease (e.g., proteinuria):

1. Normal kidney function – GFR above 90 (mL/min)/(1.73 m^2) and no proteinuria
2. CKD1 – GFR above 90 (mL/min)/(1.73 m^2) with evidence of kidney damage
3. CKD2 (mild) – GFR of 60 to 89 (mL/min)/(1.73 m^2) with evidence of kidney damage
4. CKD3 (moderate) – GFR of 30 to 59 (mL/min)/(1.73 m^2)
5. CKD4 (severe) – GFR of 15 to 29 (mL/min)/(1.73 m^2)
6. CKD5 kidney failure – GFR less than 15 (mL/min)/(1.73 m^2) Some people add CKD5D for those stage 5 patients requiring dialysis; many patients in CKD5 are not yet on dialysis.

Note: others add a "T" to patients who have had a transplant regardless of stage.

The aforementioned classification is not universally accepted by clinicians, with some arguing that it may incorrectly diagnose individuals, particularly the elderly, with mildly reduced kidney function as an illness. Kidney Disease: Improving Global Outcomes (KDIGO) organized a conference in 2009 to discuss these issues and to gather information on the prognosis of CKD to improve the staging and definition of the disease.

5.3.8. Ways to Keep the Kidneys Healthy

Kidney issues may be avoided by leading an active lifestyle and eating a healthy diet. However, there are some things you can do to raise your risk of kidney disease or damage. Your kidneys are the fist-sized organs on both sides of your spine that are situated at the base of your rib cage. They serve a variety of purposes. Above all, they clean your blood by removing impurities, excess water, and waste products. Urine is the subsequent method by which these waste products are released from your bladder. Your kidneys also control potassium, salt, and pH levels in your body. They also generate the hormones that control red blood cell production and blood pressure. To help your body absorb calcium for bone growth and muscle regulation, your kidneys also activate a form of vitamin D. Your general health and well-being depend on maintaining kidney health. Your body will properly filter and eliminate waste, as well as produce hormones to support proper bodily function, if your kidneys are kept in good health.

Here are some tips to help keep your kidneys healthy.

1. **Keep Active and Fit:** Exercise on a regular basis benefits your health in more ways than one. The risk of chronic kidney disease may be reduced by it. Additionally, it can lower blood pressure and improve heart health, both of which are critical in preventing kidney damage. Running marathons is not a requirement to enjoy the benefits of exercise. Exercises like walking, running, cycling, and even dancing are very beneficial to your health. Find something enjoyable to do and keep yourself occupied. You'll find it easier to maintain and get excellent outcomes.
2. **Manage Your Blood Sugar:** Kidney damage can occur in people with diabetes or other conditions that result in high blood sugar. Your kidneys have to work harder to filter your blood when the glucose (sugar) in it cannot be used by your body's cells. Years of exertion may cause potentially fatal consequences from this. Nonetheless, you lessen the chance of harm if you can control your blood sugar. Additionally, a doctor can take action to lessen or stop further damage if the damage is discovered early.
3. **Monitor Blood Pressure:** Kidney damage can result from high blood pressure. Your body may experience major effects if high blood pressure coexists with other conditions like diabetes, heart disease, or high cholesterol. 120/80 is a healthy blood pressure reading. The range of prehypertension is 139/89 and that point. At this point, dietary and lifestyle modifications may help lower your blood pressure. You may have high blood pressure if your readings are routinely higher than 140/90. You should consult a physician about changing your lifestyle, taking medication, and routinely checking your blood pressure.
4. **Monitor Weight and Eat a Balanced Diet:** Obesity and being overweight put a person at risk for several illnesses that can harm the kidneys. Diabetes, heart disease, and kidney disease are a few of these. Kidney damage may be prevented with a balanced diet low in processed meats, sodium, and other foods that damage the kidneys. Eat as much fresh food as possible that is naturally low in sodium, such as whole grains, cauliflower, blueberries, and fish.
5. **Drink Plenty of Fluids:** The cliched recommendation to drink eight glasses of water a day is not magical, but it is a good goal because it motivates you to stay hydrated. Consuming water on a regular basis is beneficial to your kidneys. Water aids in the kidneys' removal of toxins and sodium. It also lessens the chance of developing chronic renal disease. At least 1.5 to 2 liters should be your daily goal. How much water you actually need depends largely

on your lifestyle and state of health. When planning your daily water intake, it's important to take into account factors like climate, exercise, gender, general health, and whether you're nursing or pregnant. To help avoid future stone deposits, people who have previously had kidney stones should drink a little bit more water.

6. **Don't Smoke:** Smoking damages your body's blood vessels. This leads to slower blood flow throughout your body and to your kidneys.

Smoking also puts your kidneys at an increased risk for cancer. If you smoke and stop smoking, your risk will drop. However, it'll take many years Trusted Source to return to the risk level of a person who's never smoked.

7. **Be Aware of the Amount of OTC Pills You Take:** You might be harming your kidneys if you take over-the-counter (OTC) painkillers regularly. If you take nonsteroidal anti-inflammatory drugs (NSAIDs) regularly for arthritis, headaches, or chronic pain, such as ibuprofen and naproxen, you run the risk of kidney damage. The National Kidney Foundation states that these drugs shouldn't be taken for more than three days in the case of a fever or more than 10 days in the case of pain. If you take more than eight aspirin tablets daily, your kidney function may be temporarily or permanently reduced. Individuals who take the medication occasionally and don't have kidney problems should be safe. But if you take these drugs regularly, you might be endangering the health of your kidneys. If you're managing pain, see a doctor about kidney-safe treatments.

8. **Have Your Kidney Function Tested if You're at High Risk:** If you're at high risk of kidney damage or kidney disease, it's a good idea to have regular kidney function tests. The following people may benefit from regular screening:
   - people who are over 60 years old
   - people who were born with a low birth weight
   - people who have cardiovascular disease or have family members with it
   - people who have or have a family history of high blood pressure
   - people who have obesity
   - people who believe they may have kidney damage

A regular kidney function test is a great way to know your kidney's health and to check for possible changes. Getting ahead of any damage can help slow or prevent future damage (Lote, 2012).

A Closer Look

Glomerular Filtration Rate (GFR)

Glomerular filtration rate (GFR) is a key indicator of kidney function that measures the volume of blood filtered by the glomeruli in the kidneys per minute. The glomeruli are tiny, intricate networks of capillaries within the nephrons, the functional units of the kidney. GFR reflects how well the kidneys are cleaning the blood and removing waste products and excess fluids. It is a critical parameter used in diagnosing and monitoring kidney diseases, particularly chronic kidney disease (CKD). A normal GFR varies by age, sex, and body size, but generally, a GFR of 90 mL/min/1.73 m^2 or higher is considered normal.

To estimate GFR, healthcare providers commonly use equations that factor in serum creatinine levels, age, sex, and race. Serum creatinine, a waste product of muscle metabolism, is filtered out by the kidneys, and its level in the blood provides an indirect measure of kidney function. The most widely used equations include the Modification of Diet in Renal Disease (MDRD) study equation and the Chronic Kidney Disease Epidemiology Collaboration (CKD-EPI) equation. The CKD-EPI equation is often preferred because it provides more accurate estimates across a wider range of GFR values and demographic groups.

GFR is categorized into different stages to assess the severity of kidney dysfunction. For instance, a GFR between 60 and 89 mL/min/1.73 m^2 may indicate mild kidney damage, especially if other markers such as proteinuria are present. A GFR between 30 and 59 mL/min/1.73 m^2 indicates moderate kidney damage, while a GFR between 15 and 29 mL/min/1.73 m^2 suggests severe kidney damage. A GFR below 15 mL/min/1.73 m^2 typically indicates kidney failure, where the kidneys can no longer maintain their necessary functions without medical intervention such as dialysis or a kidney transplant.

Monitoring GFR over time is crucial for individuals at risk of or diagnosed with CKD, as it helps in tracking the progression of the disease, guiding treatment decisions, and adjusting medication dosages. Regular assessment of GFR allows for early intervention, which can slow the progression of kidney disease and improve patient outcomes. Additionally, GFR is an important factor in managing other conditions that affect kidney health, such as diabetes and hypertension, as these conditions can accelerate the decline in kidney function.

Despite its importance, GFR estimation has limitations. The equations used can be less accurate in certain populations, such as those with extreme muscle mass variations, the elderly, or those with acute kidney injury (AKI). In such cases, direct measurement of GFR using exogenous markers like inulin, iohexol, or radiolabeled substances can be more accurate but are less commonly used due to their complexity and cost.

Summary

- Assessing kidney function is a crucial aspect of diagnosing and managing renal diseases, as well as monitoring overall health. The primary functions of the kidneys include filtering waste products from the blood, regulating fluid and electrolyte balance, and maintaining acid-base homeostasis.
- The glomerular filtration rate (GFR) is considered the best overall indicator of kidney function. GFR measures how much blood is filtered by the glomeruli (the tiny filtering units in the kidneys) each minute.
- In humans, the kidneys are two reddish-brown bean-shaped blood-filtering organs that are a multilobar, multipapillary form of mammalian kidneys, usually without signs of external lobulation.
- In humans, the kidneys are located high in the abdominal cavity, one on each side of the spine, and lie in a retroperitoneal position at a slightly oblique angle. The asymmetry within the abdominal cavity, caused by the position of the liver, typically results in the right kidney being slightly lower and smaller than the left, and being placed slightly more to the middle than the left kidney.
- The kidney and nervous system communicate via the renal plexus, whose fibers course along the renal arteries to reach each kidney.
- The kidneys excrete a variety of waste products produced by metabolism into the urine. The microscopic structural and functional unit of the kidney is the nephron. It processes the blood supplied to it via filtration, reabsorption, secretion and excretion; the consequence of those processes is the production of urine.
- Reabsorption is the transport of molecules from this ultrafiltrate and into the peritubular capillary. It is accomplished via selective receptors on the luminal cell membrane. Water is 55% reabsorbed in the proximal tubule.
- Secretion is the reverse of reabsorption: molecules are transported from the peritubular capillary through the interstitial fluid, then through the renal tubular cell and into the ultrafiltrate.
- Dialysis is a treatment that substitutes for the function of normal kidneys. Dialysis may be instituted when approximately 85%–90% of kidney function is lost, as indicated by a glomerular filtration rate (GFR) of less than 15.

References

1. Boga, M. S., & Sönmez, M. G. (2019). Long-term renal function following zero ischemia partial nephrectomy. *Research and Reports in Urology, 11*, 43–52.
2. Damiati, S. (2019). A pilot study to assess kidney functions and toxic dimethyl-arginines as risk biomarkers in women with low vitamin D levels. *Journal of Medical Biochemistry, 38*(2), 145–152.
3. Gai, Z., Wang, T., Visentin, M., Kullak-Ublick, G. A., Fu, X., & Wang, Z. (2019). Lipid accumulation and chronic kidney disease. *Nutrients, 11*(4). https://doi.org/10.3390/nu11040936.

4. Hounkpatin, H. O., Fraser, S. D., Glidewell, L., Blakeman, T., Lewington, A., & Roderick, P. J. (2019). Predicting risk of recurrent acute kidney injury: A systematic review. *Nephron, 142*(2), 83–90. https://doi.org/10.1159/000501749.
5. Kamianowska, M., Szczepański, M., & Wasilewska, A. (2019). Tubular and glomerular biomarkers of acute kidney injury in newborns. *Current Drug Metabolism, 20*(5), 332–349. https://doi.org/10.2174/1389201020666190723092 3.
6. Levey, A. S., Coresh, J., Tighiouart, H., Greene, T., & Inker, L. A. (2020). Measured and estimated glomerular filtration rate: Current status and future directions. *Nature Reviews Nephrology, 16*(1), 51–64. https://doi.org/10.1038/s41581-019-0191-y.
7. Lote, C. J. (2012). *Principles of Renal Physiology* (5th ed.). Springer.
8. Nwose, E. U., Obianke, J., Richards, R. S., Bwitit, P. T., & Igumbor, E. O. (2019). Prevalence and correlations of hepatorenal functions in diabetes and cardiovascular disease among stratified adults. *Acta Biomedica, 90*(1), 97–103.
9. Okoro, R. N., & Farate, V. T. (2019). The use of nephrotoxic drugs in patients with chronic kidney disease. *International Journal of Clinical Pharmacy, 41*(3), 767–775. https://doi.org/10.1007/s11096-019-00897-6.
10. Rodríguez-Cubillo, B., Carnero-Alcázar, M., Cobiella-Carnicer, J., Rodríguez-Moreno, A., Alswies, A., Velo-Plaza, M., Pérez-Camargo, D., Sánchez Fructuoso, A., & Maroto-Castellanos, L. (2019). Impact of postoperative acute kidney failure in long-term survival after heart valve surgery. *Interactive Cardiovascular and Thoracic Surgery, 29*(1), 35–42. https://doi.org/10.1093/icvts/ivz096.
11. Thomas, S. R. (2005). Modelling and simulation of the kidney. *Journal of Biological Physics and Chemistry, 5*(2/3), 70–83. https://doi.org/10.4024/230503.jbpc.05.02.
12. Wiles, K., Bramham, K., Seed, P. T., Nelson-Piercy, C., Lightstone, L., & Chappell, L. C. (2019). Serum creatinine in pregnancy: A systematic review. *Kidney International Reports, 4*(3), 408–419. https://doi.org/10.1016/j.ekir.2018.12.013.

Chapter 6

ACUTE KIDNEY INJURY (AKI)

Contents

Introduction

Acute Kidney Injury (AKI) is defined as an abrupt increase in serum creatinine and/or a decrease in urine output, accompanied by a sudden and frequently reversible decline in renal function. Because of its high incidence—particularly in hospitalized patients—and correlation with higher rates of morbidity and mortality, this condition poses a serious clinical challenge. Numerous factors, broadly classified as prerenal, intrinsic, and postrenal factors, can lead to AKI. Prerenal causes are illnesses that lower renal perfusion without endangering the kidneys directly. Desiccation, bleeding, heart failure, and sepsis are typical cases. These illnesses cause the kidneys' blood flow to be reduced, which sets off compensatory mechanisms like the renin-angiotensin-aldosterone system, which tries to maintain renal function by preserving water and salt. Damage to the kidney tissues directly is the cause of intrinsic renal causes. The most frequent intrinsic cause is acute tubular necrosis (ATN), which is frequently brought on by extended ischemia or exposure to nephrotoxins such as certain drugs (e.g., aminoglycosides, contrast agents used in radiography) and internal poisons (e.g., in rhabdomyolysis, myoglobin). Vasculitis, glomerulonephritis, and acute interstitial nephritis are additional intrinsic causes. These illnesses harm the renal parenchyma, which impairs filtration and causes waste materials to build up in the blood.

Urine flow obstruction from the renal pelvis to the urethra can be caused by postrenal causes. Kidney stones, tumors, and benign prostatic hyperplasia are common causes. If the obstruction is not immediately cleared, it can result in hydronephrosis and kidney damage by lowering the glomerular filtration rate (GFR) and increasing intratubular pressure. AKI can present with a variety of clinical symptoms but frequently involves oliguria (a urine output of less than 400 mL per day), anuria, edema, and electrolyte imbalances like metabolic acidosis and hyperkalemia. To determine the underlying cause and evaluate kidney function, the diagnosis process combines a patient's medical history, physical examination, laboratory testing (serum creatinine, blood urea nitrogen, electrolytes), and imaging studies (ultrasound, CT scans).

The underlying cause of AKI must be quickly identified and treated to manage the condition. Hemodynamic support and fluid resuscitation usually have a positive effect on prerenal AKI. Depending on the etiology, intrinsic renal AKI may need the stopping of corticosteroids, immunosuppressive therapy, or nephrotoxic medications. Relief of the blockage by catheterization, stenting, or surgery is required for postrenal AKI. In cases of AKI, supportive care is really important. Renal function, electrolyte levels, and fluid balance must all be closely monitored. Renal replacement therapy (RRT), such as dialysis, may be required in severe cases or when conservative measures are ineffective in managing complications and maintaining renal function until recovery takes place. AKI is a complicated illness that needs to be diagnosed and treated using a multimodal approach to improve patient outcomes and stop the condition from developing into chronic kidney disease.

Orientation and Directional Terms

Terms	Definition	Illustration
Acute tubular necrosis	Acute tubular necrosis (ATN) is a kidney disorder involving damage to the tubule cells of the kidneys, which can lead to acute kidney failure.	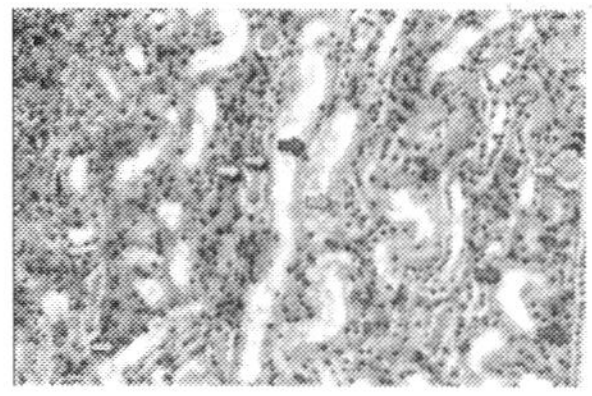
Chronic kidney disease	Chronic kidney disease (CKD) is when the kidneys have become damaged over time (for at least 3 months) and have a hard time doing all their important jobs.	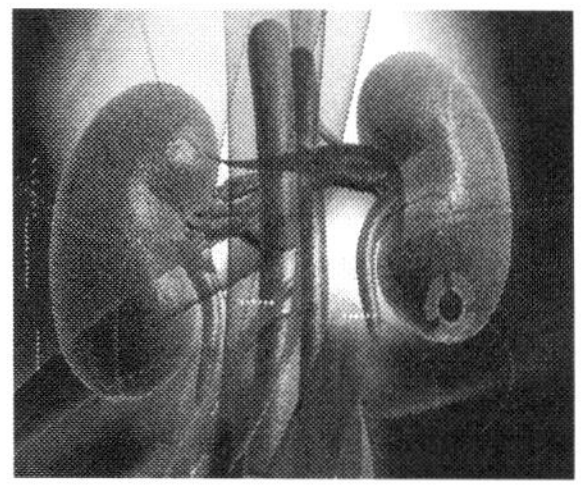
Renal replacement therapy	Renal replacement therapy is a term used to encompass life-supporting treatments for renal failure.	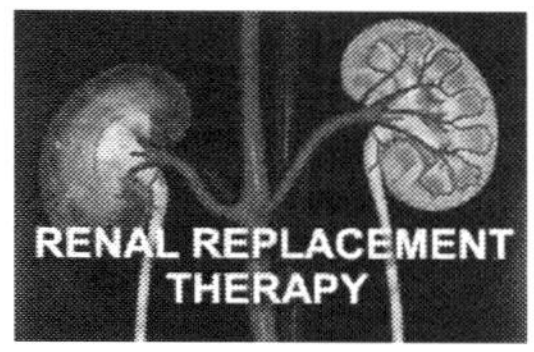
Glomerular filtration rate	Glomerular filtration rate (GFR) is a test used to check how well the kidneys are working.	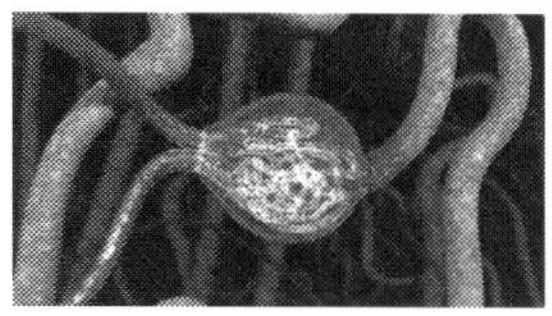
Endoplasmic reticulum	The endoplasmic reticulum (ER) is a part of the transportation system of the eukaryotic cell and has many other important functions such as protein folding.	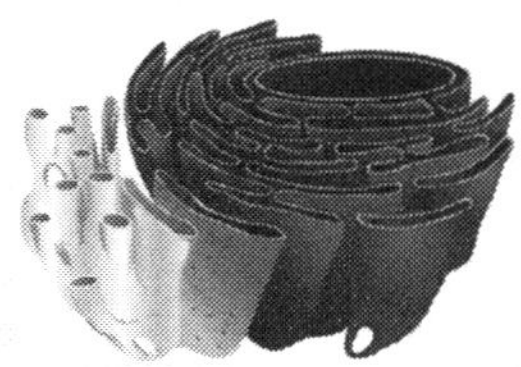

6.1. Overview of Acute Kidney Injury (AKI)

Acute kidney injury (AKI) is linked to elevated rates of morbidity, mortality, and healthcare expenses, making it a significant public health concern. AKI has been more common recently, both in hospital and community settings. With an incidence of 21.6% in adults and 33.7% in children during a single hospital episode of care, AKI is thought to affect over 13 million people annually. The estimated death rate from AKI is still very high, at 23.9% in adults and 13.8% in children, despite all the advancements in the field. AKI is linked to high morbidity and high costs, in addition to its high mortality rate of 1 in 7 million per year. AKI-related hospital expenses total at least $5 billion in the United States, but only 1% of the National Health Service budget is allocated to AKI in England. AKI primarily affects elderly patients and those in critical care units in the developed world; in developing nations, however, adults and women are disproportionately more likely to be affected. Contrary to popular belief, not all AKI patients fully recover from the illness; many go on to experience worsening preexisting chronic kidney disease (CKD), end-stage renal disease (ESRD), or chronic kidney disease (CKD). To improve renal function recovery and lower the high morbidity and mortality, AKI treatment is required. Other than dialysis, no other intervention has been shown to consistently increase survival, reduce injury, or promote recovery. The search for an effective pharmacological therapy has been made more difficult by the multifactorial etiology, heterogeneous patient population, and complex clinical course of AKI patients. The onset of AKI can be predicted in certain situations, such as surgery or intravenous contrast administration, giving clinicians a window of opportunity for intervention and prevention. Intervention is typically initiated subsequent to the onset of AKI, with the objective of expediting the recuperation of renal function (Alkhunaizi, 2019).

6.1.1. Definition and Staging of Acute Kidney Injury

The terms acute renal failure and acute renal insufficiency, which were once used to refer to the same clinical condition, have been replaced by the term AKI. AKI encompasses not only failure but the whole spectrum of the syndrome, from mild variations in renal function to the most severe form that may necessitate renal replacement therapy (RRT).

The term "AKI" has been defined in over 35 ways over the past few decades. The most widely used definition is predicated on criteria related to serum creatinine and/or urine output. The Acute Kidney Injury Network (AKIN) and "risk, injury, failure, loss of kidney function, and end-stage kidney disease" (RIFLE) classifications are the most widely used ones for AKI.

The RIFLE classification takes into account two outcome classes (loss of kidney function and end-stage kidney disease) and three severity classes of AKI (risk, injury, and failure), based on variations in serum creatinine and/or urine output. It is based on these determinants. The patient ought to be categorized based on Table 6.1, which results in the worst classification (maximum RIFLE). However, as Table 6.2 illustrates, the AKIN has classified/staged the AKI into three phases.

Table 6.1. Risk, Injury, Failure, Loss of Kidney Function and End-Stage Kidney Disease (RIFLE) Classification of Acute Kidney Injury

Class	GFR	Urine Output
Risk	↑ SCr × 1.5 or ↓ GFR >25%	<0.5 mL/kg/h × 6 h
Injury	↑ SCr × 2 or ↓ GFR >50%	<0.5 mL/kg/h × 12 h
Failure	↑ SCr × 3 or ↓ GFR >75% or if baseline SCr ≥353.6 µmol/L (≥4 mg/dL) ↑ SCr >44.2 µmol/L (>0.5 mg/dL)	<0.3 mL/kg/h × 24 h or anuria × 12 h
Loss of kidney function	Complete loss of kidney function >4 weeks	–
End-stage kidney disease	Complete loss of kidney function >3 months	–

GFR, glomerular filtration rate; SCr, serum creatinine.

Source: M. Alkhunaizi, A. (2019). Acute Kidney Injury. IntechOpen. doi: 10.5772/intechopen.80625.

Table 6.2. Acute Kidney Injury Network (AKIN) Classifications of Acute Kidney Injury

Stage	Change in Serum Creatinine	Urine Output
1	Increase ≥0.3 mg/dL (26.52 µmol/L) or ≥150–200% from baseline	<0.5 mL/kg/h for more than 6 h
2	Increase >200–300% from baseline	<0.5 mL/kg/h for more than 12 h
3	Increase >300% from baseline or ≥4.0 mg/dL (353.60 µmol/L) with an acute rise of at least 0.5 mg/dL (44.20 µmol/L)	<0.3 mL/kg/h for 24 h or anuria for 12 h

Source: M. Alkhunaizi, A. (2019). Acute Kidney Injury. IntechOpen. doi: 10.5772/intechopen.80625.

RIFLE and AKIN classifications have been combined by the Kidney Disease Improving Global Outcomes (KDIGO) work group to create a single AKI classification for use in public health, research, and practice. This means that AKI is now defined as an abrupt reduction in renal function (within 48 hours) based on an increase of more than or equal to 0.3 mg/dL (≥26.4 µmol/L) in serum creatinine, a percentage increase of more than or equal to 50% (1.5-fold from baseline) in serum creatinine, or a combination of these factors.

6.1.2. Etiology of Acute Kidney Injury

The kidney's ability to filter and eliminate nitrogenous waste from the blood is one of its most vital roles. Raised blood urea nitrogen (BUN) and creatinine levels are markers of reduced renal function, which in turn indicates a reduction in the removal of waste products from the body. The current definition of acute kidney injury (AKI) is a sharp decrease in glomerular filtration rate (GFR) that leads to the retention of nitrogenous wastes, mainly blood urea nitrogen and creatinine. As a result, the diagnosis is currently based on the serial measurement of these substances in patients' blood over time. The rate of this decline usually happens within hours to days, but it can happen over a period of hours to months. Because of the relative imprecision of these measurements as a surrogate marker of GFR, better techniques for assessing GFR and a direct assessment of renal injury are desperately needed in medical practice.

A sufficient level of renal perfusion is necessary to maintain a normal GFR. A decrease in GFR brought on by a drop in renal perfusion pressure without any harm to the renal parenchyma is the hallmark of prerenal azotemia. Renal perfusion can be significantly impacted by any failure of the general circulation or a single intrarenal circulation failure, as the kidneys receive up to 25% of the cardiac output. Prerenal azotemia can be caused by hypovolemia from illnesses like bleeding, vomiting, diarrhea, "third spacing," poor oral intake, burns, excessive perspiration, and renal losses (e.g., diuresis); reduced cardiac output states (e.g., congestive heart failure); and impaired cardiac output. (e.g., severe pulmonary hypertension, pericardial tamponade); reduced vascular resistance (peripheral vasodilation) brought on by illnesses like anaphylaxis, autonomic neuropathy, sepsis, or vasodilator drugs; and renal vasoconstriction brought on by hypercalcemia or vasoconstrictive drugs.

When prerenal conditions arise, the kidney's natural reaction is to maximally concentrate urine and avidly reabsorb sodium in an attempt to maintain or increase intravascular volume and restore normal renal perfusion. Renal function will typically improve quickly with therapy targeted at quickly restoring renal perfusion. There is a spectrum from prerenal azotemia to ischemic AKI, so it's crucial to understand that prolonged or severe prerenal azotemia can cause ischemia damage to the kidney.

Urinary flow obstruction that is acute is a characteristic of AKI caused by postrenal causes. Blockage of the urinary tract raises intratubular pressure, which lowers GFR. Furthermore, inflammatory processes and reduced renal blood flow can result from acute urinary tract obstruction, both of which lower GFR. Any degree of urinary tract obstruction can result in AKI. Usually, for obstruction to cause substantial renal failure, it has to affect one or both kidneys. On the other hand, AKI can occur in a patient with pre-existing renal insufficiency even if there is only one kidney blocked.

In addition to nocturia or nonoliguric AKI, urinary obstruction can also manifest as anuria or intermittent urine flow (such as polyuria alternating with oliguria). Acyclovir or indinavir precipitation, retroperitoneal fibrosis, ureteral stones, papillary necrosis, neurogenic bladder, benign prostatic hyperplasia and prostate cancer in men, gynecologic cancers, particularly cervical cancer in women, and intratubular obstruction are among the causes of postrenal AKI.

The etiology of AKI can be divided into three categories, Table 6.3:

1. Prerenal (caused by decreased renal perfusion, often due to volume depletion)

2. Intrinsic renal (caused by a process within the kidneys)
3. Postrenal (caused by a process distal to the kidneys such as obstruction)

Table 6.3. Etiology of Acute Kidney Injury

Prerenal
Intrarenal Vasoconstriction (Hemodynamically Mediated):
Medications: nonsteroidal anti-inflammatory drugs, angiotensin system blockers, calcineurin inhibitors
Cardiorenal syndrome: advanced heart failure
Hepatorenal syndrome: liver cirrhosis
Abdominal compartment syndrome
Hypercalcemia
Systemic vasodilation: sepsis
Volume depletion:
Renal loss: diuretics, osmotic diuresis (severe hyperglycemia), salt wasting
Extrarenal loss: blood loss, gastrointestinal loss (vomiting, diarrhea), skin (burns, sweating)
Intrinsic renal
Glomerulonephritis (isolated or a part of systemic diseases)
Interstitial nephritis:
Medications: antibiotics (β lactams, sulfonamides, quinolones, rifampin), phenytoin, antiretrovirals, proton pump inhibitors, nonsteroidal anti-inflammatory drugs
Infections: viruses (Epstein-Barr virus, cytomegalovirus, human immunodeficiency virus), bacteria (tuberculosis, legionella species), fungi (candidiasis, histoplasmosis)
Systemic disease: sarcoidosis, connective tissue diseases
Tubular necrosis:
Ischemic: prolonged hypotension
Nephrotoxic: exogenous toxins (radiographic contrast agents, aminoglycosides, cisplatin, methotrexate, amphotericin B)
Endogenous toxins: pigment-induced (hemolysis and rhabdomyolysis), tumor lysis syndrome, multiple myeloma
Vascular
Renal artery and vein thrombosis, malignant hypertension, scleroderma renal crisis, atheroembolic disease, microangiopathies
Post Renal
Extrarenal obstruction: outlet obstruction (prostate hypertrophy, neurogenic bladder; malignancy of the urogenital tract), retroperitoneal fibrosis
Intrarenal obstruction: stones, crystals (acyclovir, indinavir, ethylene glycol), blood clots, tumors

Source: M. Alkhunaizi, A. (2019). Acute Kidney Injury. IntechOpen. doi: 10.5772/intechopen.80625.

Only "intrinsic" AKI is a true kidney disease among these three categories; pre- and postrenal AKI result from extrarenal processes that lower glomerular filtration rate (GFR). If left untreated, pre- and postrenal conditions have the potential to progress into intrinsic renal damage. AKI is more common in patients with CKD and those admitted to the intensive care unit (ICU). According to the AKI-EPI study, AKI affected over 50% of ICU patients; it was primarily brought on by sepsis, hypovolemia, and nephrotoxic drugs.

6.1.3. Pathophysiology of Acute Kidney Injury

Although many cellular mechanisms implicated in the development of AKI have been identified, the pathophysiology of AKI remains largely unclear. Understanding the pathophysiology of acute kidney injury (AKI) in humans has been made possible by the use of animal models of ischemia-reperfusion injury and drug nephrotoxicity. The complexity of the disease in humans, which is characterized by population heterogeneity and preexisting comorbidities like diabetes, hypertension, and CKD, is not reflected in the current in vivo models of AKI in healthy rodents, although these models offer important insights into the pathophysiological mechanisms of renal injury. We will talk about a few of the AKI mechanisms, but not all of them (Alkhunaizi, 2019).

6.1.3.1. Microvascular Injury

One of the main players in the pathophysiology of AKI is the renal microvasculature. The kidney is a vascular organ that receives 25% of the heart's output. It extracts oxygen (O_2) with comparatively little energy demand. The O_2 supply to the kidney is well regulated in a normal steady-state. For the mitochondria to produce adenosine triphosphate (ATP), nitric oxide (NO), and reactive oxygen species (ROS), which are essential for the homeostatic regulation of renal function, there must be an adequate supply of oxygen. Because the outer medulla receives relatively little oxygen, its vascular architecture is especially vulnerable to ischemia injury.

Damage impairs microcirculation, which causes an imbalance in the supply and consumption of NO, ROS, and O_2. Pathogenic events such as oxidative stress and hypoxia ensue. Further alterations in perfusion and O_2 delivery, as well as more endothelial cell injury and inflammation, result from damage to the microvascular endothelium and modifications to the glycocalyx. These events also cause endothelial cell activation and the expression of cell surface markers that encourage leukocyte and platelet recruitment and adhesion. Consequently, heightened vascular permeability and the emergence of interstitial edema cause additional blood flow compromise, intensifying the original injury. Furthermore, oxidative stress and damaged tubular cellular generation of vasoactive prostaglandins worsen local microvascular occlusion, which further reduces O_2 delivery. Reduced peritubular capillary density is the primary long-term effect of microvascular injury. This is a reaction to decreased vascular endothelial growth factor (VEGF) and increased transforming growth factor beta (TGF-β) signaling, which exacerbates ongoing hypoxia and leads to the development of renal fibrosis.

6.1.3.2. Changes in Endoplasmic Reticulum

The endoplasmic reticulum (ER) is crucial in maintaining protein balance by regulating the concentration, structure, folding, and movement of client proteins. When endothelial or epithelial cells are under stress, improperly folded proteins can build up in the ER, leading to the unfolded protein response (UPR). While the UPR initially helps cells adapt to stress, it can also lead to cell death if the stress is severe or prolonged. Research suggests that the UPR plays a role in causing cell death in tubules due to damage to epithelial cells. Therefore, targeting the UPR could be a potential strategy to prevent or treat acute kidney injury (AKI).

6.1.3.3. Mitochondrial Dysfunction

The mitochondrial-ER-associated membrane (MAM) refers to the multiple contact sites between the ER and mitochondria. On electron micrographs, the MAM is seen as ER tubules that are closely positioned to the mitochondria and contain proteins from both organelles. Cell stress conditions, such as a changed cellular redox state, cause the MAM to modify the regulatory proteins it has on hand, which in turn modifies the MAM's function. Because they rely on aerobic metabolism and have more oxidized mitochondria than distal tubular cells, which can use glycolysis, proximal tubules are particularly susceptible to mitochondrial dysfunction in the pathophysiology of AKI. Mitochondrial fragmentation was seen in rat renal tubular cells after either ATP depletion or cisplatin treatment, before cytochrome c release and apoptosis. A new approach to treating AKI may involve addressing mitochondrial dysfunction in conjunction with gaining additional knowledge about the regulation of mitochondrial dynamics and the pathogenic alterations that result from it.

6.1.3.4. Autophagy

Proteins, organelles, and cytoplasmic elements are transported to lysosomes for breakdown and recycling during the catabolic process of autophagy. During AKI, renal tubular cells are stimulated to undergo autophagy. It starts with the encapsulation of organelles and cytoplasmic proteins in autophagosomes, which subsequently fuse with lysosomes to be degraded. Once triggered, it can eliminate aberrant proteins from the ER and/or remove ER membranes that contain UPR sensors to reduce cellular stress. In animal models, it was discovered that autophagy activation protected against cisplatin-induced AKI, whereas blocking the autophagic flux increased AKI. Additionally, during the AKI recovery phase, the resolution of autophagy may encourage tubular cell proliferation and regeneration. An inflammatory modulator that targets autophagy may be used to treat a variety of kidney diseases.

6.1.3.5. Inflammation

One of the main contributing factors to the pathophysiology of ischemia-induced AKI is inflammation. The innate immune response is influenced by modifications in protein folding and mitochondrial function, which leads to inflammation. AKI also involves the activation of multiple inflammatory pathways and cytokines. Furthermore, after ischemia–reperfusion injury, immune cells from both the innate and adaptive immune systems, including neutrophils, dendritic cells, macrophages, and lymphocytes, contribute to the pathophysiology of renal injury and some also aid in its repair. T and B lymphocytes are significant in the progression phase of renal injury, while neutrophils and monocytes mediate the acute phase during the first 24 hours of injury. Reduction of renal injury, cell death, and chronic fibrosis are all lessened when leukocyte infiltration into the kidney is inhibited. Experimental evidence suggests that tubular injury during AKI may be facilitated by inducible nitric oxide synthase (iNOS). It has been demonstrated that ischemia kidneys express more iNOS protein and that hypoxia in isolated proximal tubules increases nitric oxide release. In rat models, the in vivo administration of an antisense oligonucleotide to inhibit the up-regulation of iNOS provided protection against ischemia-induced renal damage. Similarly, iNOS knockout mice's tubules were shielded from hypoxic damage.

Phospholipase A2 (PLA2) is a group of enzymes that remove the acyl group from the sn-2 position of phospholipids, resulting in the production of free fatty acids. During hypoxic injury to the renal tubules, the activity of PLA2 is elevated. Studies have shown that inhibiting PLA2 with exogenous fatty acids like arachidonic acid can protect against hypoxia-induced damage in isolated proximal renal tubules (Alkhunaizi, 2019).

6.1.4. Sepsis and Acute Kidney Injury

A severe inflammatory reaction to infection, sepsis is marked by an inflammatory state throughout the body and can have serious repercussions, such as multiple organ failure. AKI is a common, severe sepsis-related complication that affects ICU patients frequently and is linked to high in-hospital and long-term mortality. More than half of ICU patients had AKI, according to the multinational AKI-EPI study, and higher AKI severity was linked to higher mortality.

6.1.4.1. Pathogenesis of Sepsis-Induced Acute Kidney Injury

Despite being one of the main causes of AKI, septic shock's underlying mechanisms are not fully understood. AKI in sepsis has a complicated and multifactorial pathophysiology that involves many processes, such as endothelial dysfunction, intrarenal hemodynamic perturbations, inflammatory cell infiltration, inflammatory cytokine upregulation, intraglomerular thrombosis, induction of apoptosis, and tubular obstruction with necrotic cells and debris. A major factor in the development of sepsis is thought to be the activation of pro- and anti-inflammatory mechanisms.

Following the initial host-microbial encounter, the innate immune response is triggered, coordinating a defensive response involving both humoral and cellular components. This results in the release and stimulation of multiple cytokines, chief among them interleukin-1 (IL-1), tumor necrosis factor-α (TNF-α), and IL-6. These eventually cause hemodynamic instability, cytokine storm, organ failure, and sepsis.

In Gram-negative bacteria, the outer membrane contains a substance called lipopolysaccharide (LPS), which can quickly and powerfully activate a wide range of cell types, including macrophages, monocytes, and leukocytes. Gram-negative sepsis manifests as a result of a series of events that begin with the activation of inflammatory cells by LPS. LPS triggers several intracellular signaling processes, such as nuclear factor-κB (NF-κB) activation, which in turn causes the production and release of several pro-inflammatory mediators, such as IL-1, IL-6, IL-8, and TNF-a. It has been demonstrated that the toll-like receptor (TLR) family of transmembrane proteins, which is crucial for the immune system's defense against pathogenic microbial infection, mediates the pathway that triggers NF-κB. TLRs, specifically TLR-2 and TLR-4 expression, are markedly up-regulated in the sepsis context. LPS activates both TLR-2 and TLR-4, and the response is dependent on the LPS-binding protein and is amplified by CD14. Figure 6.1 shows an overview of the TLR signaling pathway. The major pathways implicated in the pathophysiology of sepsis-induced AKI are illustrated in Figure 6.2, which also has implications for the clinical course of sepsis.

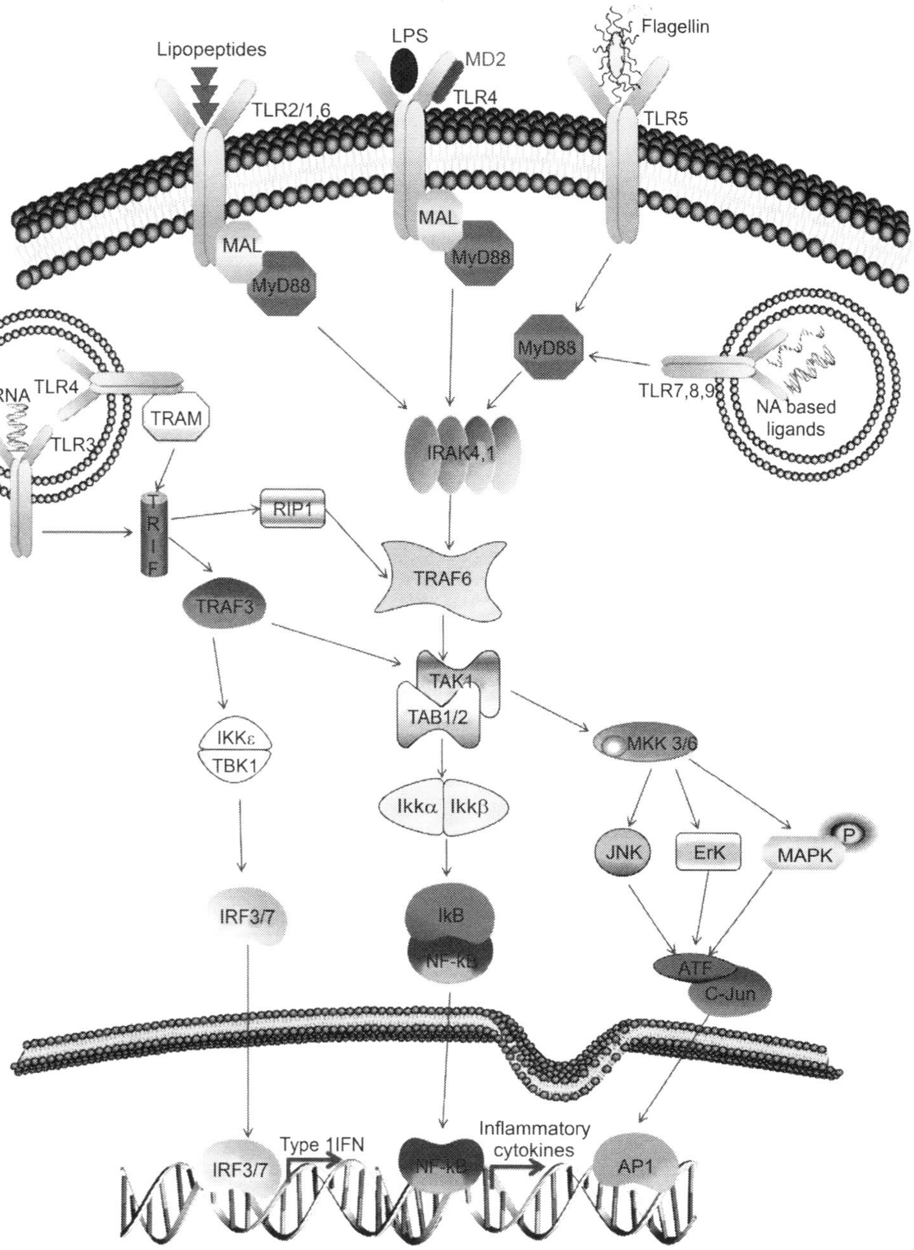

Figure 6.1. *Toll-like receptor (TLR) signaling pathway. When TLRs are stimulated by their respective ligands, they dimerize and recruit downstream adaptor molecules, such as myeloid differentiation primary-response protein 88 (MyD88), MyD88-adaptor-like (MAL), toll/interleukin (IL)-1 receptor (TIR)-domain-containing adaptor-inducing interferon-β (TRIF), TRIF-related adaptor molecule (TRAM), which activate other downstream molecules leading to the activation of signaling cascades that converge at the nuclear factor-κB (NF-κB), interferon (IFN) response factors (IRFs), and mitogen-activated protein (MAP) kinases. These molecules induce the transcription of several pro-inflammatory molecules, such as interleukin (IL)-6, IL-8, IL-12, and tumor necrosis factor-α (TNF-α). AP1, activator protein 1;*

ATF, activating transcription factor; dsRNA, double-stranded RNA; ERK, extracellular signal-regulated kinase; IKK, inhibitor of kappa light polypeptide gene enhancer in B-cell kinase; IRAK, IL-1 receptor-associated kinase; JNK, c-Jun N-terminal kinase; LPS, lipopolysaccharide; MD, myeloid differentiation factor; MKK, MAPK kinase; NA, nucleic acid; TAB, transforming growth factor-β-activated kinase 1/ MAP3K7-binding protein; TAK, transforming growth factor-activated kinase; TRAF, tumor necrosis factor receptor-associated factor; RIP1, receptor-interacting protein 1.

Source: M. Alkhunaizi, A. (2019). Acute Kidney Injury. IntechOpen. doi: 10.5772/intechopen.80625.

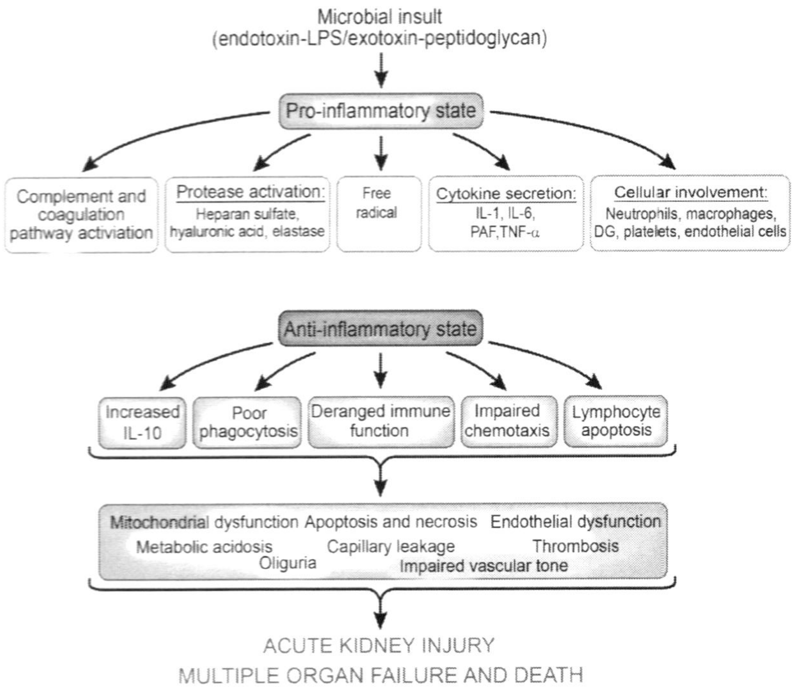

Figure 6.2. *Key pathogenic pathways involved in sepsis that also have implications in the pathophysiology of sepsis-induced acute kidney injury.*

Source: M. Alkhunaizi, A. (2019). Acute Kidney Injury. IntechOpen. doi: 10.5772/intechopen.80625.

TLR modulation may develop into a novel therapeutic target for the management of sepsis-related organ dysfunction, including AKI. In patients with sepsis and AKI, cytokine adsorption to the membrane during continuous renal replacement therapy may also become a therapeutic option.

6.1.5. Clinical Presentation of Acute Kidney Injury

The type and degree of renal damage determine how AKI manifests clinically. Patients with mild to moderate AKI are identified through laboratory testing; this condition is asymptomatic. On the other hand, many symptoms, such as exhaustion, anorexia, nausea, vomiting, restlessness, confusion, fluid retention, and weight gain, are frequently seen in patients with severe AKI. Severe and protracted AKI can result in severe anemia, bleeding tendency owing to platelet malfunction, and central nervous system symptoms like uremic encephalopathy with asterixis, confusion, and seizures. Patients with AKI may have normal urine output, oliguria (urine output less than 400 mL/24 h) or anuria (urine output less than 100 mL/24 h).

6.2. Diagnosis of Acute Kidney Injury

To identify the cause of AKI, a patient's history and physical examination are essential. Particular attention should be paid to evaluating the patient's volume status. The use of nephrotoxic drugs and the existence of systemic diseases that could reduce renal perfusion or directly affect renal function should be discussed in the history. The intravascular volume status and any skin rashes that might point to systemic diseases should be evaluated during a physical examination. Urinalysis, urine microscopy, complete blood count, electrolytes, serum creatinine or cystatin C level, and fractional excretion of sodium (FENa) should all be part of the initial laboratory evaluation. When diagnosing AKI, urine microscopy and urinalysis are crucial. The results of urine microscopy and urinalysis guide the differential diagnosis and further research. Ultrasonography in particular can be useful for imaging studies when working up AKI initially. For older men with AKI who may have bladder outlet obstruction due to prostate hypertrophy, ultrasonography is especially important. When a patient has AKI and its cause is unknown, renal biopsy is the treatment of choice. When an underlying condition, such as glomerulonephritis or interstitial nephritis, is suspected and specific therapy is needed, a renal biopsy is especially crucial. When glomerulonephritis progresses quickly, as evidenced by elevated serum creatinine or cystatin C levels and the presence of dysmorphic or cast-like red blood cells on urine microscopy, renal biopsy ought to be carried out immediately.

6.2.1. New Biomarkers for the Quick Detection of Acute Kidney Injury

While the RIFLE and AKIN criteria have improved the diagnosis of AKI by utilizing serum creatinine and urine output, there is still a lack of a reliable tool to differentiate between true parenchymal and prerenal azotemia in clinical settings. Recently, several studies have explored new urinary and serum biomarkers for diagnosing and predicting the prognosis of AKI, aiming to facilitate earlier diagnosis and treatment. Some of these biomarkers are listed in Table 6.4. However, their current utility in preventing and treating AKI is very limited (Alkhunaizi, 2019).

Table 6.4. Urinary and Serum Biomarkers for the Diagnosis of Acute Kidney Injury

Acronym	Legend	Main Source
AP	Alkaline phosphatase	Liver, bone, intestine, placenta, brush border proximal convoluted tubules
α_1MG	Alpha 1 microglobulin	Liver. Reabsorption by renal proximal tubular cells
$\alpha_1$acidGP	Alpha 1 acid glycoprotein	Liver. Reabsorption by renal proximal tubular cells
B_2MG	Beta 2 microglobulin	All nucleated cells. Reabsorption by renal proximal tubular cells

Cystatin C	Cystatin C	All nucleated cells. Reabsorption by renal proximal tubular cells
FENA	Fractional excretion of sodium	
GGTP	Gamma-glutamyl transpeptidase	All cells except myocytes. Mainly liver and kidney (brush border proximal convoluted tubules and loop of Henle)
αGST	Alpha-glutathione S-transferase	Expressed in almost all tissues. Kidney: proximal tubular cells (cytoplasmatic)
πGST	Pi glutathione S-transferase	Expressed in almost all tissues. Kidney: distal tubular cells (cytoplasmatic)
HGF	Hepatocyte growth factor	Mesenchymal cells
IL-6	Interleukin 6	T lymphocytes, macrophages, endothelial cells, monocytes
IL-8	Interleukin 8	Monocytes, macrophages, epithelial cells, endothelial cells
IL-10	Interleukin 10	Monocytes, lymphocytes, macrophages
IL-18	Interleukin 18	Monocytes, dendritic cells, macrophages and epithelial cells
KIM-1	Kidney injury molecule 1	Kidney: proximal tubular cells
LFABP	Liver-type fatty acid-binding protein	Hepatocytes, kidney: proximal tubular cells
NGAL	Neutrophil gelatinase-associated lipocalin	Leucocytes, loop of Henle and collecting ducts
NAG	*N*-Acetyl beta glucosaminidase	Several tissues (liver, brain, spleen, etc.). Kidney: proximal tubular cells (lysosomal)
PAI-1	Plasminogen activator inhibitor 1	Endothelium
PCX	Podocalyxin	Podocytes
RBP	Retinol-binding protein	Liver. Reabsorption by renal proximal tubular cells
sTNFR-I	Soluble tumor necrosis factor receptor I	Most cells and tissues (cytotoxic, apoptotic, and pro-inflammatory effects)

sTNFR-II	Soluble tumor necrosis factor receptor II	Most cells and tissues (proliferative and anti-apoptotic effects)
TNF-α	Tumor necrosis factor-alpha	Macrophages, lymphoid cells, renal parenchymal cells
11 k-TXB_2	11-keto-Thromboxane B_2	Platelets
vWF	Von Willebrand factor	Endothelium, megakaryocytes, subendothelial connective tissue
TIMP-2	Tissue inhibitor of metalloproteinase-2	Ubiquitous expression. Renal tubular cells
IGFBP7	Insulin-like growth factor-binding protein 7	Ubiquitous expression. Renal tubular cells

Source: M. Alkhunaizi, A. (2019). Acute Kidney Injury. IntechOpen. doi: 10.5772/intechopen.80625.

6.3. Management And Treatment Approaches for AKI

Acute Kidney Injury (AKI) is a life-threatening illness marked by an abrupt reduction in kidney function. Timely and efficient management is essential to prevent negative consequences. Recognizing and treating the underlying etiology is the cornerstone of managing AKI. To differentiate between pre-renal, intrinsic renal, and post-renal causes, a comprehensive clinical evaluation that includes a history, physical examination, and pertinent laboratory tests is typically the first step in this process.

Ensuring adequate renal perfusion and optimizing hemodynamic status are the primary goals of initial management. This entails stopping nephrotoxic medications like NSAIDs and some antibiotics in addition to performing fluid resuscitation with isotonic saline to restore intravascular volume in cases of pre-renal AKI. Diuretics should be used carefully when there is a risk of fluid overload, such as in heart failure, or inotropic support may be necessary. Treatment for intrinsic renal causes, such as glomerulonephritis or acute tubular necrosis, focuses on the particular underlying pathology. Corticosteroids and other immunosuppressive treatments may be beneficial for immune-mediated or inflammatory conditions. Antimicrobial therapy that is appropriate for infectious etiologies is needed. It is also essential to manage complications like acidosis, hyperkalemia, and volume overload. In severe cases, this may entail the use of bicarbonate therapy, dialysis, or other renal replacement therapies (RRT). Relief of the obstruction is necessary for post-renal AKI, which is usually caused by obstructive uropathy. The treatment plan may include catheterization, stenting, or surgery, contingent upon the type and extent of obstruction. Urologists should often be consulted early to guide these interventions.

Throughout the management of AKI, supportive care and monitoring are essential. Ongoing treatment is guided by routine evaluations of renal function, electrolytes, and fluid balance. RRT might be required for patients who do not respond to first treatments or who experience serious side effects. RRT modalities include peritoneal dialysis, continuous renal replacement therapy (CRRT), and intermittent hemodialysis. The selection of each modality is contingent upon the patient's hemodynamic stability and the particular clinical circumstances.

To manage patients who are at risk of AKI, preventative measures are also essential. This includes taking precautions to avoid contrast-induced nephropathy in patients undergoing radiographic procedures, as well as closely monitoring renal function in high-risk groups, such as those undergoing major surgery or receiving nephrotoxic drugs. A multimodal approach that takes into account the patient's unique circumstances, severity, and underlying cause is necessary for the management of AKI. To enhance results and lower the chance of developing chronic kidney disease, early detection, timely intervention, and ongoing monitoring are crucial (Alkhunaizi, 2019).

6.3.1. Fluid Management and Renal Replacement Therapy

To ensure proper renal perfusion, avoid fluid overload, and treat the consequences of impaired kidney function, fluid management and renal replacement therapy (RRT) are essential elements in the management of acute kidney injury (AKI).

6.3.1.1. Fluid Management

Restoring and maintaining optimal intravascular volume is the main objective of fluid management in AKI to guarantee sufficient renal perfusion. A comprehensive evaluation of the patient's volume status is the first step, which includes a clinical examination, vital signs, urine output, and laboratory testing for electrolytes, creatinine, and blood urea nitrogen.

This comprehensive evaluation helps to distinguish between hypovolemia, euvolemia, and hypervolemia.

- **Fluid Resuscitation:** In hypovolemic patients, prompt fluid resuscitation with isotonic crystalloids, such as normal saline or lactated Ringer's solution, is crucial. The amount and rate of fluid administration should be carefully tailored to the patient's needs, considering factors like underlying cardiac function and the risk of fluid overload. The goal is to restore perfusion pressure and urine output without causing pulmonary edema or worsening fluid balance.
- **Maintenance Fluids:** Once adequate intravascular volume is achieved, maintenance fluids may be required to sustain hydration and electrolyte balance. This involves calculating daily fluid requirements based on ongoing losses (urine, insensible losses) and adjusting for any additional needs due to fever, diarrhea, or other factors. Close monitoring of fluid status through daily weight, input-output charts, and frequent reassessment of clinical signs is essential.
- **Fluid Overload:** In patients with fluid overload, careful fluid restriction and the use of diuretics, such as furosemide, may be necessary to manage volume status. Diuretics can help mobilize excess fluid, but their use should be balanced against the risk of worsening renal perfusion and electrolyte imbalances.

6.3.1.2. Renal Replacement Therapy

When conservative treatments for AKI are ineffective in treating complications such as refractory hyperkalemia, severe metabolic acidosis, volume overload that is not responsive to diuretics, and uremic symptoms, RRT is recommended.

The choice of RRT modality depends on the patient's hemodynamic stability, the severity of AKI, and the clinical setting:

- **Intermittent Hemodialysis (IHD):** IHD is a common form of RRT that involves periodic sessions, typically lasting 3–4 hours, during which blood is filtered through a dialysis machine. It is effective for rapid removal of toxins and excess fluid but may not be suitable for hemodynamically unstable patients due to the risk of hypotension.
- **Continuous Renal Replacement Therapy (CRRT):** CRRT is often preferred in critically ill patients with hemodynamic instability. It provides slow and continuous removal of solutes and fluid over 24 hours, minimizing the risk of hemodynamic fluctuations. CRRT includes modalities like continuous venovenous hemofiltration (CVVH) and continuous venovenous hemodiafiltration (CVVHDF).
- **Peritoneal Dialysis (PD):** PD is another option, particularly useful in settings where vascular access is challenging or in patients with contraindications to hemodialysis. It involves the infusion of dialysis fluid into the peritoneal cavity, allowing waste products to diffuse across the peritoneal membrane.

Careful fluid management is necessary for the effective treatment of AKI to guarantee sufficient renal perfusion and avoid complications resulting from fluid imbalance. RRT is an essential tool for managing the severe metabolic disturbances associated with AKI when conservative measures prove insufficient. The clinical status and unique requirements of the patient should be taken into consideration when selecting the RRT modality (Alkhunaizi, 2019).

6.3.2. Management of Acute Kidney Injury

Nephrologists and other medical professionals involved in the patient's care must work closely together in the management of AKI. A detailed physical examination and a close history are part of the clinical evaluation of AKI. Herbal remedies, recreational drugs, and over-the-counter medications should all be included in the drug history. After it is established, AKI management primarily provides support. Unless AKI is mild and has a readily treatable cause, the majority of patients should be admitted to the hospital. Assessment of the contributing causes of the kidney injury, assessment of the clinical course including comorbidities, careful assessment of volume status, and implementation of appropriate therapeutic measures aimed at reversing or preventing the worsening of functional or structural kidney abnormalities should all be part of the evaluation and initial management of patients with AKI. Separating prerenal, renal, and postrenal causes should be part of the initial evaluation of patients with AKI. For the majority of cases, the established method of using ultrasonography to rule out postrenal causes is sufficient for the initial assessment. It is more difficult to distinguish between prerenal and renal causes because renal hypoperfusion can occur at any stage of AKI.

The first line of treatment for AKI must focus on preventing hypovolemia, achieving and maintaining hemodynamic stability, and ensuring appropriate renal perfusion. If determining intravascular volume is difficult, measuring central venous pressure may be useful. Prerenal azotemia can be quickly treated if the underlying cause is addressed. It is crucial to note that there are diagnostic restrictions on some components of the prerenal azotemia definition. Compensation mechanisms designed to sustain GFR may come into action in the event of renal hypoperfusion. These compensatory mechanisms result in increased tubular reabsorption of water and solutes through neuro/hormonal changes, efferent arteriolar dilation, and efferent arteriolar vasoconstriction. This suggests that urine output criteria may identify patients with renal hypoperfusion as having AKI even in the absence of a discernible shift in serum creatinine concentration.

Absolute or relative hypovolemia can cause prerenal conditions that can be corrected with volume resuscitation. Fluid administration, however, is not always effective in correcting renal hypoperfusion brought on by low cardiac output (severe cardiomyopathy) or reduced renal perfusion pressure (sepsis, or end-stage liver disease). How about isotonic solutions? since these solutions have a negative impact, (e.g., 0.9 sodium chloride) are recommended over hyperoncotic solutions. (e.g., albumin, dextrans, and hydroxyethyl starch). In patients with severe sepsis or septic shock, the use of hydroxyethyl starch as a plasma-volume expander has been demonstrated to be an independent risk factor for AKI. Vasopressors may be required in patients with persistent hypotension to keep their mean blood pressure at 65 mmHg.

6.3.3. Pharmacologic Interventions for Management of Acute Kidney Injury

Numerous pharmacologic strategies for the early management of AKI have been studied. While some aim to modify intrarenal pathophysiology, others are intended to increase renal perfusion. Both terlipressin and norepinephrine were successful in increasing mean arterial blood pressure (MAP) in patients with hyperdynamic septic shock, which improved renal function. Since low-dose (renal-dose) dopamine is thought to have renoprotective effects, it was commonly used in the intensive care unit. On the first day of use, low-dose dopamine may cause an increase in urine output; however, prospective, retrospective, and multiple meta-analyzes have not demonstrated any beneficial effects in preventing AKI or improving renal function in AKI patients. On the other hand, it has been demonstrated that low-dose dopamine deteriorates renal perfusion in individuals with confirmed AKI. Consequently, it is best to stop giving critically ill patients low-dose dopamine on a regular basis.

Fenoldopam is a selective dopamine A1 agonist; however, studies on early AKI and contrast nephropathy using randomized controlled trials have shown that it is not useful in protecting renal function or lowering the need for renal replacement. However, some meta-analyzes have demonstrated that fenoldopam reduces the risk of AKI in patients undergoing major surgery and cardiac procedures, without affecting hospital mortality or renal replacement. The majority of these studies linked fenoldopam to hypotension.

Fluids with high chloride content may raise the risk of AKI and mortality in sepsis patients. In patients admitted to the intensive care unit with sepsis, early goal-directed therapy with close monitoring of central venous pressure, mean arterial pressure, and oxygen saturation has been demonstrated to be protective against AKI.

When atrial distension or elevated atrial pressure occurs, cardiac atrial myocytes release atrial natriuretic peptide (ANP). It increases glomerular filtration and sodium excretion from the urine by inducing afferent dilatation and efferent vasoconstriction. Similar effects are primarily produced by the cardiac ventricles when producing B-type (brain) natriuretic peptide (BNP). Low dosages of recombinant human ANP improved dialysis-free survival in early, ischemic acute renal dysfunction following complex cardiac surgery, reduced the likelihood of dialysis, and enhanced renal excretory function. Patients receiving liver transplants experienced similar outcomes. However, in large randomized clinical trials, higher doses of ANP did not improve dialysis-free survival or reduce the need for dialysis.

Adenosine antagonist theophylline has been demonstrated in many preliminary reports to help prevent cisplatin nephrotoxicity and contrast nephropathy. A few supplemental substances, like carotenoids (lycopene) and flavonoids (silymarin), have been tried in pilot studies with cancer patients receiving cisplatin, with varying degrees of success. There aren't enough well-powered, controlled trials to back up these agents' effectiveness.

Levosimendan is a calcium sensitizer with anti-inflammatory, inodilator, and cardioprotective properties. According to two meta-analyzes, patients who are critically ill or undergoing cardiac surgery may require less renal replacement therapy when levosimendan is used. Small and diverse studies were included in both meta-analyzes, and AKI was not always a predetermined endpoint.

Although osmotic agents and loop diuretics can reduce tubular oxygen consumption and relieve intratubular obstruction in animal models, their efficacy in the prevention and management of acute kidney injury (AKI) in humans has been found wanting. In addition to raising concerns about the increased risk of ototoxicity associated with high doses, a meta-analysis has demonstrated that frusemide was not linked to any significant clinical benefits in the prevention and treatment of AKI in adults.

A thiol-containing antioxidant called N-acetyl-cysteine has been studied in many studies, primarily for the prevention of nephropathy brought on by contrast. It is still debatable whether N-acetyl-cysteine has any protective effects, despite some encouraging reports. Similarly, N-acetyl-cysteine was not found to be protective against other causes of AKI, especially in hypotensive patients in the intensive care unit or patients undergoing heart surgery. Studies have demonstrated that sodium bicarbonate hydration is more effective than normal saline at preventing contrast-induced nephropathy. Other research has not demonstrated that sodium bicarbonate is any better than saline at preventing contrast-induced nephropathy. The best way to avoid contrast-induced nephropathy is to use low osmolar contrast agents in conjunction with hydration with isotonic solutions, such as sodium bicarbonate or normal saline.

For high-risk patients undergoing contrast administration for angiography, statins might be helpful. Short-term rosuvastatin use was found to be protective against contrast nephropathy in diabetic patients with concurrent CKD who underwent coronary/peripheral arterial angiography in a randomized multicenter clinical trial. Another single-center trial found that giving statin-naïve patients with acute coronary syndrome who were scheduled for an early invasive procedure high-dose rosuvastatin (40 mg on admission followed by 20 mg daily) protected against contrast-induced AKI and improved the short-term clinical outcome. Compared to 15% of patients in the control group, 6.7% of patients in the early high-dose rosuvastatin group experienced AKI. The rosuvastatin group also experienced a decrease in the 30-day rate of adverse cardiovascular and renal events (3.6 versus 7.9%). Rosuvastatin showed a protective effect among female diabetic patients with CKD in a subgroup analysis of this study. Similarly, in diabetic patients with renal failure, a single high dose of atorvastatin (80 mg) given within 24 hours of exposure to intravenous contrast was successful in lowering the rate of AKI. Numerous meta-analyzes have confirmed the protective effect of statins. Nevertheless, patients undergoing cardiac surgery did not benefit from statins in the same way that patients receiving coronary interventions did. The use of statins was either harmful or showed no benefit in this group of patients.

6.3.4. Renal Replacement Therapy for Acute Kidney Injury

Regarding the indication and timing of RRT for patients with AKI, clinical practice varies greatly. Additionally, there is disagreement over the choice of RRT modality and recommended therapy intensity. Continuous renal replacement therapy has grown in popularity among the various RRT modalities, particularly in the intensive care unit (ICU) context where patients may be too hemodynamically unstable to tolerate intermittent hemodialysis. Regarding the various RRT modalities, there doesn't seem to be a significant difference in terms of either mortality or renal function recovery (Alkhunaizi, 2019).

6.3.5. Prevention of Acute Kidney Injury

More than 50% of ICU patients experience acute kidney injury, which is linked to higher rates of morbidity and mortality. The European Society of Intensive Care Medicine's Working Group on Prevention has released recommendations for preventing AKI. These recommendations specifically address the use of care bundles, diuretics, inotropes, vasopressors/vasodilators, hormonal and nutritional interventions, sedatives, statins, remote ischemic preconditioning, and fluids. Table 6.5 illustrates these recommendations. The guidelines can be summed up as follows: the mainstay of AKI prevention continues to be prompt resuscitation using fluids, vasopressors, and inotropic agents. Isotonic crystalloid volume expansion is only used in cases of confirmed or suspected hypovolemia. It is best to stay away from using dextrans and starches. Vasoconstrictors, ideally norepinephrine, should be given with or after volume expansion to patients who are hypotensive. For the majority of patients, a mean arterial pressure (MAP) of 65–70 mmHg is sufficient; however, in those with preexisting chronic hypertension, a higher MAP of 80–85 mmHg should be the goal. It is essential to review all prescriptions and stop using nephrotoxic drugs. Diuretics may be helpful in situations of volume overload and congestion, but they should not be used to prevent AKI. Avoiding hyperglycemia is advised. Statins' effects seem to vary depending on the situation; they show promise when used in conjunction with contrast, but have no effect or even cause harm in patients undergoing cardiac surgery (Alkhunaizi, 2019).

Table 6.5. Expert Opinion of the Working Group on Prevention, AKI Section, European Society of Intensive Care Medicine

Volume Expansion
Controlled fluid resuscitation in volume depletion, while, however, avoiding volume overload (1 C)
Avoidance of starches, gelatine, and dextrans (2C)
Correction of hypovolemia/dehydration using isotonic crystalloids in patients receiving intravascular contrast media (1 B)
Regular monitoring of chloride levels and acid–base status in situations where chloride-rich solutions are used (BPS)
Use of balanced crystalloids for large-volume resuscitation (2C)
Use of human albumin if necessary for the treatment of patients with septic shock (2C).
Use of Diuretics
No loop diuretics for the prevention of AKI (Grade 1B)
Diuretics to control or avoid fluid overload in patients that are diuretic-responsive (Grade 2D)
Use of Vasopressors
Titrating vasopressors to a MAP of 65–70 mmHg (Grade 1B) in patients with septic shock and to (80–85 mmHg) for patients with chronic HTN (Grade 1C).
lowering SBP to 140–190 mmHg in patients with acute cerebral hemorrhage with severe admission hypertension (Grade 1C)
Norepinephrine as the first-choice vasopressor to protect kidney function (Grade 1B) and vasopressin in patients with vasoplegic shock after cardiac surgery (Grade 2C).
Individualizing target pressure when premorbid blood pressure is available (BPS)
Use of Vasodilators
No low-dose dopamine for protection against AKI (Grade 1A)
No levosimendan for renal protection in patients with sepsis and in cardiac surgery patients with poor preoperative left ventricular function (Grade 1B).
No fenoldopam or natriuretic peptides for renal protection in critically ill or cardiovascular surgery patients at risk of AKI (Grade 2B).
Sedatives
Shorter sedation using propofol or dexmedetomidine (BPS)
Hormonal Manipulation
Target a blood glucose level of at least below 180 mg/dL (10 mmol/l) (Grade 2B).
Use of erythropoietin or steroids (Grade 2 B)
Metabolic Interventions
Avoid using high-dose IV selenium for renal protection in critically ill patients (1B)

Avoid using N-acetylcysteine to prevent contrast-associated AKI in critically ill patients (Grade 2B)
Provide adequate nutritional support preferably through the enteral route (BPS)
Statins
Avoid the use of high-dose statins to prevent postoperative AKI in cardiac surgery (Grade 1A)
Use atorvastatin or rosuvastatin to prevent contrast-associated AKI in high-risk patients undergoing coronary contrast angiography (Grade 2B)
Remote Ischemic Preconditioning
Do not use remote ischemic preconditioning for prevention of AKI in critically ill patients
AKI Care Bundles
Use of the KDIGO recommendations to reduce the incidence of AKI after cardiac surgery (Grade 2C).
Use of AKI care bundles outside the intensive care unit has some benefits, including the potential to improve the outcome of AKI (BPS).

AKI, acute kidney injury; HTN, hypertension; MAP, mean arterial pressure; BPS, best practice statement.

Source: M. Alkhunaizi, A. (2019). Acute Kidney Injury. IntechOpen. doi: 10.5772/intechopen.80625.

6.3.6. Prognosis of Acute Kidney Injury

With the advent of agreed definition and classification of AKI based on changes in serum creatinine and urine output, there is now increasing awareness of the poor prognosis following AKI. Multiple studies have shown that patients with AKI are at high risk for progression to advanced-stage CKD and death following hospital discharge. In a meta-analysis of 13 cohort studies comparing the risk of CKD, ESRD, and death in patients with and without AKI, the pooled incidence of CKD and ESRD were 25.8/100 person-years and 8.6/100 person-years, respectively. Patients with AKI had higher risks of developing CKD (pooled adjusted hazard ratio 8.8), ESRD (pooled adjusted HR 3.1), and mortality (pooled adjusted HR 2.0) than patients without AKI. In another meta-analysis of 48 studies containing 47,107 patients between 1985 and 2007, the incidence rate of mortality was 8.9 deaths/100 person-years in survivors of AKI compared to 4.3 deaths/100 patient-years in survivors without AKI (rate ratio 2.59). The incidence rate of CKD after an episode of AKI was 7.8 events/100 patient-years, and the rate of ESRD was 4.9 events/100 patient-years. In an observational cohort study with a median follow-up of 9 years the intermediate-term (30–364 days) adjusted mortality HRs for AKI versus no AKI were 2.48, 2.50, 1.90, and 1.63 for baseline eGFRs ≥60, 45–59, 30–44, and <30 mL/min/1.73 m^2, respectively. This indicates that baseline renal function is an important determinant factor for outcome following an episode of AKI. A retrospective cohort study showed that patients who developed AKI during hospitalization were at substantial risk for the development of CKD in the following year, and the timing of recovery was a strong predictor, even for the mildest forms of AKI. The multinational AKI-EPI study on ICU patients in 97 centers showed that increasing AKI severity was associated with increased mortality, and AKI patients had worse renal function at the time of hospital discharge (Alkhunaizi, 2019).

A Closer Look

Chronic Kidney Disease

The progressive loss of kidney function over time is the hallmark of chronic kidney disease (CKD). The kidneys are essential for eliminating waste materials and extra fluid from the blood, controlling electrolyte levels, and generating hormones that raise the production of red blood cells and lower blood pressure. These essential processes are jeopardized when kidney function is low, which can result in a buildup of toxins in the body and other issues.

Early-stage CKD is frequently asymptomatic, making diagnosis difficult until considerable damage has been done. Obesity, diabetes, hypertension, and a family history of kidney disease are common risk factors for CKD. As the illness worsens, symptoms like weariness, edema in the ankles and legs, irregular urination, nausea, and itching may appear.

The goals of CKD management are to control symptoms, avoid complications, and slow down the disease's progression. This usually entails changing one's diet, exercising frequently, and taking medicine to regulate one's blood pressure and blood sugar levels. Treatments like kidney transplantation or dialysis may be required in advanced stages to restore lost kidney function and enhance quality of life. Effective CKD management and lowering the risk of complications depend on early detection and intervention. Frequent screening for high-risk individuals can aid in the early detection of CKD when interventions are most successful.

Summary

- Acute Kidney Injury (AKI) is a sudden and often reversible decline in renal function, characterized by an abrupt rise in serum creatinine and/or a decrease in urine output.
- Treatment of AKI is needed to reduce the high morbidity and mortality and improve recovery of renal function. As part of dialysis, there are no other interventions that reliably improve survival, limit injury, or enhance recovery.
- One of the most important functions of the kidney is the filtration and excretion of nitrogenous waste products from the blood. The measurements of elevated blood urea nitrogen (BUN) and creatinine serve as indicators of decreased renal function indicative of the decreased clearance of these waste products.
- Maintaining a normal GFR is dependent on adequate renal perfusion. Prerenal azotemia is characterized by a decrease in GFR due to a decrease in renal perfusion pressure without damage to the renal parenchyma.
- Autophagy is a catabolic process in which proteins, organelles, and cytoplasmic components are delivered to lysosomes for degradation and recycling.
- Inflammation plays a major role in the pathophysiology of AKI resulting from ischemia. Changes in protein folding and mitochondrial function influence the innate immune response, contributing to inflammation.
- Lipopolysaccharide (LPS), a component of the outer membrane of Gram-negative bacteria, is a potent and rapid activator of a variety of cell types such as leukocytes, monocytes, and macrophages.
- Fluid management and renal replacement therapy (RRT) are critical components in the management of Acute Kidney Injury (AKI), aimed at ensuring adequate renal perfusion, preventing fluid overload, and addressing the complications of impaired kidney function.
- RRT is indicated in AKI when conservative measures fail to manage complications like refractory hyperkalemia, severe metabolic acidosis, volume overload unresponsive to diuretics, and uremic symptoms.

References

1. Akamatsu, N., Sugawara, Y., Tamura, S., Kaneko, J., Togashi, J., Kishi, Y., et al. (2005). Prevention of renal impairment by continuous infusion of human atrial natriuretic peptide after liver transplantation. *Transplantation, 80*(8), 1093–1098.
2. Aksu, U., Demirci, C., & Ince, C. (2011). The pathogenesis of acute kidney injury and the toxic triangle of oxygen, reactive oxygen species and nitric oxide. *Contributions to Nephrology, 174*, 119–128.
3. Albanese, J., Leone, M., Delmas, A., & Martin, C. (2005). Terlipressin or norepinephrine in hyperdynamic septic shock: A prospective, randomized study. *Critical Care Medicine, 33*(9), 1897–1902.

4. Alkhunaizi, A. M., Yaqoob, M. M., Edelstein, C. L., Gengaro, P. E., Burke, T. J., Nemenoff, R. A., et al. (1996). Arachidonic acid protects against hypoxic injury in rat proximal tubules. *Kidney International, 49*(3), 620–625.
5. Alkhunaizi, M. A. (2019). *Acute Kidney Injury*. IntechOpen. https://doi.org/10.5772/intechopen.80625.
6. Allgren, R. L., Marbury, T. C., Rahman, S. N., Weisberg, L. S., Fenves, A. Z., Lafayette, R. A., et al. (1997). Anaritide in acute tubular necrosis. Auriculin Anaritide Acute Renal Failure Study Group. *The New England Journal of Medicine, 336*(12), 828–834.
7. Anwar, M. A., Basith, S., & Choi, S. (2013). Negative regulatory approaches to the attenuation of toll-like receptor signaling. *Experimental & Molecular Medicine, 45*, e11.
8. Armstrong, L., Medford, A. R., Hunter, K. J., Uppington, K. M., & Millar, A. B. (2004). Differential expression of toll-like receptor (TLR)-2 and TLR-4 on monocytes in human sepsis. *Clinical and Experimental Immunology, 136*(2), 312–319.
9. Atan, R., Crosbie, D., & Bellomo, R. (2012). Techniques of extracorporeal cytokine removal: A systematic review of the literature. *Blood Purification, 33*(1–3), 88–100.
10. Badr, K. F., & Ichikawa, I. (1988). Prerenal failure: A deleterious shift from renal compensation to decompensation. *The New England Journal of Medicine, 319*(10), 623–629.
11. Bagshaw, S. M., & Ghali, W. A. (2005). Theophylline for prevention of contrast-induced nephropathy: A systematic review and meta-analysis. *Archives of Internal Medicine, 165*(10), 1087–1093.
12. Bagshaw, S. M., Lapinsky, S., Dial, S., Arabi, Y., Dodek, P., Wood, G., et al. (2009). Acute kidney injury in septic shock: Clinical outcomes and impact of duration of hypotension prior to initiation of antimicrobial therapy. *Intensive Care Medicine, 35*(5), 871–881.
13. Bagshaw, S. M., McAlister, F. A., Manns, B. J., & Ghali, W. A. (2006). Acetylcysteine in the prevention of contrast-induced nephropathy: A case study of the pitfalls in the evolution of evidence. *Archives of Internal Medicine, 166*(2), 161–166.
14. Barbieri, L., Verdoia, M., Schaffer, A., Nardin, M., Marino, P., & De Luca, G. (2014). The role of statins in the prevention of contrast-induced nephropathy: A meta-analysis of 8 randomized trials. *Journal of Thrombosis and Thrombolysis, 38*(4), 493–502.
15. Basile, D. P., Donohoe, D., Roethe, K., & Osborn, J. L. (2001). Renal ischemic injury results in permanent damage to peritubular capillaries and influences long-term function. *American Journal of Physiology: Renal Physiology, 281*(5), F887–F899.
16. Bedford, M., Farmer, C., Levin, A., Ali, T., & Stevens, P. (2012). Acute kidney injury and CKD: Chicken or egg? *American Journal of Kidney Diseases, 59*(4), 485–491.
17. Bellomo, R., Ronco, C., Kellum, J. A., Mehta, R. L., & Palevsky, P. (2004). Acute renal failure—Definition, outcome measures, animal models, fluid therapy and information technology needs: The Second International Consensus Conference of the Acute Dialysis Quality Initiative (ADQI) Group. *Critical Care, 8*(4), R204–R212.
18. Benoehr, P., Krueth, P., Bokemeyer, C., Grenz, A., Osswald, H., & Hartmann, J. T. (2005). Nephroprotection by theophylline in patients with cisplatin chemotherapy: A randomized, single-blinded, placebo-controlled trial. *Journal of the American Society of Nephrology, 16*(2), 452–458.

19. Billings, F. T., Hendricks, P. A., Schildcrout, J. S., Shi, Y., Petracek, M. R., Byrne, J. G., et al. (2016). High-dose perioperative atorvastatin and acute kidney injury following cardiac surgery: A randomized clinical trial. *Journal of the American Medical Association, 315*(9), 877–888.

20. Bonventre, J. V., & Zuk, A. (2004). Ischemic acute renal failure: An inflammatory disease? *Kidney International, 66*(2), 480–485.

21. Bove, T., Matteazzi, A., Belletti, A., Paternoster, G., Saleh, O., Taddeo, D., et al. (2015). Beneficial impact of levosimendan in critically ill patients with or at risk for acute renal failure: A meta-analysis of randomized clinical trials. *Heart Lung Vessel, 7*(1), 35–46.

22. Bove, T., Zangrillo, A., Guarracino, F., Alvaro, G., Persi, B., Maglioni, E., et al. (2014). Effect of fenoldopam on use of renal replacement therapy among patients with acute kidney injury after cardiac surgery: A randomized clinical trial. *Journal of the American Medical Association, 312*(21), 2244–2253.

23. Brezis, M., Agmon, Y., & Epstein, F. H. (1994). Determinants of intrarenal oxygenation. I. Effects of diuretics. *The American Journal of Physiology, 267*(6 Pt 2), F1059–F1062.

24. Briguori, C., Airoldi, F., D'Andrea, D., Bonizzoni, E., Morici, N., Focaccio, A., et al. (2007). Renal Insufficiency Following Contrast Media Administration Trial [REMEDIAL]: A randomized comparison of 3 preventive strategies. *Circulation, 115*(10), 1211–1217.

25. Brochard, L., Abroug, F., Brenner, M., Broccard, A. F., Danner, R. L., Ferrer, M., et al. (2010). An official ATS/ERS/ESICM/SCCM/SRLF statement: Prevention and management of acute renal failure in the ICU patient: An international consensus conference in intensive care medicine. *American Journal of Respiratory and Critical Care Medicine, 181*(10), 1128–1155.

26. Brooks, C., Wei, Q., Cho, S. G., & Dong, Z. (2009). Regulation of mitochondrial dynamics in acute kidney injury in cell culture and rodent models. *The Journal of Clinical Investigation, 119*(5), 1275–1285.

27. Burke, J. E., & Dennis, E. A. (2009). Phospholipase A2 biochemistry. *Cardiovascular Drugs and Therapy, 23*(1), 49–59.

28. Cerda, J., Bagga, A., Kher, V., & Chakravarthi, R. M. (2008). The contrasting characteristics of acute kidney injury in developed and developing countries. *Nature Clinical Practice: Nephrology, 4*(3), 138–153.

29. Chawla, L. S. (2011). Acute kidney injury leading to chronic kidney disease and long-term outcomes of acute kidney injury: The best opportunity to mitigate acute kidney injury? *Contributions to Nephrology, 174*, 182–190.

30. Chawla, L. S., Eggers, P. W., Star, R. A., & Kimmel, P. L. (2014). Acute kidney injury and chronic kidney disease as interconnected syndromes. *The New England Journal of Medicine, 371*(1), 58–66.

31. Chow, J. C., Young, D. W., Golenbock, D. T., Christ, W. J., & Gusovsky, F. (1999). Toll-like receptor-4 mediates lipopolysaccharide-induced signal transduction. *The Journal of Biological Chemistry, 274*(16), 10689–10692.

32. Coca, S. G., Singanamala, S., & Parikh, C. R. (2012). Chronic kidney disease after acute kidney injury: A systematic review and meta-analysis. *Kidney International, 81*(5), 442–448.

33. Coca, S. G., Yusuf, B., Shlipak, M. G., Garg, A. X., & Parikh, C. R. (2009). Long-term risk of

mortality and other adverse outcomes after acute kidney injury: A systematic review and meta-analysis. *American Journal of Kidney Diseases, 53*(6), 961–973.

34. Denton, M. D., Chertow, G. M., & Brady, H. R. (1996). "Renal-dose" dopamine for the treatment of acute renal failure: Scientific rationale, experimental studies and clinical trials. *Kidney International, 50*(1), 4–14.
35. Devarajan, P., & Basu, R. K. (2017). Sepsis-associated acute kidney injury—Is it possible to move the needle against this syndrome? *Jornal de Pediatria (Rio J), 93*(1), 1–3.
36. Ferenbach, D. A., & Bonventre, J. V. (2015). Mechanisms of maladaptive repair after AKI leading to accelerated kidney ageing and CKD. *Nature Reviews: Nephrology, 11*(5), 264–276.
37. Friedrich, J. O., Adhikari, N. K., Herridge, M. S., & Beyene, J. (2005). Meta-analysis: Low-dose dopamine increases urine output but does not prevent renal dysfunction or death. *Annals of Internal Medicine, 142*(7), 510–524.
38. Fry, A. C., & Farrington, K. (2006). Management of acute renal failure. *Postgraduate Medical Journal, 82*(964), 106–116.
39. Gillies, M. A., Kakar, V., Parker, R. J., Honore, P. M., & Ostermann, M. (2015). Fenoldopam to prevent acute kidney injury after major surgery—A systematic review and meta-analysis. *Critical Care, 19*, 449.
40. Goldberg, R., & Dennen, P. (2008). Long-term outcomes of acute kidney injury. *Advances in Chronic Kidney Disease, 15*(3), 297–307.
41. Gosmanova, E. O., Wu, S., & O'Neill, W. C. (2009). Application of ultrasound in nephrology practice. *Advances in Chronic Kidney Disease, 16*(5), 396–404.
42. Han, Y., Zhu, G., Han, L., Hou, F., Huang, W., Liu, H., et al. (2014). Short-term rosuvastatin therapy for prevention of contrast-induced acute kidney injury in patients with diabetes and chronic kidney disease. *Journal of the American College of Cardiology, 63*(1), 62–70.
43. Hasslacher, J., Bijuklic, K., Bertocchi, C., Kountchev, J., Bellmann, R., Dunzendorfer, S., et al. (2011). Levosimendan inhibits release of reactive oxygen species in polymorphonuclear leukocytes in vitro and in patients with acute heart failure and septic shock: A prospective observational study. *Critical Care, 15*(4), R166.
44. He, L., Livingston, M. J., & Dong, Z. (2014). Autophagy in acute kidney injury and repair. *Nephron: Clinical Practice, 127*(1–4), 56–60.
45. Heung, M., Steffick, D. E., Zivin, K., Gillespie, B. W., Banerjee, T., Hsu, C. Y., et al. (2016). Acute kidney injury recovery pattern and subsequent risk of CKD: An analysis of veteran's health administration data. *American Journal of Kidney Diseases, 67*(5), 742–752.
46. Himmelfarb, J., Joannidis, M., Molitoris, B., Schietz, M., Okusa, M. D., Warnock, D., et al. (2008). Evaluation and initial management of acute kidney injury. *Clinical Journal of the American Society of Nephrology, 3*(4), 962–967.
47. Ho, K. M., & Sheridan, D. J. (2006). Meta-analysis of frusemide to prevent or treat acute renal failure. *BMJ, 333*(7565), 420.
48. Holmes, C. L., & Walley, K. R. (2003). Bad medicine: Low-dose dopamine in the ICU. *Chest, 123*(4), 1266–1275.

49. Hoste, E. A., Bagshaw, S. M., Bellomo, R., Cely, C. M., Colman, R., Cruz, D. N., et al. (2015). Epidemiology of acute kidney injury in critically ill patients: The multinational AKI-EPI study. *Intensive Care Medicine, 41*(8), 1411–1423.

50. Hotchkiss, R. S., & Karl, I. E. (2003). The pathophysiology and treatment of sepsis. *The New England Journal of Medicine, 348*(2), 138–150.

51. Hynninen, M. S., Niemi, T. T., Poyhia, R., Raininko, E. I., Salmenpera, M. T., Lepantalo, M. J., et al. (2006). N-acetylcysteine for the prevention of kidney injury in abdominal aortic surgery: A randomized, double-blind, placebo-controlled trial. *Anesthesia and Analgesia, 102*(6), 1638–1645.

52. Inagi, R. (2009). Endoplasmic reticulum stress in the kidney as a novel mediator of kidney injury. *Nephron: Experimental Nephrology, 112*(1), e1–e9.

53. Ishani, A., Xue, J. L., Himmelfarb, J., Eggers, P. W., Kimmel, P. L., Molitoris, B. A., et al. (2009). Acute kidney injury increases risk of ESRD among elderly. *Journal of the American Society of Nephrology, 20*(1), 223–228.

54. Ix, J. H., McCulloch, C. E., & Chertow, G. M. (2004). Theophylline for the prevention of radiocontrast nephropathy: A meta-analysis. *Nephrology, Dialysis, Transplantation, 19*(11), 2747–2753.

55. Jang, H. R., & Rabb, H. (2015). Immune cells in experimental acute kidney injury. *Nature Reviews: Nephrology, 11*(2), 88–101.

56. Jaynes, M. P., Murphy, C. V., Ali, N., Krautwater, A., Lehman, A., & Doepker, B. A. (2018). Association between chloride content of intravenous fluids and acute kidney injury in critically ill medical patients with sepsis. *Journal of Critical Care, 44*, 363–367.

57. Jha, V., & Parameswaran, S. (2013). Community-acquired acute kidney injury in tropical countries. *Nature Reviews: Nephrology, 9*(5), 278–290.

58. Jiang, M., Wei, Q., Dong, G., Komatsu, M., Su, Y., & Dong, Z. (2012). Autophagy in proximal tubules protects against acute kidney injury. *Kidney International, 82*(12), 1271–1283.

59. Joannidis, M., Druml, W., Forni, L. G., Groeneveld, A. B. J., Honore, P. M., Hoste, E., et al. (2017). Prevention of acute kidney injury and protection of renal function in the intensive care unit: Update 2017: Expert opinion of the Working Group on Prevention, AKI section, European Society of Intensive Care Medicine. *Intensive Care Medicine, 43*(6), 730–749.

60. Kama, A., Yilmaz, S., Yaka, E., Dervisoglu, E., Dogan, N. O., Erimsah, E., et al. (2014). Comparison of short-term infusion regimens of N-acetylcysteine plus intravenous fluids, sodium bicarbonate plus intravenous fluids, and intravenous fluids alone for prevention of contrast-induced nephropathy in the emergency department. *Academic Emergency Medicine, 21*(6), 615–622.

61. Karthik, S., & Lisbon, A. (2006). Low-dose dopamine in the intensive care unit. *Seminars in Dialysis, 19*(6), 465–471.

62. Kellum, J. A., & Lameire, N. (2013). Diagnosis, evaluation, and management of acute kidney injury: A KDIGO summary (Part 1). *Critical Care, 17*(1), 204.

63. Kidney Disease: Improving Global Outcomes (KDIGO). (2012). KDIGO clinical practice guideline for acute kidney injury. *Kidney International Supplements, 2*(1), S1–S138.

64. Kimura, T., Isaka, Y., & Yoshimori, T. (2017). Autophagy and kidney inflammation. *Autophagy, 13*(6), 997–1003.

65. Kohjimoto, Y., Kennington, L., Scheid, C. R., & Honeyman, T. W. (1999). Role of phospholipase A2 in the cytotoxic effects of oxalate in cultured renal epithelial cells. *Kidney International, 56*(4), 1432–1441.

66. Komisarof, J. A., Gilkey, G. M., Peters, D. M., Koudelka, C. W., Meyer, M. M., & Smith, S. M. (2007). N-acetylcysteine for patients with prolonged hypotension as prophylaxis for acute renal failure [NEPHRON]. *Critical Care Medicine, 35*(2), 435–441.

67. Kuhn, M. (2009). The natriuretic peptide/guanylyl cyclase—A system functions as a stress-responsive regulator of angiogenesis in mice. *Journal of Clinical Investigation, 119*(7), 2019–2030.

68. Kuhn, M. (2012). Endothelial actions of atrial and B-type natriuretic peptides. *British Journal of Pharmacology, 166*(2), 522–531.

69. Kumar, H., Kawai, T., & Akira, S. (2009). Toll-like receptors and innate immunity. *Biochemical and Biophysical Research Communications, 388*(4), 621–625.

70. Lafrance, J. P., & Miller, D. R. (2010). Acute kidney injury associates with increased long-term mortality. *Journal of the American Society of Nephrology, 21*(2), 345–352.

71. Lameire, N. H., Vanholder, R. C., & Van Biesen, W. A. (2011). How to use biomarkers efficiently in acute kidney injury. *Kidney International, 79*(10), 1047–1050.

72. Lameire, N., Van Biesen, W., & Vanholder, R. (2005). Acute renal failure. *Lancet, 365*(9457), 417–430.

73. Lauschke, A., Teichgraber, U. K., Frei, U., & Eckardt, K. U. (2006). 'Low-dose' dopamine worsens renal perfusion in patients with acute renal failure. *Kidney International, 69*(9), 1669–1674.

74. Lee, J. M., Park, J., Jeon, K. H., Jung, J. H., Lee, S. E., Han, J. K., et al. (2014). Efficacy of short-term high-dose statin pretreatment in prevention of contrast-induced acute kidney injury: Updated study-level meta-analysis of 13 randomized controlled trials. *PLoS One, 9*(11), e111397.

75. Leoncini, M., Toso, A., Maioli, M., Tropeano, F., Villani, S., & Bellandi, F. (2014). Early high-dose rosuvastatin for contrast-induced nephropathy prevention in acute coronary syndrome: Results from the PRATO-ACS study [Protective effect of rosuvastatin and antiplatelet therapy on contrast-induced acute kidney injury and myocardial damage in patients with acute coronary syndrome]. *Journal of the American College of Cardiology, 63*(1), 71–79.

76. Lewis, J., Salem, M. M., Chertow, G. M., Weisberg, L. S., McGrew, F., Marbury, T. C., et al. (2000). Atrial natriuretic factor in oliguric acute renal failure. Anaritide acute renal failure study group. *American Journal of Kidney Diseases, 36*(4), 767–774.

77. Li, J., Li, Y., Xu, B., Jia, G., Guo, T., Wang, D., et al. (2016). Short-term rosuvastatin therapy prevents contrast-induced acute kidney injury in female patients with diabetes and chronic kidney disease: A subgroup analysis of the TRACK-D study. *Journal of Thoracic Disease, 8*(5), 1000–1006.

78. Ling, H., Gengaro, P. E., Edelstein, C. L., Martin, P. Y., Wangsiripaisan, A., Nemenoff, R., et al. (1998). Effect of hypoxia on proximal tubules isolated from nitric oxide synthase knockout mice. *Kidney International, 53*(6), 1642–1646.

79. Lopes, J. A., & Jorge, S. (2013). The RIFLE and AKIN classifications for acute kidney injury: A critical and comprehensive review. *Clinical Kidney Journal, 6*(1), 8–14.

80. Mahmoodnia, L., Mohammadi, K., & Masumi, R. (2017). Ameliorative effect of lycopene on cisplatin-induced nephropathy in patients. *Journal of Nephropathology, 6*(3), 144–149.
81. Maioli, M., Toso, A., Leoncini, M., Gallopin, M., Tedeschi, D., Micheletti, C., et al. (2008). Sodium bicarbonate versus saline for the prevention of contrast-induced nephropathy in patients with renal dysfunction undergoing coronary angiography or intervention. *Journal of the American College of Cardiology, 52*(8), 599–604.
82. Marenzi, G., Assanelli, E., Marana, I., Lauri, G., Campodonico, J., Grazi, M., et al. (2006). N-acetylcysteine and contrast-induced nephropathy in primary angioplasty. *The New England Journal of Medicine, 354*(26), 2773–2782.
83. Martins, P. S., Brunialti, M. K., da Luz Fernandes, M., Martos, L. S., Gomes, N. E., Rigato, O., et al. (2006). Bacterial recognition and induced cell activation in sepsis. *Endocrine, Metabolic & Immune Disorders Drug Targets, 6*(2), 183–191.
84. Mehta, R. L., Cerda, J., Burdmann, E. A., Tonelli, M., Garcia-Garcia, G., Jha, V., et al. (2015). International Society of Nephrology's 0by25 initiative for acute kidney injury (zero preventable deaths by 2025): A human rights case for nephrology. *The Lancet, 385*(9987), 2616–2643.
85. Mehta, R. L., Kellum, J. A., Shah, S. V., Molitoris, B. A., Ronco, C., Warnock, D. G., et al. (2007). Acute kidney injury network: Report of an initiative to improve outcomes in acute kidney injury. *Critical Care, 11*(2), R31.
86. Mehta, R. L., Pascual, M. T., Soroko, S., & Chertow, G. M. (2002). Diuretics, mortality, and nonrecovery of renal function in acute renal failure. *Journal of the American Medical Association, 288*(20), 2547–2553.
87. Merten, G. J., Burgess, W. P., Gray, L. V., Holleman, J. H., Roush, T. S., Kowalchuk, G. J., et al. (2004). Prevention of contrast-induced nephropathy with sodium bicarbonate: A randomized controlled trial. *Journal of the American Medical Association, 291*(19), 2328–2334.
88. Molitoris, B. A. (2014). Therapeutic translation in acute kidney injury: The epithelial/endothelial axis. *The Journal of Clinical Investigation, 124*(6), 2355–2363.
89. Momeni, A., Hajigholami, A., Geshnizjani, S., & Kheiri, S. (2015). Effect of silymarin in the prevention of cisplatin nephrotoxicity, a clinical trial study. *Journal of Clinical and Diagnostic Research, 9*(4), OC11–OC13.
90. Nigwekar, S. U., & Kandula, P. (2009). N-acetylcysteine in cardiovascular-surgery-associated renal failure: A meta-analysis. *The Annals of Thoracic Surgery, 87*(1), 139–147.
91. Noiri, E., Peresleni, T., Miller, F., & Goligorsky, M. S. (1996). In vivo targeting of inducible NO synthase with oligodeoxynucleotides protects rat kidney against ischemia. *The Journal of Clinical Investigation, 97*(10), 2377–2383.
92. O'Neill, W. C. (2014). Renal relevant radiology: Use of ultrasound in kidney disease and nephrology procedures. *Clinical Journal of the American Society of Nephrology, 9*(2), 373–381.
93. Ozcan, E. E., Guneri, S., Akdeniz, B., Akyildiz, I. Z., Senaslan, O., Baris, N., et al. (2007). Sodium bicarbonate, N-acetylcysteine, and saline for prevention of radiocontrast-induced nephropathy. A comparison of 3 regimens for protecting contrast-induced nephropathy in patients undergoing coronary procedures. A single-center prospective controlled trial. *American Heart Journal, 154*(3), 539–544.

94. Park, J. H., Shim, J. K., Song, J. W., Soh, S., & Kwak, Y. L. (2016). Effect of atorvastatin on the incidence of acute kidney injury following valvular heart surgery: A randomized, placebo-controlled trial. *Intensive Care Medicine, 42*(9), 1398–1407.

95. Quintavalle, C., Fiore, D., De Micco, F., Visconti, G., Focaccio, A., Golia, B., et al. (2012). Impact of a high loading dose of atorvastatin on contrast-induced acute kidney injury. *Circulation, 126*(25), 3008–3016.

96. Rahman, M., Shad, F., & Smith, M. C. (2012). Acute kidney injury: A guide to diagnosis and management. *American Family Physician, 86*(7), 631–639.

97. Raturi, A., & Simmen, T. (2013). Where the endoplasmic reticulum and the mitochondrion tie the knot: The mitochondria-associated membrane (MAM). *Biochimica et Biophysica Acta, 1833*(1), 213–224.

98. Rivers, E., Nguyen, B., Havstad, S., Ressler, J., Muzzin, A., Knoblich, B., et al. (2001). Early goal-directed therapy in the treatment of severe sepsis and septic shock. *The New England Journal of Medicine, 345*(19), 1368–1377.

99. Sato, K., Sekiguchi, S., Kawagishi, N., Akamatsu, Y., Enomoto, Y., Takeda, I., et al. (2006). Continuous low-dose human atrial natriuretic peptide promotes diuresis in oliguric patients after living donor liver transplantation. *Transplantation Proceedings, 38*(10), 3591–3593.

100. Sawhney, S., Marks, A., Fluck, N., Levin, A., Prescott, G., & Black, C. (2017). Intermediate and long-term outcomes of survivors of acute kidney injury episodes: A large population-based cohort study. *American Journal of Kidney Diseases, 69*(1), 18–28.

101. Schmidt, P., Pang, D., Nykamp, D., Knowlton, G., & Jia, H. (2007). N-acetylcysteine and sodium bicarbonate versus N-acetylcysteine and standard hydration for the prevention of radiocontrast-induced nephropathy following coronary angiography. *The Annals of Pharmacotherapy, 41*(1), 46–50.

102. Schortgen, F., Lacherade, J. C., Bruneel, F., Cattaneo, I., Hemery, F., Lemaire, F., et al. (2001). Effects of hydroxyethylstarch and gelatin on renal function in severe sepsis: A multicentre randomised study. *Lancet, 357*(9260), 911–916.

103. Schrier, R. W., Wang, W., Poole, B., & Mitra, A. (2004). Acute renal failure: Definitions, diagnosis, pathogenesis, and therapy. *The Journal of Clinical Investigation, 114*(1), 5–14.

104. Shahbazi, F., Sadighi, S., Dashti-Khavidaki, S., Shahi, F., Mirzania, M., Abdollahi, A., et al. (2015). Effect of silymarin administration on cisplatin nephrotoxicity: Report from a pilot, randomized, double-blinded, placebo-controlled clinical trial. *Phytotherapy Research, 29*(7), 1046–1053.

105. Shehata, M., & Hamza, M. (2015). Impact of high loading dose of atorvastatin in diabetic patients with renal dysfunction undergoing elective percutaneous coronary intervention: A randomized controlled trial. *Cardiovascular Therapeutics, 33*(2), 35–41.

106. Silver, S. A., & Chertow, G. M. (2017). The economic consequences of acute kidney injury. *Nephron, 137*(4), 297–301.

107. Solomon, R., Werner, C., Mann, D., D'Elia, J., & Silva, P. (1994). Effects of saline, mannitol, and furosemide on acute decreases in renal function induced by radiocontrast agents. *The New England Journal of Medicine, 331*(21), 1416–1420.

108. Stone, G. W., McCullough, P. A., Tumlin, J. A., Lepor, N. E., Madyoon, H., Murray, P., et al. (2003). Fenoldopam mesylate for the prevention of contrast-induced nephropathy: A randomized controlled trial. *Journal of the American Medical Association, 290*(17), 2284–2291.

109. Susantitaphong, P., Cruz, D. N., Cerda, J., Abulfaraj, M., Alqahtani, F., Koulouridis, I., et al. (2013). World incidence of AKI: A meta-analysis. *Clinical Journal of the American Society of Nephrology, 8*(9), 1482–1493.

110. Sward, K., Valsson, F., Odencrants, P., Samuelsson, O., & Ricksten, S. E. (2004). Recombinant human atrial natriuretic peptide in ischemic acute renal failure: A randomized placebo-controlled trial. *Critical Care Medicine, 32*(6), 1310–1315.

111. Sward, K., Valsson, F., Sellgren, J., & Ricksten, S. E. (2005). Differential effects of human atrial natriuretic peptide and furosemide on glomerular filtration rate and renal oxygen consumption in humans. *Intensive Care Medicine, 31*(1), 79–85.

112. Tepel, M., van der Giet, M., Schwarzfeld, C., Laufer, U., Liermann, D., & Zidek, W. (2000). Prevention of radiographic-contrast-agent-induced reductions in renal function by acetylcysteine. *The New England Journal of Medicine, 343*(3), 180–184.

113. Thadhani, R., Pascual, M., & Bonventre, J. V. (1996). Acute renal failure. *The New England Journal of Medicine, 334*(22), 1448–1460.

114. Traub, S. J., Mitchell, A. M., Jones, A. E., Tang, A., O'Connor, J., Nelson, T., et al. (2013). N-acetylcysteine plus intravenous fluids versus intravenous fluids alone to prevent contrast-induced nephropathy in emergency computed tomography. *Annals of Emergency Medicine, 62*(5), 511–520.e25.

115. Tumlin, J. A., Finkel, K. W., Murray, P. T., Samuels, J., Cotsonis, G., & Shaw, A. D. (2005). Fenoldopam mesylate in early acute tubular necrosis: A randomized, double-blind, placebo-controlled clinical trial. *American Journal of Kidney Diseases, 46*(1), 26–34.

116. Ukaigwe, A., Karmacharya, P., Mahmood, M., Pathak, R., Aryal, M. R., Jalota, L., et al. (2014). Meta-analysis on efficacy of statins for prevention of contrast-induced acute kidney injury in patients undergoing coronary angiography. *The American Journal of Cardiology, 114*(9), 1295–1302.

117. Vanmassenhove, J., Vanholder, R., Nagler, E., & Van Biesen, W. (2013). Urinary and serum biomarkers for the diagnosis of acute kidney injury: An in-depth review of the literature. *Nephrology, Dialysis, Transplantation, 28*(2), 254–273.

118. Venkatachalam, M. A., Griffin, K. A., Lan, R., Geng, H., Saikumar, P., & Bidani, A. K. (2010). Acute kidney injury: A springboard for progression in chronic kidney disease. *American Journal of Physiology: Renal Physiology, 298*(5), F1078–F1094.

119. Wan, L., Bagshaw, S. M., Langenberg, C., Saotome, T., May, C., & Bellomo, R. (2008). Pathophysiology of septic acute kidney injury: What do we really know? *Critical Care Medicine, 36*(4 Suppl), S198–S203.

120. Yang, R. B., Mark, M. R., Gray, A., Huang, A., Xie, M. H., Zhang, M., et al. (1998). Toll-like receptor-2 mediates lipopolysaccharide-induced cellular signaling. *Nature, 395*(6699), 284–288.

121. Ysebaert, D. K., De Greef, K. E., Vercauteren, S. R., Ghielli, M., Verpooten, G. A., Eyskens, E. J., et al. (2000). Identification and kinetics of leukocytes after severe ischaemia/reperfusion renal injury. *Nephrology, Dialysis, Transplantation, 15*(10), 1562–1574.

122. Yu, L., Gengaro, P. E., Niederberger, M., Burke, T. J., & Schrier, R. W. (1994). Nitric oxide: A mediator in rat tubular hypoxia/reoxygenation injury. *Proceedings of the National Academy of Sciences of the United States of America, 91*(5), 1691–1695.

123. Zager, R. A., Schimpf, B. A., Gmur, D. J., & Burke, T. J. (1993). Phospholipase A2 activity can protect renal tubules from oxygen deprivation injury. *Proceedings of the National Academy of Sciences of the United States of America, 90*(17), 8297–8301.

124. Zangrillo, A., Biondi-Zoccai, G. G., Frati, E., Covello, R. D., Cabrini, L., Guarracino, F., et al. (2012). Fenoldopam and acute renal failure in cardiac surgery: A meta-analysis of randomized placebo-controlled trials. *Journal of Cardiothoracic and Vascular Anesthesia, 26*(3), 407–413.

125. Zarjou, A., & Agarwal, A. (2011). Sepsis and acute kidney injury. *Journal of the American Society of Nephrology, 22*(6), 999–1006.

126. Zhan, M., Brooks, C., Liu, F., Sun, L., & Dong, Z. (2013). Mitochondrial dynamics: Regulatory mechanisms and emerging role in renal pathophysiology. *Kidney International, 83*(4), 568–581.

127. Zhang, K., & Kaufman, R. J. (2008). From endoplasmic-reticulum stress to the inflammatory response. *Nature, 454*(7203), 455–462.

128. Zheng, Z., Jayaram, R., Jiang, L., Emberson, J., Zhao, Y., Li, Q., et al. (2016). Perioperative rosuvastatin in cardiac surgery. *The New England Journal of Medicine, 374*(18), 1744–1753.

129. Zhou, C., Gong, J., Chen, D., Wang, W., Liu, M., & Liu, B. (2016). Levosimendan for prevention of acute kidney injury after cardiac surgery: A meta-analysis of randomized controlled trials. *American Journal of Kidney Diseases, 67*(3), 408–416.

130. Zuk, A., & Bonventre, J. V. (2016). Acute kidney injury. *Annual Review of Medicine, 67*, 293–307.

131. Zuk, A., Gershenovich, M., Ivanova, Y., MacFarland, R. T., Fricker, S. P., & Ledbetter, S. (2014). CXCR4 antagonism as a therapeutic approach to prevent acute kidney injury. *American Journal of Physiology: Renal Physiology, 307*(7), F783–F797.

Chapter 7

CHRONIC KIDNEY DISEASE (CKD)

Contents

Introduction

Chronic Kidney Disease (CKD) is a progressive condition marked by the gradual loss of kidney function over time. This debilitating ailment affects millions of people worldwide, often remaining asymptomatic until the later stages. The kidneys play a crucial role in filtering waste products and excess fluids from the blood, regulating electrolyte balance, and producing hormones that help control blood pressure and stimulate red blood cell production. However, in CKD, the kidneys become damaged and are unable to perform these functions efficiently.

There are various causes of CKD, including diabetes, hypertension (high blood pressure), glomerulonephritis (inflammation of the kidney's filtering units), and polycystic kidney disease (a genetic disorder characterized by the growth of numerous cysts in the kidneys). Additionally, certain lifestyle factors such as smoking, obesity, and a diet high in sodium and processed foods can contribute to the development and progression of CKD. As CKD progresses, individuals may experience symptoms such as fatigue, weakness, swelling in the legs and ankles, changes in urination frequency, and difficulty concentrating. Complications can arise as the condition advances, including cardiovascular disease, anemia, bone disorders, and fluid overload.

Early detection and management are crucial in slowing the progression of CKD and preventing complications. Treatment typically involves lifestyle modifications such as maintaining a healthy diet, exercising regularly, managing blood pressure and blood sugar levels, and avoiding tobacco and excessive alcohol consumption. Medications may also be prescribed to control symptoms and prevent further kidney damage.

In advanced stages of CKD, when kidney function is significantly impaired, dialysis or kidney transplantation may be necessary to sustain life. However, these interventions come with their own challenges and limitations.

Overall, CKD represents a significant public health concern, highlighting the importance of awareness, early detection, and comprehensive management strategies to improve outcomes and enhance the quality of life for affected individuals.

Orientation and Directional Terms

Term	Definition	Illustration
Renal Disease	Renal disease, also known as kidney disease, encompasses a wide range of conditions that affect the kidneys' ability to function properly. The kidneys are vital organs responsible for filtering waste products and excess fluids from the blood, regulating electrolyte balance, and maintaining overall fluid homeostasis.	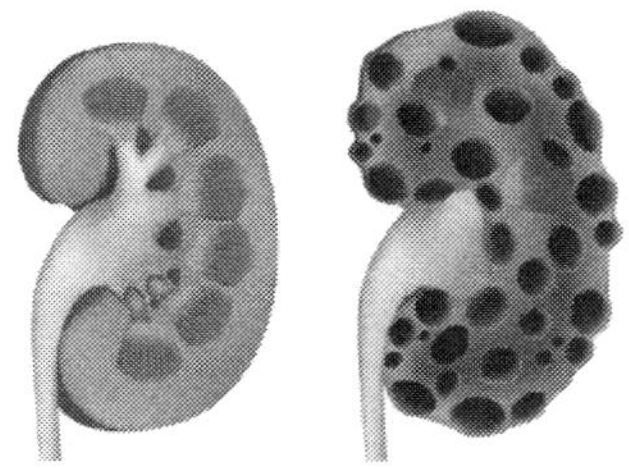
Tubulointerstitial	Tubulointerstitial nephritis is inflammation that affects the tubules of the kidneys and the tissues that surround them (interstitial tissue).	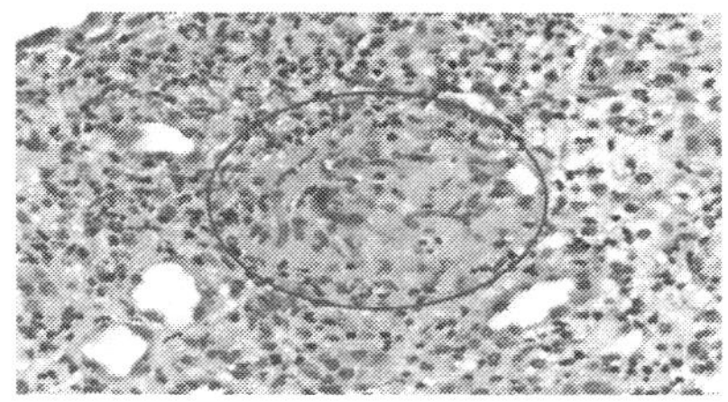
Diabetes Mellitus (DM)	Diabetes mellitus (DM) is a metabolic disease, involving inappropriately elevated blood glucose levels. DM has several categories, including type 1, type 2, maturity-onset diabetes of the young (MODY), gestational diabetes, neonatal diabetes, and secondary causes due to endocrinopathies, steroid use, etc.	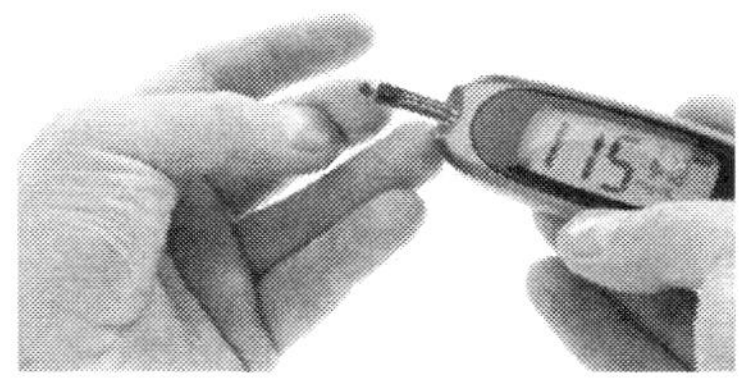
Kidney Transplant	A kidney transplant is a surgery done to replace a diseased or injured kidney with a healthy kidney from a donor.	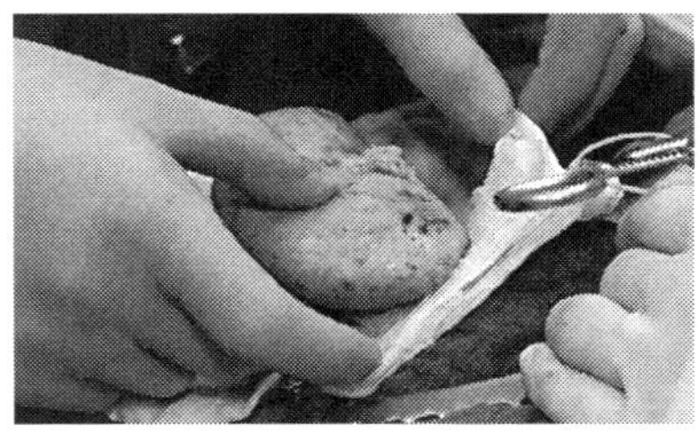
Acute Tubular Necrosis	Acute tubular necrosis is a condition that causes a lack of oxygen and blood flow to the kidneys, damaging them.	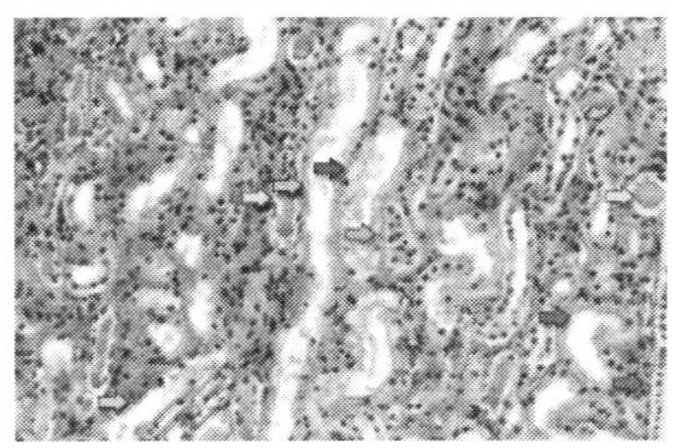

7.1. CKD Definition and Staging

The existence of an anomaly in kidney structure or function that lasts longer than three months is referred to as chronic kidney disease. This comprises one or more of the subsequent conditions: (1) GFR < 60 mL/min/1.73 m^2; (2) albuminuria (i.e., urine albumin ≥ 30 mg/24 h or urine albumin-to-creatinine ratio [ACR] ≥30 mg/g); (3) anomalies in urine sediment, histology, or imaging indicating renal damage; (4) renal tubular disorders; or (5) preceding kidney transplantation. Repeat evaluations are necessary to differentiate chronic kidney disease (CKD) from acute kidney injury, which is defined as a change in kidney function that occurs within two to seven days, and acute kidney disease, which is defined as kidney damage or decreased kidney function that persists for more than three months. Clinical history, physical examination, and urine findings should all be taken into consideration when evaluating the cause of chronic kidney disease (CKD) (Figure 7.1).

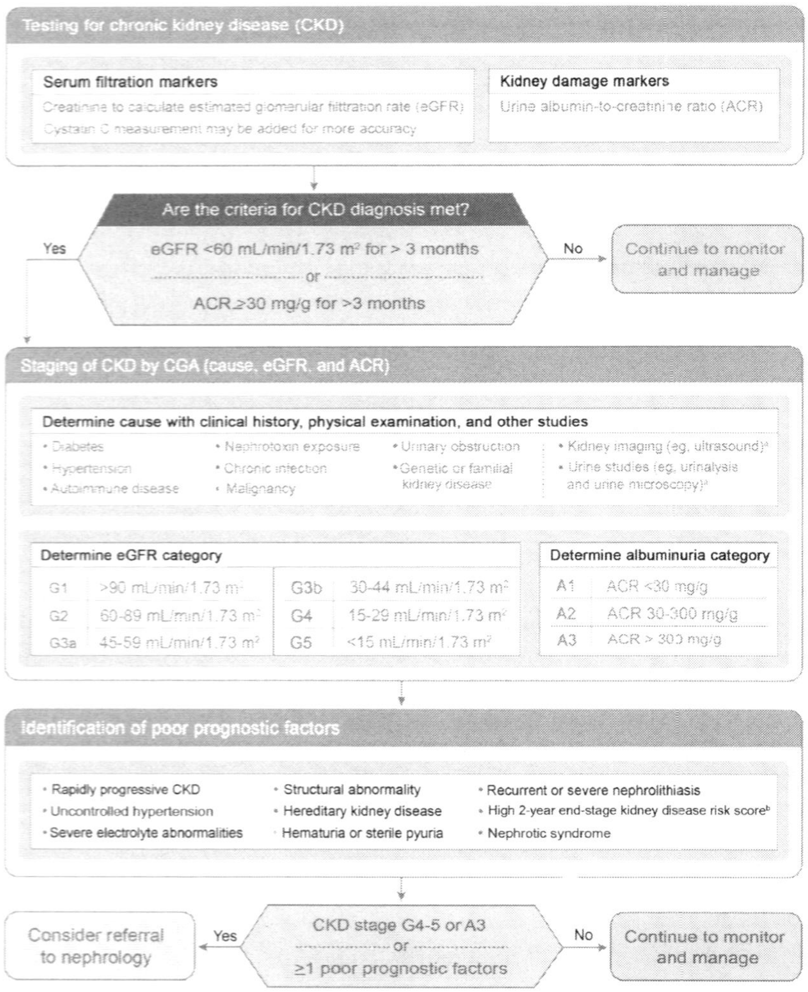

Figure 7.1. *Considerations for diagnosis, staging, and referral of patients with chronic kidney disease.*

Source: Teresa K. Chen, Daphne H. Knicely, & Morgan E. Grams, Chronic Kidney Disease Diagnosis and Management. doi: 10.1001/jama.2019.14745.

Staging is decided upon based on GFR, albuminuria, and the CKD cause after a diagnosis of CKD has been made (Figure 7.2). The levels of GFR staging are categorized as follows: G1 (GFR ≥90 mL/min/1.73 m^2), G2 (GFR 60–89 mL/min/1.73 m^2), G3a (45–59 mL/min/1.73 m^2), G3b (30–44 mL/min/1.73 m^2), G4 (15–29 mL/min/1.73 m^2), and G5 (<15 mL/min/1.73 m^2). While agents like iohexol or iothalamate can be cleared to measure GFR directly, the creation of estimating equations (e.g., The need for direct measurement in clinical practice has largely been replaced by equations (e.g., the Chronic Kidney Disease Epidemiology Collaboration [CKD-EPI] and Modification of Diet in Renal Disease Study [MDRD]). These days, clinical laboratories frequently report estimated GFR (eGFR) that is derived from filtration markers. Creatinine, a 113-dalton byproduct of creatine metabolism, is the most often used filtration marker. Since 2003, laboratory assays for this marker have been standardized. Since the CKD-EPI 2009 creatinine equation is more accurate than the previous MDRD equation, especially for eGFR values greater than 60 mL/min/1.73 m^2, it is the recommended estimating equation in the United States and most of the world. In the CKD-EPI 2012 creatinine-cystatin C equation, cystatin C can be substituted for creatinine in cases where more accuracy and precision are needed. A high-protein diet, limb amputation, excessive body size or muscle mass, use of creatinine supplements, or use of medications that affect tubular secretion of creatinine are some examples of conditions where adding cystatin C may be especially helpful.

				Persistent albuminuria categories, description, and range		
				A1	A2	A3
				Normal to mildly increased	Moderately increased	Severely increased
				<30 mg/g	30-300 mg/g	>300 mg/g
GFR categories, description, and range (mL/min/1.73 m²)	G1	Normal or high	≥90			
	G2	Mildly decreased	60-89			
	G3a	Mildly to moderately decreased	45-59			
	G3b	Moderately to severely decreased	30-44			
	G4	Severely decreased	15-29			
	G5	Kidney failure	<15			

Figure 7.2. *Definition and prognosis of chronic kidney disease by GFR and albuminuria categories, KDIGO 2012.*

Source: *Teresa K. Chen, Daphne H. Knicely, and Morgan E. Grams, Chronic Kidney Disease Diagnosis and Management, doi: 10.1001/jama.2019.14745.*

KDIGO stands for Kidney Disease Improving Global Outcomes; GFR stands for glomerular filtration rate. Groups of categories are based on the risk of progression, which includes the progression of chronic kidney disease, which is defined as a decline in GFR category along with a decline in estimated GFR of at least 25% from baseline or a sustained decline in estimated GFR of at least 5 mL/min/1.73 m^2 annually. When there are no additional kidney disease markers or chronic kidney disease (CKD), green indicates low risk; yellow, moderately elevated risk; orange, high risk; and red, extremely high risk.

Ideally, a urine ACR should be used to measure albuminuria. The staging of albuminuria is categorized as A1 (urine ACR <30 mg/g), A2 (30–300 mg/g), and A3 (> 300 mg/g). Urine ACR is preferred over urine protein-to-creatinine ratio when staging chronic kidney disease (CKD) according to guidelines because the assays for the former are more likely to be standardized and have better precision at lower albuminuria levels. Because urine albumin excretion varies greatly throughout the day due to biological variability, the most accurate measurements are obtained from a first morning sample or 24-hour collection. However, random samples can also be used for preliminary screening. Since certain urine proteins, like uromodulin, are present (and possibly even protective) in normal physiology, urine ACR is thought to be a more sensitive and specific marker of glomerular pathology than urine protein-to-creatinine ratio. Urine protein electrophoresis or testing for the particular protein can be done if tubular or overflow proteinuria is suspected (e.g., α_1-microglobulin, β_2-microglobulin, immunoglobulin heavy and light chains). In all patients with a diagnosis of chronic kidney disease (CKD), kidney ultrasonography should be considered as a means of assessing morphology and ruling out urinary obstruction.

The location of anatomic abnormality and the presence or absence of systemic disease are the two main factors that determine the cause of chronic kidney disease (CKD). Diabetes, autoimmune diseases, chronic infections, cancer, and genetic disorders affecting multiple organs in addition to the kidney are examples of systemic diseases. The categories of anatomic locations include vascular, tubulointerstitial, glomerular, and cystic/congenital diseases. The prognosis and course of treatment for CKD may be significantly impacted by the cause's identification. For instance, polycystic kidney disease (PKD) can lead to end-stage kidney disease (ESKD) more quickly than other causes. It is often necessary to assess for extrarenal manifestations and to explore targeted therapies like tolvaptan, a vasopressin V2 receptor antagonist that slows the decline in GFR. Patients with CKD causes that are unknown ought to be referred to nephrologists.

7.1.1. Etiology

The causes of CKD vary globally, and the most common primary diseases causing CKD and, ultimately, end-stage renal disease (ESRD) are as follows:

- Diabetes mellitus type 2 (30% to 50%)
- Diabetes mellitus type 1 (3.9%)
- Hypertension (27.2%)
- Primary glomerulonephritis (8.2%)
- Chronic Tubulointerstitial nephritis (3.6%)
- Hereditary or cystic diseases (3.1%)
- Secondary glomerulonephritis or vasculitis (2.1%)
- Plasma cell dyscrasias or neoplasm (2.1)
- Sickle Cell Nephropathy (SCN) which accounts for less than 1% of ESRD patients in the United States

Any of the three disease processes that cause chronic kidney disease (CKD) can be prerenal (lower renal perfusion pressure), intrinsic (vessel, glomerular, or tubule-interstitium pathology), or postrenal (obstructive).

- **Prerenal Disease:** Patients with chronic heart failure or cirrhosis who have persistently reduced renal perfusion are at a higher risk of experiencing multiple episodes of intrinsic kidney injury, such as acute tubular necrosis (ATN), if they have chronic prerenal disease. Over time, this causes a progressive loss of renal function.

Intrinsic Renal Vascular Disease: Nephrosclerosis, the most prevalent chronic renal vascular disease, damages blood vessels, glomeruli, and the tubulointerstitium over time. Renal artery stenosis from atherosclerosis or fibro-muscular dysplasia are the other renal vascular diseases. These conditions can cause ischemic nephropathy, which is characterized by glomerulosclerosis and tubulointerstitial fibrosis, over the course of months or years.

Intrinsic Glomerular Disease (Nephritic or Nephrotic): Abnormal urine microscopy with dysmorphic red blood cells and red blood cell casts, occasionally white blood cells (WBCs), and varying degrees of proteinuria suggest a nephritic pattern. The most frequent causes include vasculitis, lupus nephritis, IgA nephropathy, shunt nephritis, post-streptococcal GN, and infective endocarditis.

Proteinuria, typically in the nephrotic range (greater than 3–5 gm per 24 hours), and an inactive urine microscopic analysis with few cells or casts are linked to a nephrotic pattern. The most common causes are amyloidosis, diabetic nephropathy, membranous GN, membranoproliferative GN (Type 1 and 2 and associated with cryoglobulinemia), minimal change disease, and focal segmental glomerulosclerosis.

Some patients may be assigned to one of these two categories.

1. *Intrinsic Tubular and Interstitial Disease:* Polycystic kidney disease is the most prevalent chronic tubulointerstitial disease (PKD). Other causes include reflux nephropathy in children and young adults, sarcoidosis, Sjogren syndrome, and nephrocalcinosis (which is typically brought on by hypercalcemia and hypercalciuria). Mesoamerican nephropathy, a relatively high prevalence of chronic kidney disease (CKD) of unknown cause among agricultural workers from Central America and parts of Southeast Asia, is becoming more widely recognized (Madero et al., 2017).
2. *Postrenal (Obstructive Nephropathy):* Common causes of chronic obstruction include nephrolithiasis, prostatic disease, and abdominal/pelvic tumors with mass effects on the ureter(s). Chronic ureteral obstruction is infrequently caused by retroperitoneal fibrosis.

7.1.2. Epidemiology

Due to the asymptomatic nature of early to moderate CKD, it is challenging to ascertain the actual incidence and prevalence of CKD. In the general population, CKD prevalence ranges from 10% to 14%. Similarly, the prevalence of GFR less than 60 ml/min/1.73 mt^2 and albuminuria (microalbuminuria, or A2) is 3 to 5% and 7%, respectively.

Worldwide, CKD accounted for 2,968,600 (1%) of disability-adjusted life-years and 2,546,700 (1% to 3%) of life-years lost in 2012 (Webster et al., 2017).

According to the Kidney Disease Outcomes Quality Initiative (KDOQI), patients must be tested three times in three months, with two of the three results consistently being positive, to be labeled as having chronicity or CKD.

7.1.3. Natural History and Progression of CKD

The natural history and course of progression of community-discharged chronic kidney disease (CKD) differ markedly from those of patients referred to nephrology practices (referred to CKD).

Community-onset CKD primarily affects the elderly population. These people have lived their entire lives with diabetes, hypertension, and cardiovascular risk factors—all of which can have an adverse effect on the kidneys. After the age of 40 to 50, the average rate of decline in GFR in this population is approximately 0.75–1 ml/min/year. In a substantial study by Kshirsagar et al. community-based CKD renal replacement therapy (RRT) was only necessary in 1% and 20% of patients with CKD stages G3 and G4, respectively. However, the majority of deaths (24 and 45%, respectively) were due to cardiovascular disease (CVD), indicating that cardiac events—rather than ESRD progression—are the most common consequence of community-based CKD.

Patients with referred CKD often present earlier than those with community CKD due to either an acquired (such as tubulointerstitial disease, diabetic nephropathy, or glomerulonephritis) or hereditary (such as autosomal dominant polycystic kidney disease, ADPKD) nephropathy that causes progressive renal damage and loss of function. Referred patients' rates of progression in chronic kidney disease (CKD) differ depending on the underlying disease process and each patient. It has been demonstrated that GFR declines quickly in diabetic nephropathy, on average by 10 ml/min/year. Patients with chronic proteinuric GN typically experience a faster rate of progression in nondiabetic nephropathies compared to those with low proteinuria. Compared to other nephropathies, patients with ADPKD and renal impairment, CKD stage G3b and above, may progress more quickly. A very slow progression of hypertensive nephrosclerosis is linked to patients with minimal proteinuria and well-controlled blood pressure.

7.1.4. Risk Factors for Progression of CKD

7.1.4.1. Non-Modifiable CKD Risk Factors

The advancement of CKD is negatively impacted by older age, male gender, and non-white ethnicity, which includes African Americans, Afro-Caribbean people, Hispanics, and Asians (South Asians and Pacific Asians).

There are genetic variables that influence the course of CKD in a variety of kidney diseases. Luttropp et al. conducted a population-based cohort study of single nucleotide polymorphisms in the MTHFS and TCF7L2 genes were linked to the development of CKD and diabetic nephropathy. Polymorphisms of the renin-angiotensin-aldosterone system (RAAS) and mediators of renal scarring were found to have an impact on the progression of chronic kidney disease (CKD) in the same study (Luttropp et al., 2009).

7.1.4.2. Modifiable CKD Risk Factors

Among them are metabolic variables, proteinuria, and systemic hypertension. One of the primary causes of end-stage renal disease (ESRD) globally and the second most common cause in the US after diabetes is systemic hypertension. It is thought that one of the factors influencing the development of glomerulosclerosis is the transmission of systemic hypertension into glomerular capillary beds and the subsequent glomerular hypertension. The 24-hour blood pressure measurement (ABPM) and nighttime readings seem to have the strongest correlation with the advancement of CKD. In addition to being linked to CKD complications, systolic blood pressure (as opposed to diastolic blood pressure) appears to be predictive of the course of CKD.

Significant proteinuria (albuminuria A3) has been linked to a quicker rate of chronic kidney disease (CKD) progression in both diabetic and nondiabetic kidney disease patients, according to numerous studies. Additionally, a better prognosis for the kidneys is linked to reducing marked proteinuria through diet or RAS blockade. However, despite a notable decrease in albuminuria, significant declines in GFR were observed in large intervention studies such as the Ongoing Telmisartan Alone and in Combination with Ramipril Global End Point Trial (ONTARGET) and Avoiding Cardiovascular Events Through Combination Therapy in Patients Living with Systolic Hypertension (ACCOMPLISH). As a result, albuminuria at a moderate level (A2) is not a valid proxy for the advancement of chronic kidney disease (CKD), and a decrease in albuminuria may actually worsen the course of the disease.

Numerous investigations have connected the pathophysiology of renal fibrosis, proteinuria, and hypertension in chronic kidney disease (CKD) to the RAAS system. Interventions aimed at RAAS have thus shown promise in delaying the advancement of CKD. As a result, RAAS blockers are now frequently used to treat proteinuric and diabetic kidney disease.

Smoking and obesity have been linked to the onset and course of chronic kidney disease. Additionally, the onset and course of chronic kidney disease (CKD) have been linked to metabolic variables such as insulin resistance, dyslipidemia, and hyperuricemia.

7.1.5. Recommendations for CKD Screening

Across the world, screening is being used, primarily on high-risk individuals. Screening high-risk populations, such as those with diabetes mellitus, hypertension, and those over 65, is advised by the KDOQI guidelines. A urinalysis, a urine albumin-creatinine ratio (ACR), a serum creatinine measurement, and an estimation of GFR—ideally using the chronic kidney disease epidemiology collaboration (CKD-EPI) equation—should all be part of this. It is the most economical method, and there is no evidence to support CKD screening of asymptomatic members of the general public.

7.2. Pathophysiology

In contrast to acute kidney injury (AKI), which results in full functional kidney recovery after the healing process is finished, chronic and sustained insults from progressive nephropathies lead to progressive kidney fibrosis and the destruction of the kidney's normal architecture. This has an impact on the kidney's three compartments: the glomeruli, tubules, interstitium, and vessels. Histologically, glomerulosclerosis, tubulointerstitial fibrosis, and vascular sclerosis are the manifestations.

The sequence of events that lead to scarring and fibrosis are complex, overlapping, and multistage phenomena.

- Infiltration of damaged kidneys with extrinsic inflammatory cells
- Activation, proliferation, and loss of intrinsic renal cells (through apoptosis, necrosis, mesangiolysis, and podocytopenia)
- Activation and proliferation of extracellular matrix (ECM) producing cells including myofibroblasts and fibroblasts
- Deposition of ECM replacing the normal architecture

Mechanisms of Accelerated Progression of CKD

- Systemic and intraglomerular hypertension
- Glomerular hypertrophy
- Intrarenal precipitation of calcium phosphate
- Altered prostanoid metabolism

All these mechanisms lead to a histological entity called focal segmental glomerulosclerosis.

Black racial background, hypertension, proteinuria, and hyperglycemia are clinical risk factors for accelerated CKD progression. Environmental exposures like obesity, smoking, lead, metabolic syndrome, and maybe some analgesic medications have also been connected to a faster course of chronic kidney disease (CKD).

7.3. History and Physical

In the early stages of CKD, there are no symptoms; in stages 4 or 5, symptoms do appear. Regular testing of the blood or urine is commonly used to detect it. Some common symptoms and signs at these stages of CKD are:

- Nausea
- Vomiting
- Loss of appetite
- Fatigue and weakness
- Sleep disturbance
- Oliguria
- Decreased mental sharpness
- Muscle twitches and cramps
- Swelling of feet and ankles
- Persistent pruritus
- Chest pain due to uremic pericarditis
- Shortness of breath due to pulmonary edema from fluid overload
- Hypertension that's difficult to control
- Physical examination is often not helpful, but patients may have
- Skin pigmentation
- Scratch marks from pruritus
- Pericardial friction rub due to uremic pericarditis
- Uremic frost, where high levels of BUN result in urea in sweat
- Hypertensive fundal changes suggesting chronicity

7.4. Evaluation

7.4.1. Establishing Chronicity

If a patient has an eGFR of less than 60 ml/min/1.73 m, it is important to consider the patient's clinical history, past blood and urine test results, and AKI or CKD that has been present but asymptomatic. The following factors would be helpful.

1. History of long-standing chronic hypertension, proteinuria, microhematuria, and symptoms of the prostatic disease
2. Skin pigmentation, scratch marks, left ventricular hypertrophy, and hypertensive fundal changes.
3. Blood test results of other conditions like multiple myeloma and systemic vasculitis would be helpful.
4. Low serum calcium and high phosphorus levels have little discriminatory value, but normal Parathyroid hormone levels suggest AKI rather than CKD.
5. Individuals who appear relatively well and still pass normal volumes

of urine, but have very high blood urea nitrogen (BUN) values greater than 140 mg/dl and serum creatinine greater than 13.5 mg/dl are much more likely to have CKD than acute kidney disease.

7.4.2. Assessment of Glomerular Filtration Rate

Kidney function tests should be repeated two weeks after the initial diagnosis of low eGFR below 60 ml/min/1.73 m^2 in patients in whom the distinction between AKI and CKD is unclear. When repeat blood tests conducted over a period of three months yield consistent results, or when prior testing indicates that the low eGFR is chronic, CKD is confirmed. Measurements using other markers, such as cystatin-c or isotope-clearance, can be made if eGFR based on serum creatinine is known to be less accurate.

7.4.3. Assessment of Proteinuria

KDIGO advises measuring the albumin-creatinine ratio (ACR) after collecting a urine sample in the early morning to evaluate proteinuria. Former terms like microalbuminuria have been replaced with an A1–A3 grading system for albuminuria. Urine protein-creatinine ratio (PCR) testing may be more helpful for specific conditions because some patients may excrete proteins other than albumin.

7.4.4. Imaging of Kidneys

An ultrasound examination of the kidneys that reveals small kidneys with numerous cysts, scarring, increased echogenicity, and decreased cortical thickness points to a chronic process. Diagnosing chronic hydronephrosis in ADPKD patients with obstructive uropathy and renal cystic enlargement may also be beneficial.

- Renal ultrasound Doppler can be used in suspected renal artery stenosis to evaluate the renal vascular flow.
- Computerized tomography: Renal stone disease is diagnosed with low-dose non-contrast CT. Additionally, since ultrasonography cannot detect suspected ureteric obstruction, it is used to diagnose the condition.
- Renal angiography has its role in the diagnosis of polyarteritis nodosa, where multiple aneurysms and irregular areas of constriction are seen.
- Voiding cystourethrography is generally utilized in cases where CKD is suspected to be caused by chronic vesicourethral reflux. It is employed to evaluate the degree of reflux and validate the diagnosis.
- Renal scans can provide adequate details regarding the structure and operation of the kidneys. Since they are associated with a lower radiation exposure than CT scans, they are primarily used on children. Renal function differences are measured by radionuclide renal scans.

7.4.5. Establishing an Accurate Diagnosis

A precise etiology for CKD must be identified, such as in cases of underlying treatable conditions like ANCA vasculitis or lupus nephritis that need to be managed appropriately. Additionally, accurate diagnosis will impact later management because certain diseases have a higher frequency of kidney recurrence in the kidney after transplantation. In addition to providing information about the degree of kidney fibrosis, a kidney biopsy is used to diagnose the cause of CKD.

7.5. Symptoms of Chronic Kidney Disease

The kidneys play a vital role in maintaining overall health by filtering waste products and excess fluids from the blood, regulating electrolyte balance, and producing hormones that help control blood pressure and stimulate red blood cell production. When kidney function is impaired, waste products and fluids can accumulate in the body, leading to various symptoms and complications associated with CKD.

7.5.1. Early Stage CKD Symptoms

In the early stages of CKD, when kidney function is only mildly reduced, individuals may not experience any noticeable symptoms. This is because the kidneys have a remarkable ability to compensate for decreased function, and symptoms may not become apparent until kidney damage is more advanced. However, some early signs and symptoms of CKD may include:

1. **Fatigue**: Feeling tired or lethargic despite adequate rest and sleep.
2. **Changes in Urination**: Increased or decreased frequency of urination, particularly at night (nocturia).
3. **Fluid Retention**: Mild swelling (edema) in the legs, ankles, or around the eyes due to fluid retention.
4. **Changes in Appetite**: Loss of appetite or changes in taste sensation.
5. **Difficulty Concentrating**: Difficulty focusing or experiencing brain fog.
6. **Muscle Cramps**: Painful muscle cramps, particularly in the legs.
7. **Itching**: Pruritus or persistent itching, often due to the buildup of waste products in the blood.
8. **Dry Skin**: Skin may become dry, flaky, or irritated.

7.5.2. Progression to Advanced Stage CKD Symptoms

As chronic kidney disease progresses and kidney function further declines, symptoms may become more pronounced and debilitating. Advanced-stage CKD symptoms may include:

1. **Severe Fatigue**: Overwhelming fatigue that interferes with daily activities and quality of life.
2. **Persistent Swelling**: Swelling in the legs, ankles, feet, or face due to fluid retention (edema).
3. **Shortness of Breath**: Dyspnea or difficulty breathing, particularly during physical exertion or lying flat.
4. **High Blood Pressure**: Hypertension, which may be difficult to control despite medication.
5. **Nausea and Vomiting**: Persistent nausea, vomiting, or loss of appetite.
6. **Unexplained Weight Loss**: Weight loss without trying or significant changes in body composition.

7. **Changes in Urine Output**: Decreased urine output or changes in the color, odor, or appearance of urine.
8. **Increased Risk of Infections**: Weakened immune system and increased susceptibility to infections.
9. **Bone Pain**: Bone pain or fractures due to mineral and bone disorders associated with CKD.
10. **Easy Bruising and Bleeding**: Due to impaired blood clotting function.
11. **Cognitive Impairment**: Memory loss, confusion, or difficulty concentrating.
12. **Restless Legs Syndrome**: Uncontrollable urge to move the legs, often accompanied by uncomfortable sensations.
13. **Sleep Disturbances**: Insomnia, restless sleep, or frequent waking during the night.
14. **Skin Changes**: Yellowish discoloration of the skin (jaundice) or pale skin due to anemia.
15. **Depression and Anxiety**: Feelings of sadness, anxiety, or hopelessness, often associated with the burden of managing a chronic illness.

7.5.3. Symptoms of Complications Associated With CKD

In addition to the symptoms directly related to kidney dysfunction, chronic kidney disease can lead to various complications that further exacerbate symptoms and impact overall health. These complications may include:

1. **Cardiovascular Disease**: CKD increases the risk of heart disease, heart attack, stroke, and peripheral artery disease.
2. **Anemia**: Reduced production of red blood cells leading to fatigue, weakness, pale skin, and shortness of breath.
3. **Bone Disease**: Mineral and bone disorders such as renal osteodystrophy, causing bone pain, fractures, and skeletal deformities.
4. **Fluid and Electrolyte Imbalances**: Imbalance of fluids, electrolytes (sodium, potassium, calcium), and acid-base levels, leading to complications such as high blood pressure, swelling, and muscle cramps.
5. **Malnutrition**: Inadequate intake of nutrients due to loss of appetite, nausea, vomiting, or dietary restrictions.
6. **Peripheral Neuropathy**: Nerve damage leading to numbness, tingling, or burning sensations, especially in the hands and feet.
7. **Pericarditis**: Inflammation of the membrane surrounding the heart, causing chest pain, fever, and difficulty breathing.
8. **Uremic Syndrome**: Buildup of uremic toxins in the blood, causing a wide range of symptoms such as confusion, seizures, coma, and eventually death if left untreated.

7.5.4. Underlying Mechanisms of Symptoms in CKD

The symptoms of chronic kidney disease arise from various underlying mechanisms associated with impaired kidney function and the body's attempts to compensate for it. These mechanisms may include:

1. **Fluid and Electrolyte Imbalance**: Dysfunction of the kidneys' ability to regulate fluid balance and electrolyte levels can lead to fluid retention, electrolyte imbalances, and high blood pressure.
2. **Uremic Toxins**: Accumulation of waste products such as urea, creatinine, and uric acid in the blood due to decreased filtration by the kidneys can cause systemic toxicity and various symptoms.
3. **Anemia**: Reduced production of erythropoietin (a hormone produced by the kidneys) leads to decreased red blood cell production and anemia, resulting in fatigue, weakness, and shortness of breath.
4. **Mineral and Bone Disorders**: Imbalance of calcium, phosphorus, and parathyroid hormone levels can lead to bone disease, fractures, and skeletal abnormalities.
5. **Hypertension**: Chronic kidney disease can lead to hypertension through mechanisms involving fluid retention, activation of the renin-angiotensin-aldosterone system, and impaired sodium excretion.
6. **Inflammation and Oxidative Stress**: CKD is associated with chronic inflammation and oxidative stress, which contribute to the development of cardiovascular disease, anemia, and other complications.
7. **Metabolic Acidosis**: Impaired kidney function can lead to metabolic acidosis, a condition characterized by an excess of acid in the blood, causing symptoms such as fatigue, muscle weakness, and bone demineralization.

7.5.5. Impact of Symptoms on Quality of Life

Chronic kidney disease and its associated symptoms can have a profound impact on patients' quality of life, physical health, and emotional well-being. Symptoms such as fatigue, pain, nausea, and depression can interfere with daily activities, work, social interactions, and relationships. Moreover, managing symptoms and complications of CKD often requires significant lifestyle modifications, dietary restrictions, complex medication regimens, and frequent medical appointments, adding to the burden experienced by patients and their caregivers.

7.6. Routine Treatment and Management

The care of CKD patients includes:

- Slowing the progression of CKD;
- Treat complications related to the pathology, such as anemia, mineral and bone disorder, electrolyte disorders, metabolic acidosis, and cardiovascular disease;
- Prepare the patient for renal replacement therapy (RRT);
- Establish an immunization routine, especially for hepatitis B.

It is critical to emphasize that a multidisciplinary team, including members with expertise in nutrition, nursing, psychology, and social assistance, is required at all treatment levels.

7.6.1. Routine for the Assessment and Management of CKD Progression

The assessment of the progression of chronic kidney disease (CKD) is based on the evaluation of three factors: the decline in renal function in patients who were followed up on over time using similar techniques; the occurrence of renal failure, as indicated by the start of renal replacement therapy (RRT); any symptoms or complications resulting from this decline in renal function; and the onset or worsening of proteinuria, especially in cases of diabetic nephropathy.

Data from the literature with approximately two years of follow-up of patients with CKD show that the average decrease in the glomerular filtration rate was 4–5 mL/min/year and that 85% of the patients had this average decline. Therefore, we must periodically evaluate the decrease of the glomerular filtration rate (GFR), and consider a decrease greater than 5 ml/min/1.73 m^2 /$year^2$ to be an indicator of accelerated progression. In Table 7.1, we suggest a frequency of monitoring; however, this scheme should be tailored according to the clinical status of the patient and the underlying renal disease.

Table 7.1. Frequency of Follow-up (Number of Times Per Year), According to the GFR and Level of Albuminuria (Adapted from 3); GFR: Glomerular Filtration Rate in ml/min/1.73 m^2

Albuminuria				
	GFR	<30 mg/g	30-300 mg/g	>300 mg/g
Stage 1	≥90	1 if CKD	1	2
Stage 2	60-89	1 if CKD	1	2
Stage 3A	45-59	1	2	3
Stage 3B	30-44	2	3	3
Stage 4	15-29	3	3	4 or more
Stage 5	<15	4 or more	4 or more	4 or more

Source: *https://doi.org/10.1590/1806-9282.66.S1.3.*

In general, the strategies used to reduce the progression of CKD are:

- use of angiotensin-converting enzyme inhibitors or angiotensin receptor blockers for patients with proteinuria above 500 mg/24 hours;
- reach target blood pressure below 130 × 80 mmhg;
- reach levels of glycated hemoglobin lower than 7% for diabetic patients;
- protein restriction indicated and managed by a nutritionist;
- correction of metabolic acidosis;
- stimulation for smoking cessation.

Evaluation of the presence of CKD exacerbation factors is also crucial. These include volume depletion, use of nephrotoxic substances like iodinated contrast, antibiotics, non-steroidal anti-inflammatory drugs, and urinary tract obstruction.

7.6.2. Routine for the Evaluation of Anemia in CKD

Erythropoietin deficiency, along with iron, folic acid, and vitamin B12 deficiency, is the most common cause of anemia, a common complication in people with chronic kidney disease (CKD). As a result, determining the existence of anemia and monitoring its treatment are standard procedures for CKD patients.

The hemoglobin concentration should be obtained for patients without anemia when clinically warranted or following Table 7.2 recommendation. Hemoglobin concentration tests should be ordered for patients with anemia, which is defined as hemoglobin levels less than 13 g/dl for men and 12 for women. Patients in stages III to V of CKD should have these tests done every three months. The measurement of hemoglobin and iron levels must be performed at each patient consultation or, at the very least, every three months for patients receiving treatment for anemia with iron replacement or erythropoiesis-stimulating agents.

7.6.3. Routine for the Evaluation of Mineral and Bone Disorder in CKD

Renal osteodystrophy, a histological sign of the disease, is one of the changes in the mineral metabolism that are referred to as "mineral and bone disorder" in patients with chronic kidney disease (CKD). In addition to venous blood gas, the serum levels of calcium, phosphorus, intact parathyroid hormone (PTH), and alkaline phosphatase must be measured to diagnose mineral and bone disorders in patients with chronic kidney disease (CKD). All patients with CKD whose GFR is less than 60 ml/min/1.73 m^2 should have these tests done. As indicated in Table 7.2, the frequency of exams should be determined by the stage and risk of progression of CKD.

Since vitamin D deficiency is common in chronic kidney disease (CKD) patients receiving conservative treatment and is linked to the advancement of hyperparathyroidism, decreased bone mineral density, and an increased risk of fractures, testing for it could also be a routine part of treatment. Additionally, insulin resistance, vascular function abnormalities, immunological response changes, and cardiomyopathy have all been linked to vitamin D deficiency (Ravani et al., 2009).

7.6.4. Routine for the Evaluation of Metabolic Acidosis and Electrolytic Changes in CKD

Most CKD patients experience metabolic acidosis when their glomerular filtration rate is less than 30 milliliters per minute. It typically ranges from 12 to 22 mEq/L for bicarbonate, making it mild to moderate. The literature has detailed the advantages of reversing metabolic acidosis. To be precise, BritoAshurst et al. observed that supplementing with bicarbonate slowed the progression of CKD to its final stages and improved the nutritional status of 134 patients with CKD (creatinine clearance of 15 to 30 ml/min/1.73 m^2) and serum bicarbonate between 16 and 20 mmol/L.

The target level of bicarbonate must be greater than or equal to 22 mEq/L, and alkaline salts should be used to reach this target. The determination of bicarbonate should be performed routinely in accordance with the stage of CKD.

Hyperkalemia is the primary electrolyte imbalance seen in CKD patients receiving conservative treatment. Every patient consultation should include a measurement of potassium levels. If hyperkalemia is found, it's critical to evaluate dietary mistakes, medications that may cause hyperkalemia, metabolic acidosis, and the use or dosage increase of potassium-sparing diuretics.

7.6.5. Routine for the Evaluation of Cardiovascular Disease in CKD

The primary cause of morbidity and death in the CKD population is cardiovascular disease (CVD). All patients with CKD should be regarded as having a high risk of cardiovascular disease (CVD) based on data from the literature. They should be assessed for both "traditional" and "non-traditional" (related to uremia) risk factors for CVD, and their treatment should aim to reduce modifiable cardiovascular risk factors.

A yearly electrocardiogram and echocardiogram, as well as non-invasive testing like stress echocardiography or myocardial scintigraphy, can be established as routine methods of identifying CVD in these patients. These tests should be reserved for patients who exhibit symptoms or changes in segmental motility, have three or more traditional risk factors, or have a history of cerebral vascular accident and peripheral vascular insufficiency. When invasive or non-invasive exams yield positive results along with clinical symptoms, it is advised to refer the patient to a specialized cardiac assessment.

Apart from recognizing cardiovascular disease (CVD), it's crucial to devise tactics to mitigate risk factors. These tactics include managing hypertension and diabetes, evaluating dyslipidemia, quitting smoking, encouraging physical activity, treating anemia, and lowering proteinuria levels.

7.6.6. Routine for Hepatitis B Immunization in CKD

According to the 2012 dialysis census by the SBN, the prevalence of hepatitis B in patients undergoing hemodialysis in Brazil is 1%. The correct application of a vaccination scheme is one of the main factors responsible for the reduction in the incidence of this infection in dialysis. It is worth pointing out that the response to vaccination in this population varies from 40% to 60%, and that the maintenance of the antibodies titer is not sustained. It is important to establish a routine vaccination for non-immune patients. One of the proposed schemes carried out in basic health units is to make four applications with a double dose (4 ml) of Engedrix B© on the deltoid muscle in months 0, 1, 2, and 6. After 30 days of the end of the scheme, the AntiHbs are monitored – if lower than 10 miu/ml, a booster dose is recommended with a double dose (4 ml) of Engedrix B©; the maximum booster doses allowed are three.

7.6.7. Routine to Prepare for Renal Replacement Therapy

When a patient with chronic kidney disease (CKD) decides when to begin dialysis, both the patient and the doctor evaluate both objective and subjective factors. There are no precise lab results that specify when starting dialysis is necessary. A patient's quality of life, psychological factors related to anxiety about undergoing complex therapy, the nephrologist's assessment of the patient's health, the patient's declining renal function, and the risks of renal replacement therapy are all taken into account when determining whether to start renal replacement therapy (RRT).

It is crucial to discuss the various types of RRT, as well as their indications, benefits, and drawbacks when monitoring CDK patients who exhibit a progressive decline in renal function or who have a GFR of less than 20 ml/min. It is imperative to initiate the necessary preparations, such as manufacturing the arteriovenous fistula for hemodialysis, training in peritoneal dialysis, implanting the Tenckhoff catheter, and serology for HIV, hepatitis B, and C, once the patient has chosen a specific type of RRT and there are no medical contraindications. The patient may also be referred to outpatient clinics that specialize in pre-renal transplantation evaluation if they are interested and meet the clinical requirements.

We must request RRT from the appropriate Single Health System organs or through supplemental medical services as soon as the patient exhibits a significantly decreased GFR and/or compatible symptoms, such as nausea, vomiting, drowsiness, weight loss, or hiccups, among others. It is crucial to stress that the patient needs to be referred for an immediate start of RRT if these symptoms worsen or if there are changes in the laboratory results that point to a high risk.

In Table 7.2, we suggest a model of test grouping according to the risk of progression of CKD.

Table 7.2. Routine of Exams According to the Risk of Progression of CKD

Department	Low	Moderate	High	Very High
Renal function	–	–	–	–
GFR	Every consultation	Every consultation	Every consultation	Every consultation
Urine 1	Yearly	Every six months	Every six months	Every six months
Proteinuria	Yearly	Every six months	Every six months	Every six months
Anemia				
Complete blood count	Yearly	Every six months	Every consultation	Every consultation
Iron	–	Every six months	Quarterly #	Quarterly #
Transferrin	–	Every six months	Quarterly #	Quarterly #
Ferritin	–	Every six months	Quarterly #	Quarterly #
Bone disease	–	–	–	–
Ionized calcium	Yearly	Every six months	Quarterly	Every consultation
Phosphorus	Yearly	Every six months	Quarterly	Every consultation
PTH	–	Yearly	Every six months	Quarterly #
Metabolism	–	–	–	–
Cholesterol	Yearly	CV Risk*	CV Risk*	CV Risk*
Triglycerides	Yearly	CV Risk*	CV Risk*	CV Risk*

Uric acid	Yearly	Every six months	Every six months	Every six months
Venous blood gas	–	Yearly	Quarterly	Every consultation
Glycemia	Yearly	If diabetes	Quarterly	Every consultation
Hb1Ac	–	If diabetes	Quarterly	Quarterly
TGO, TGP; CPK	Consultation&	Consultation&	Consultation&	Consultation&
Nutrition	–	–	–	–
Urea clearance	–	Every six months	Quarterly	Bimonthly
Urine Sodium	Yearly	Every six months	Every six months	Every six months
Potassium	Yearly	Every consultation	Every consultation	Every consultation
Viral profile	–	–	–	–
HbsAg	–	Yearly	Yearly	Dialysis**
Anti-HbsAg	–	Yearly	Yearly	Dialysis**
Anti-Hbc	–	Yearly	Yearly	Dialysis**
Anti-HIV	–	–	–	Dialysis**
Anti-HCV	–	–	–	Dialysis**
Others	–	–	–	–
Echocardiogram	Yearly	Yearly	Yearly	Yearly

GFR = estimated glomerular filtration rate or by 24-hour urine creatinine clearance; # if treatment; * according to the cardiovascular risk; ** at the moment of referral to dialysis; & if under treatment with statins or fibrates.

Source: *https://doi.org/10.1590/1806-9282.66.S1.3.*

7.7. Monitoring of Established CKD and Treatment of Complications

Following the diagnosis of CKD, the KDIGO guidelines advise yearly monitoring of albuminuria and eGFR. Patients who pose a high risk should have these measures checked at least twice a year, and those who pose a very high risk should have them checked at least three times a year (Figure 7.2). Anemia, mineral and bone disorders, and electrolyte abnormalities are more common in patients with moderate to severe chronic kidney disease (CKD). The stage of chronic kidney disease determines the screening and frequency of evaluation for laboratory abnormalities, which includes measurements of the lipid panel, parathyroid hormone, serum albumin, phosphate, basic metabolic panel, complete blood count, and 25-hydroxyvitamin D.

Table 7.3. Screening, Monitoring, and Management of the Complications of Chronic Kidney Disease (CKD)

Complication	Relevant Tests	Frequency of Repeat Testing	Management
Anemia	Hemoglobin	No anemia: CKD stages G1-G2: when clinically indicated CKD stage G3: at least once per year CKD stages G4-G5: at least twice per year With anemia: CKD stages 3–5: at least every 3 months	Rule out other causes of anemia: iron deficiency, vitamin B_{12} deficiency, folate deficiency, occult bleeding Consider iron supplementation and referral to a nephrologist for erythropoietin-stimulating agent therapy when hemoglobin <10 g/dL
Mineral and bone disorder	Serum calcium, phosphate, parathyroid hormone, 25-hydroxyvitamin D	Calcium/phosphate: CKD stage G3: every 6–12 months CKD stage G4: every 3–6 months CKD stage G5: every 1–3 months Parathyroid hormone: CKD stage G3: at baseline, then as needed CKD stage G4: every 6–12 months CKD stage G5: every 3–6 months Vitamin D: CKD stages 3–5: at baseline, then as needed	Consider phosphate-lowering therapy (eg, calcium acetate, sevelamer, iron-based binders) and vitamin D supplementation

Hyperkalemia	Serum potassium	At baseline and as needed	Low-potassium diet, correction of hyperglycemia and acidemia, consider potassium binders
Metabolic acidosis	Serum bicarbonate	At baseline and as needed	Oral bicarbonate supplementation (e.g., sodium bicarbonate, baking soda, or sodium citrate/citric acid) for values persistently <22 mmol/L
Cardiovascular disease	Lipid panel	At baseline and as needed	Low- to moderate-dose statin therapy for patients aged ≥50 years with CKD Statin therapy for patients aged 18–49 years with CKD and coronary artery disease, diabetes, prior ischemic stroke, or high risk of myocardial infarction or cardiovascular death

Source: Teresa K. Chen, Daphne H. Knicely, and Morgan E. Grams, Chronic Kidney Disease Diagnosis and Management, doi: 10.1001/jama.2019.14745.

7.7.1. Anemia and the Role of Erythropoietin in CKD

One of the most typical side effects of CKD is anemia 41% of the 209 311 participants in a study with 19 CKD cohorts from around the globe had low hemoglobin levels, which are defined as <13 g/dL for men and <12 g/dL for women. An evaluation of iron stores should be part of the initial workup for anemia; individuals with low iron levels may benefit from oral or intravenous iron replacement therapy. Referrals to a nephrologist for further medical therapy, such as erythropoietin-stimulating agents, may be necessary for patients whose hemoglobin levels remain consistently below 10 g/dL after reversible causes have been addressed. However, the risks of erythropoietin-stimulating agents, such as increased risk of stroke, venous thromboembolism, and death, must be carefully considered against any potential benefits.

7.7.2. Electrolyte, Mineral, and Bone Abnormalities in CKD

Between 3 and 11% of patients with CKD have abnormalities related to electrolytes. Dietary restrictions and supplement prescriptions are common components of initial treatment plans.

For instance, patients with hyperkalemia and hyperphosphatemia should be prescribed low-potassium and low-phosphorus diets, respectively, by primary care physicians. Studies have shown that chronic metabolic acidosis is linked to a faster progression of chronic kidney disease (CKD), so oral bicarbonate supplementation should be taken into consideration for patients whose serum bicarbonate level is consistently below 22 mmol/L (Mahajan, Simoni, & Sheather, 2010).

Bone and mineral disorders are also prevalent. Of the 42,985 CKD patients in the study, 58% had intact parathyroid hormone levels higher than 65 pg/mL. Most nephrologists concur that concurrent hyperphosphatemia, hypocalcemia, and vitamin D deficiency should be treated, for example with a low-phosphate diet, phosphate binders, adequate elemental calcium intake, and vitamin D supplementation, even though the ideal intact parathyroid hormone level CKD is still unknown.

7.8. Diagnosis

Diagnosing CKD involves a series of steps aimed at assessing kidney function and identifying any underlying causes or complications. Here's an overview of the diagnostic process:

1. **Medical History and Physical Examination**: A healthcare provider will begin by taking a detailed medical history, including any symptoms the individual may be experiencing, past medical conditions, medications, family history of kidney disease, and lifestyle factors such as diet and exercise. A physical examination may also be conducted to look for signs of kidney damage, such as swelling in the legs or high blood pressure.
2. **Laboratory Tests**: Blood and urine tests are essential for diagnosing CKD and assessing kidney function. Common tests include:
   i. **Serum Creatinine**: Elevated levels of creatinine in the blood can indicate decreased kidney function.
   ii. **Glomerular Filtration Rate (GFR)**: This is a calculated value based on creatinine levels, age, gender, and other factors. A lower GFR indicates poorer kidney function.
   iii. **Urine Albumin/Creatinine Ratio (ACR)**: Increased levels of albumin (a protein) in the urine can be a sign of kidney damage.
   iv. **Complete Blood Count (CBC)**: This helps assess for anemia, a common complication of CKD.
   v. **Electrolyte Levels**: Imbalances in electrolytes such as potassium, sodium, and calcium can occur in CKD and may require monitoring.
3. **Imaging Studies**: Imaging tests such as ultrasound, CT scan, or MRI may be performed to evaluate the size, shape, and structure of the kidneys and identify any abnormalities such as cysts or blockages.
4. **Kidney Biopsy**: In some cases, a kidney biopsy may be recommended to obtain a small sample of kidney tissue for microscopic examination. This procedure is typically reserved for cases where the cause of CKD is unclear or if there is suspicion of a specific kidney disease that requires confirmation.

5. **Staging CKD**: Once a diagnosis is confirmed, CKD is staged based on the level of kidney function, as determined by the GFR, and the presence of kidney damage, as indicated by urine tests. Staging helps guide treatment and monitoring recommendations.

Overall, diagnosing CKD involves a comprehensive approach that combines medical history, physical examination, laboratory tests, and imaging studies to assess kidney function, identify underlying causes, and determine the appropriate management plan for the individual. Early detection and intervention are key to slowing the progression of CKD and preventing complications.

7.9. Staging

The 6 categories include:

- G1: GFR 90 ml/min per 1.73 m^2 and above
- G2: GFR 60 to 89 ml/min per 1.73 m^2
- G3a: GFR 45 to 59 ml/min per 1.73 m^2
- G3b: GFR 30 to 44 ml/min per 1.73 m^2
- G4: GFR 15 to 29 ml/min per 1.73 m^2
- G5: GFR less than 15 ml/min per 1.73 m^2 or treatment by dialysis

The 3 levels of albuminuria include albumin-creatinine ratio (ACR):

- A1: ACR less than 30 mg/gm (less than 3.4 mg/mmol)
- A2: ACR 30 to 299 mg/gm (3.4 to 34 mg/mmol)
- A3: ACR greater than 300 mg/gm (greater than 34 mg/mmol)

7.10. Prognosis

There are notable disparities in the incidence and prevalence rates of ESRD between racial and ethnic groups. African Americans have the highest incidence, followed by American Indians and Alaska Natives, Asian Americans, Native Hawaiians and other Pacific Islanders, and White people. Compared to non-Hispanics, Hispanics have higher incidence rates of ESRD.

Early-stage CKD and ESRD are associated with increased morbidity and healthcare utilization rates. A review of the USRDS 2009 annual data report suggests that the number of hospitalizations in ESRD patients is 1.9% per patient-year. In a study by Khan SS et al., the prevalence of cardiovascular disease, cerebrovascular disease, and peripheral vascular disease in earlier stages of CKD was comparable to those in the US dialysis population. It was also found that patients with CKD had 3-fold higher rates of hospitalization and hospital days spent per patient-year compared to the general US population. CKD patients are at a higher risk of hospitalization and cardiovascular diseases, and the risk increases with a decline in GFR.

Patients with CKD, particularly end-stage renal disease (ESRD), are at increased risk of mortality, particularly from cardiovascular disease. A review of USRDS 2009 data suggests that the 5-year survival probability in a patient on dialysis is only around 34%.

7.11. Complications

7.11.1. Treatment of Complications of Chronic Kidney Disease

The inability of CKD patients to maintain a fluid balance following a fast sodium load is more pronounced in stages IV and V of the disease. A loop diuretic and sodium restriction work for these patients. All patients with CKD are advised by the 2012 KDIGO guidelines to limit their daily sodium intake to less than 2 grams. Particularly in patients with oliguric symptoms and reduced aldosterone secretion, hyperkalemia in CKD can happen. Hyperkalemia may be caused by hypoaldosteronism, tissue deterioration, and potassium intake in the diet. Hyperkalemia may also be brought on by medications like nonselective beta-blockers and ACE inhibitors.

Because of the kidneys' heightened propensity to retain H, metabolic acidosis is a frequent consequence of advanced chronic kidney disease (CKD). Osteopenia, increased protein catabolism, and secondary hyperparathyroidism would be the outcomes of chronic metabolic acidosis in chronic kidney disease. Bicarbonate supplementation should be used in these patients' treatment to achieve a target serum bicarbonate of 23.

A substantial risk factor for CVD is chronic kidney disease (CKD), and the risk rises with CKD severity. Epicardial adipose tissue (EAT) thickness and the incidence of CVD events in patients with chronic kidney disease (CKD) are significantly correlated, according to a substantial body of evidence. The evaluation of EAT may be a valid measure for assessing cardiovascular risk in patients with chronic kidney disease.

7.11.2. Bone and Mineral Disorders

A common CKD consequence brought on by a lower phosphorus-filtered load is hyperphosphatemia. This results in secondary hyperparathyroidism and increased parathyroid hormone (PTH) secretion. Normalization of calcium and phosphorus occurs in hyperparathyroidism, but at the expense of bone. Reproductive osteodystrophy is the outcome. Thus, dietary phosphorus restriction and phosphorus binders are used to treat secondary hyperparathyroidism.

One sign of volume expansion in CKD is hypertension. Not all CKD patients have enough edema to warrant volume expansion. Therefore, to control blood pressure and prevent it from rising before considering an increase in antihypertensive therapy, a loop diuretic should be added to all patients with CKD.

Typically, normocytic normochromic anemia is seen in CKD. It is mainly caused by decreased red cell survival as well as decreased erythropoietin production from decreased functioning renal mass. Testing for hemoglobin should occur every three months for dialysis patients, every six months for those with CKD IV and V, and at least once a year for those with CKD 3. When hemoglobin is less than 10, iron saturation is at least 25%, and ferritin is more than 200 ng/mL, erythropoietin stimulating agents (ESA) should be taken into consideration for patients with CKD. The target hemoglobin concentration for dialysis patients is between 10 and 11 pg/dl.

7.11.3. Treatment of Complications of ESRD

Poor protein intake and anorexia are the main causes of malnutrition in ESRD. In an ESRD, the daily calorie intake should be at least 30 to 35 Kcal/kg. One of the complications of low platelet function is uremic bleeding. The bleeding period is extended as a result. Patients with no symptoms are not given any care. On the other hand, uremic platelet dysfunction must be corrected to perform surgery or during active bleeding. Desmopressin (dDAVP), cryoprecipitate, estrogen, and starting dialysis are a few of the interventions that are used. Uremia can present as uremic pericarditis and is an indication for initiation of dialysis. Uremic pericarditis is treated with dialysis and responds well.

7.11.4. Complications of Renal Transplantation

Complications about the gastrointestinal, neurological, renal, and cardiovascular systems. Hypertension, dyslipidemia, heart failure, arrhythmias, left ventricular hypertrophy, coronary artery disease from recently diagnosed diabetes mellitus, and renal failure are common side effects. Neurologic complications encompass neoplastic disease, neuromuscular disease, central nervous system (CNS) infections, stroke, and posterior reversible encephalopathy syndrome. The following are examples of GI complications: infection, cancer (posttransplant lymphoproliferative disorder), mucosal injury, ulceration, perforation, pancreatitis, biliary tract disease, and diverticular disease.

7.12. Deterrence and Patient Education

Patients in high-risk categories, such as those with diabetes or hypertension, ought to receive counseling regarding the warning signs and symptoms of chronic kidney disease (CKD) in addition to being screened for it. The following at-home interventions should be taught to patients with CKD.

80 to 85% of patients with CKD have hypertension; therefore, it is important to teach them to take their blood pressure every day and to record it along with their daily weight. As part of an antihypertensive regimen, a diuretic ought to be prescribed to them. Assist patients with advanced chronic kidney disease (CKD) in administering subcutaneous erythropoietin-stimulating agents at home. Physicians or nutritionists should talk to patients about low-protein diets, which can slow the progression of chronic kidney disease (CKD), and foods high in potassium.

The necessity of managing phosphorus levels should be explained to all patients with advanced chronic kidney disease. Phosphate binders should be given to them with every meal. Pregnant CKD patients should be informed about the potential for their condition to worsen and the negative effects that reduced kidney function can have on pregnancy.

7.13. Pearls and Other Issues

1. Chronic kidney disease (CKD) is defined as kidney damage or an estimated glomerular filtration rate (eGFR) less than 60 ml/min/1.73 $m^{2,}$ persisting for three months or more, irrespective of the cause.
2. CKD is usually asymptomatic till stages IV and V.
3. The KDOQI guidelines recommend screening high-risk populations, which include individuals with hypertension, diabetes mellitus, and those older than 65 years with a urinalysis, a urine albumin-creatinine ratio (ACR), measurement of serum creatinine, and estimation of GFR preferably by chronic kidney disease epidemiology collaboration (CKD-EPI) equation.
4. Calcium and phosphorus are not useful to distinguish AKI from CKD. However, normal PTH suggests AKI rather than CKD.
5. Systemic hypertension, proteinuria, hyperlipidemia, and metabolic acidosis cause the progression of CKD and need to be treated aggressively.
6. Bicarbonate supplementation to reach a serum bicarbonate target equal to 23 delays the progression of CKD.

7. All CKD patients need to be evaluated for anemia, hypertension, metabolic acidosis, and bone and mineral disorders.

7.14. Enhancing Healthcare Team Outcomes

An interdisciplinary team of medical professionals who work in one place, like a CKD clinic, is best suited to manage the many symptoms of chronic kidney disease (CKD). These clinics emphasize kidney care guided by guidelines; they assess and manage complications; they recommend lifestyle changes to patients; and they adequately educate them about the different types of dialysis. Fishbane and associates contrasted a healthy transitions program, which uses a standard care model, with a nurse care manager working with an informatics system driven by protocol to generate daily reports with all the steps needed to complete the process for each patient. It revealed lower rates of catheter use, less emergent dialysis, more AV fistula use, and fewer hospitalizations. By saving billions of dollars, these models lower the total cost of healthcare.

A nutritionist who creates meal plans and evaluates patients' nutritional status is available to the interprofessional CKD clinics. In a similar vein, a pharmacist checks a patient's medications, looks for ones that could be harmful to the kidneys, and modifies non-toxic ones based on the patient's renal function. After assessing the blood pressure, the nurse practitioner modifies the medication as necessary. The patient receives education from the primary care physician regarding the significance of quitting smoking, eating a nutritious diet, and keeping a healthy body weight. By instructing the team on how to maintain the AV fistulas or dialysis catheters, the dialysis nurse helps the team. A vascular access nurse assesses patients who are suitable for hemodialysis access as well. Lastly, details regarding the process and patient selection criteria are given by a renal transplantation nurse.

Research indicates that treating chronic renal failure with an interprofessional approach ensures better outcomes, reduces patient morbidity, avoids redundant studies, and is cost-effective.

A Closer Look

Classified Stages of Chronic Kidney Disease

Chronic Kidney Disease (CKD) is typically classified into five stages based on the severity of kidney damage and the glomerular filtration rate (GFR), a measure of how well the kidneys are filtering blood. These stages help healthcare providers assess the progression of the disease and determine appropriate management strategies for patients.

- **Stage 1 CKD:** In this initial stage, kidney function is mildly reduced, but the kidneys are still able to perform their essential functions effectively. The GFR is greater than or equal to 90 milliliters per minute per 1.73 square meters of body surface area. Despite the presence of kidney damage, individuals with stage 1 CKD often do not experience significant symptoms, and the condition may go undiagnosed without routine screening.
- **Stage 2 CKD:** Kidney function is moderately reduced in stage 2 CKD, with a GFR ranging from 60 to 89 milliliters per minute per 1.73 square meters of body surface area. While kidney damage may progress, individuals may still not experience noticeable symptoms. Healthcare providers focus on managing underlying risk factors, such as hypertension and diabetes, to slow the progression of the disease.
- **Stage 3 CKD:** Stage 3 CKD is further divided into two sub-stages:
  - **Stage 3a CKD:** Kidney function is moderately to severely reduced, with a GFR ranging from 45 to 59 milliliters per minute per 1.73 square meters of body surface area.
  - **Stage 3b CKD:** Kidney function is severely reduced, with a GFR ranging from 30 to 44 milliliters per minute per 1.73 square meters of body surface area. Individuals in stage 3 CKD may begin to experience symptoms such as fatigue, swelling, and changes in urination frequency or appearance.
- **Stage 4 CKD:** Kidney function is significantly reduced in stage 4 CKD, with a GFR ranging from 15 to 29 milliliters per minute per 1.73 square meters of body surface area. Symptoms become more pronounced, and individuals are at increased risk of developing complications such as anemia, bone disease, and cardiovascular disease. Healthcare providers intensify management strategies to delay the progression of the disease and prepare for potential renal replacement therapy, such as dialysis or kidney transplantation.
- **Stage 5 CKD (End-Stage Renal Disease, ESRD):** In the final stage of CKD, kidney function is severely impaired, with a GFR of less than 15 milliliters per minute per 1.73 square meters of body surface area. Individuals with stage 5 CKD, also known as end-stage renal disease (ESRD), experience significant symptoms and complications. Renal replacement therapy, such as dialysis or kidney transplantation, is typically necessary to sustain life.

Summary

- Kidney disease means your kidneys aren't working properly and are beginning to lose their function. Chronic kidney disease (CKD) worsens over time. High blood pressure and diabetes are two common causes of CKD. There's no cure for CKD, but you can take steps to preserve function for as long as possible. Late-stage kidney disease requires dialysis or a kidney transplant.
- Chronic prerenal disease occurs in patients with chronic heart failure or cirrhosis with persistently decreased renal perfusion, which increases the propensity for multiple episodes of an intrinsic kidney injury, such as acute tubular necrosis (ATN). This leads to progressive loss of renal function over time.
- A nephritic pattern is suggested by abnormal urine microscopy with red blood cell (RBC) casts and dysmorphic red cells, occasionally white blood cells (WBCs), and a variable degree of proteinuria. The most common causes are post-streptococcal GN, infective endocarditis, shunt nephritis, IgA nephropathy, lupus nephritis, Goodpasture syndrome, and vasculitis.
- Genetic factors that affect CKD progression have been found in different Kidney diseases. In a population-based cohort study by Luttropp et al., single nucleotide polymorphisms in the genes *TCF7L2* and *MTHFS* were associated with diabetic nephropathy and CKD progression.
- Unlike acute kidney injury (AKI), where the healing process is complete with complete functional kidney recovery, chronic and sustained insults from chronic and progressive nephropathies evolve into progressive kidney fibrosis and destruction of the normal architecture of the kidney. This affects all the 3 compartments of the kidney, namely the glomeruli, the tubules, the interstitium, and the vessels. It manifests histologically as glomerulosclerosis, tubulointerstitial fibrosis, and vascular sclerosis.
- The evaluation of CKD progression is based on the evaluation of three aspects: decline in renal function in patients who were monitored longitudinally with comparable methods; occurrence of renal failure, defined by the initiation of RRT; symptoms or complications of decrease of renal function and the development or worsening of proteinuria, particularly in diabetic nephropathy.
- Anemia is a frequent complication in individuals with CKD, and the erythropoietin deficiency is its most common factor, together with iron, folic acid, and vitamin B12 deficiency. Therefore, it is part of the routine treatment of CKD patients to investigate the presence of anemia and indicate and follow up its treatment.
- Cardiovascular disease (CVD) is the main cause of morbidity and mortality among the population with CKD. Based on data from the literature, all patients with CKD should be considered at high risk for CVD, evaluated based on "traditional" and "non-traditional" (related to uremia) risk factors for CVD and treated for the reduction of modifiable cardiovascular risk factors.

References

1. Aeddula, N. R., & Baradhi, K. M. (2023). Reflux nephropathy. In *StatPearls* [Internet]. StatPearls Publishing. Retrieved from: https://www.statpearls.com (accessed on 31 July 2024).
2. Aeddula, N. R., Bardhan, M., & Baradhi, K. M. (2023). Sickle cell nephropathy. In *StatPearls* [Internet]. StatPearls Publishing. Retrieved from: https://www.statpearls.com (accessed on 31 July 2024).
3. Aeddula, N. R., Cheungpasitporn, W., Thongprayoon, C., & Pathireddy, S. (2019). Epicardial adipose tissue and renal disease. *Journal of Clinical Medicine, 8*(3). doi: 10.3390/jcm8030375.
4. Anderson, S., Rennke, H. G., & Brenner, B. M. (1986). Antihypertensive therapy must control glomerular hypertension to limit glomerular injury. *Journal of Hypertension Supplements, 4*(5), S242–S244.
5. Astor, B. C., Matsushita, K., Gansevoort, R. T., et al.; Chronic Kidney Disease Prognosis Consortium. (2011). Lower estimated glomerular filtration rate and higher albuminuria are associated with mortality and end-stage renal disease: A collaborative meta-analysis of kidney disease population cohorts. *Kidney International, 79*(12), 1331–1340. doi: 10.1038/ki.2010.550.
6. Coresh, J., Astor, B. C., Greene, T., Eknoyan, G., & Levey, A. S. (2003). Prevalence of chronic kidney disease and decreased kidney function in the adult US population: Third National Health and Nutrition Examination Survey. *American Journal of Kidney Diseases, 41*(1), 1–12.
7. Coresh, J., Selvin, E., Stevens, L. A., et al. (2007). Prevalence of chronic kidney disease in the United States. *Journal of the American Medical Association, 298*(17), 2038–2047. doi: 10.1001/jama.298.17.2038.
8. de Brito-Ashurst, I., Varagunam, M., Raftery, M. J., & Yaqoob, M. M. (2009). Bicarbonate supplementation slows progression of CKD and improves nutritional status. *Journal of the American Society of Nephrology, 20*(9), 2075–2084.
9. Diabetes Control and Complications Trial Research Group. (1993). The effect of intensive treatment of diabetes on the development and progression of long-term complications in insulin-dependent diabetes mellitus. *New England Journal of Medicine, 329*(14), 977–986.
10. Fishbane, S., Agoritsas, S., Bellucci, A., Halinski, C., Shah, H. H., Sakhiya, V., & Balsam, L. (2017). Augmented nurse care management in CKD stages 4 to 5: A randomized trial. *American Journal of Kidney Diseases, 70*(4), 498–505.
11. Genovese, G., Friedman, D. J., Ross, M. D., et al. (2010). Association of trypanolytic ApoL1 variants with kidney disease in African Americans. *Science, 329*(5993), 841–845. doi: 10.1126/science.1193032.
12. Ghimire, S., Lee, K., Jose, M. D., Castelino, R. L., & Zaidi, S. T. R. (2019). Adherence assessment practices in hemodialysis settings: A qualitative exploration of nurses and pharmacists' perspectives. *Journal of Clinical Nursing, 28*(11–12), 2197–2205.
13. Grams, M. E., Chow, E. K., Segev, D. L., & Coresh, J. (2013). Lifetime incidence of CKD stages 3–5 in the United States. *American Journal of Kidney Diseases, 62*(2), 245–252. doi: 10.1053/j.ajkd.2013.03.009.

14. Grams, M. E., Rebholz, C. M., Chen, Y., et al. (2016). Race, APOL1 risk, and eGFR decline in the general population. *Journal of the American Society of Nephrology, 27*(9), 2842–2850. doi: 10.1681/ASN.2015070763.

15. Hallan, S. I., & Orth, S. R. (2011). Smoking is a risk factor in the progression to kidney failure. *Kidney International, 80*(5), 516–523.

16. Hsu, C. Y., Vittinghoff, E., Lin, F., & Shlipak, M. G. (2004). The incidence of end-stage renal disease is increasing faster than the prevalence of chronic renal insufficiency. *Annals of Internal Medicine, 141*(2), 95–101. doi: 10.7326/0003-4819-141-2-200407200-00007.

17. Hyperfiltration in remnant nephrons: A potentially adverse response to renal ablation. (2001). *Journal of the American Society of Nephrology, 12*(6), 1315–1325.

18. Inker, L. A., Astor, B. C., Fox, C. H., Isakova, T., Lash, J. P., Peralta, C. A., Kurella Tamura, M., & Feldman, H. I. (2014). KDOQI US commentary on the 2012 KDIGO clinical practice guideline for the evaluation and management of CKD. *American Journal of Kidney Diseases, 63*(5), 713–735.

19. Jamerson, K., Weber, M. A., Bakris, G. L., Dahlöf, B., Pitt, B., Shi, V., Hester, A., Gupte, J., Gatlin, M., & Velazquez, E. J., ACCOMPLISH Trial Investigators. (2008). Benazepril plus amlodipine or hydrochlorothiazide for hypertension in high-risk patients. *New England Journal of Medicine, 359*(23), 2417–2428.

20. Jha, V., Garcia-Garcia, G., Iseki, K., et al. (2013). Chronic kidney disease: Global dimension and perspectives. *Lancet, 382*(9888), 260–272. doi: 10.1016/S0140-6736(13)60687-X.

21. Johnson, R. J., Nakagawa, T., Jalal, D., Sánchez-Lozada, L. G., Kang, D. H., & Ritz, E. (2013). Uric acid and chronic kidney disease: Which is chasing which? *Nephrology Dialysis Transplantation, 28*(9), 2221–2228. doi: 10.1093/ndt/gft260.

22. Khan, S. S., Kazmi, W. H., Abichandani, R., Tighiouart, H., Pereira, B. J., & Kausz, A. T. (2002). Health care utilization among patients with chronic kidney disease. *Kidney International, 62*(1), 229–236. doi: 10.1046/j.1523-1755.2002.00376.x.

23. Khanna, R. (2011). Clinical presentation & management of glomerular diseases: Hematuria, nephritic & nephrotic syndrome. *Missouri Medicine, 108*(1), 33–36.

24. Kidney Disease: Improving Global Outcomes (KDIGO) CKD Work Group. (2013). KDIGO 2012 clinical practice guideline for the evaluation and management of chronic kidney disease. *Kidney International Supplements, 3*(1), 1–150. doi: 10.1038/kisup.2012.73.

25. Kitamoto, Y., Tomita, M., Akamine, M., Inoue, T., Itoh, J., Takamori, H., & Sato, T. (1993). Differentiation of hematuria using a uniquely shaped red cell. *Nephron, 64*(1), 32–36. doi: 10.1159/000187204.

26. Kshirsagar, A. V., Bang, H., Bomback, A. S., Vupputuri, S., Shoham, D. A., Kern, L. M., Klemmer, P. J., Mazumdar, M., & August, P. A. (2008). A simple algorithm to predict incident kidney disease. *Archives of Internal Medicine, 168*(22), 2466–2473. doi: 10.1001/archinte.168.22.2466.

27. Levey, A. S., & Coresh, J. (2012). Chronic kidney disease. *Lancet, 379*(9811), 165–180. doi: 10.1016/S0140-6736(11)60178-5.

28. Luttropp, K., Lindholm, B., Carrero, J. J., Glorieux, G., Schepers, E., Vanholder, R., Schalling, M., Stenvinkel, P., & Nordfors, L. (2009). Genetics/Genomics in chronic kidney disease—Towards personalized medicine? *Seminars in Dialysis, 22*(4), 417–422. doi: 10.1111/j.1525-139X.2009.00647.x.

29. Madero, M., García-Arroyo, F. E., & Sánchez-Lozada, L. G. (2017). Pathophysiologic insight into Mesoamerican nephropathy. *Current Opinion in Nephrology and Hypertension, 26*(4), 296–302. doi: 10.1097/MNH.0000000000000325.

30. Mahajan, A., Simoni, J., Sheather, S. J., Broglio, K. R., Rajab, M. H., & Wesson, D. E. (2010). Daily oral sodium bicarbonate preserves glomerular filtration rate by slowing its decline in early hypertensive nephropathy. *Kidney International, 78*(3), 303–309. doi: 10.1038/ki.2010.129.

31. Matsushita, K., Coresh, J., Sang, Y., et al.; CKD Prognosis Consortium. (2015). Estimated glomerular filtration rate and albuminuria for prediction of cardiovascular outcomes: A collaborative meta-analysis of individual participant data. *Lancet Diabetes & Endocrinology, 3*(7), 514–525. doi: 10.1016/S2213-8587(15)00040-6.

32. Methven, S., Traynor, J. P., Hair, M. D., St J O'Reilly, D., Deighan, C. J., & MacGregor, M. S. (2011). Stratifying risk in chronic kidney disease: An observational study of UK guidelines for measuring total proteinuria and albuminuria. *QJM: An International Journal of Medicine, 104*(8), 663–670. doi: 10.1093/qjmed/hcr059.

33. Mills, K. T., Xu, Y., Zhang, W., et al. (2015). A systematic analysis of worldwide population-based data on the global burden of chronic kidney disease in 2010. *Kidney International, 88*(5), 950–957. doi: 10.1038/ki.2015.230.

34. Moorhead, J. F., Chan, M. K., El-Nahas, M., & Varghese, Z. (1982). Lipid nephrotoxicity in chronic progressive glomerular and tubulo-interstitial disease. *Lancet, 2*(8311), 1309–1311. doi: 10.1016/S0140-6736(82)91685-3.

35. Muntner, P. (2009). Longitudinal measurements of renal function. *Seminars in Nephrology, 29*(6), 650–657. doi: 10.1016/j.semnephrol.2009.07.007.

36. Naik, R. P., Derebail, V. K., Grams, M. E., et al. (2014). Association of sickle cell trait with chronic kidney disease and albuminuria in African Americans. *Journal of the American Medical Association, 312*(20), 2115–2125. doi: 10.1001/jama.2014.15063.

37. National Kidney Foundation. (2002). K/DOQI clinical practice guidelines for chronic kidney disease: Evaluation, classification, and stratification. *American Journal of Kidney Diseases, 39*(2 Suppl 1), S1–S266.

38. O'Seaghdha, C. M., Parekh, R. S., Hwang, S. J., et al. (2011). The MYH9/APOL1 region and chronic kidney disease in European-Americans. *Human Molecular Genetics, 20*(12), 2450–2456. doi: 10.1093/hmg/ddr118.

39. Peralta, C. A., Vittinghoff, E., Bansal, N., et al. (2013). Trajectories of kidney function decline in young black and white adults with preserved GFR: Results from the Coronary Artery Risk Development in Young Adults (CARDIA) study. *American Journal of Kidney Diseases, 62*(2), 261–266. doi: 10.1053/j.ajkd.2013.01.012.

40. Plantinga, L. C., Boulware, L. E., Coresh, J., et al. (2008). Patient awareness of chronic kidney disease: Trends and predictors. *Archives of Internal Medicine, 168*(20), 2268–2275. doi: 10.1001/archinte.168.20.2268.

41. Ravani, P., Malberti, F., Tripepi, G., Pecchini, P., Cutrupi, S., Pizzini, P., et al. (2009). Vitamin D levels and patient outcome in chronic kidney disease. *Kidney International, 75*(1), 88–95. doi: 10.1038/ki.2008.453.

42. Sachdeva, B., Zulfiqar, H., & Aeddula, N. R. (2023). Peritoneal dialysis. In *StatPearls* [Internet]. StatPearls Publishing. Retrieved from: https://www.statpearls.com (accessed on 31 July 2024).

43. Sen, A., Callisen, H., Libricz, S., & Patel, B. (2019). Complications of solid organ transplantation: Cardiovascular, neurologic, renal, and gastrointestinal. *Critical Care Clinics, 35*(1), 169–186. doi: 10.1016/j.ccc.2018.09.002.

44. Textor, S. C. (2004). Ischemic nephropathy: Where are we now? *Journal of the American Society of Nephrology, 15*(8), 1974–1982. doi: 10.1097/01.ASN.0000137812.52489.3E.

45. Thongprayoon, C., Chokesuwattanaskul, R., Bathini, T., Khoury, N. J., Sharma, K., Ungprasert, P., Prasitlumkum, N., Aeddula, N. R., Watthanasuntorn, K., Salim, S. A., Kaewput, W., Koller, F. L., & Cheungpasitporn, W. (2018). Epidemiology and prognostic importance of atrial fibrillation in kidney transplant recipients: A meta-analysis. *Journal of Clinical Medicine, 7*(10). doi: 10.3390/jcm7100374.

46. Tzur, S., Rosset, S., Shemer, R., et al. (2010). Missense mutations in the APOL1 gene are highly associated with end stage kidney disease risk previously attributed to the MYH9 gene. *Human Genetics, 128*(3), 345–350. doi: 10.1007/s00439-010-0861-0.

47. Vidt, D. G. (2008). Telmisartan, ramipril, or both in patients at high risk for vascular events. *Current Hypertension Reports, 10*(5), 343–344. doi: 10.1007/s11906-008-0064-4.

48. Webster, A. C., Nagler, E. V., Morton, R. L., & Masson, P. (2017). Chronic kidney disease. *Lancet, 389*(10075), 1238–1252. doi: 10.1016/S0140-6736(16)32064-5.

49. Yu, H. T. (2003). Progression of chronic renal failure. *Archives of Internal Medicine, 163*(12), 1417–1429. doi: 10.1001/archinte.163.12.1417.

Chapter 8

GLOMERULAR DISEASES

Contents

Introduction

A collection of disorders known as glomerular diseases affect the kidney's small filtration units, or glomeruli, which are in charge of eliminating waste materials and extra fluid from the blood. These conditions can impair the glomeruli's normal function, which can result in hematuria, proteinuria, a drop in the glomerular filtration rate (GFR), and eventually worsened kidney function. The variety of etiology, manifestations, and prognoses of glomerular diseases make diagnosis and treatment extremely difficult.

Multiple factors, including immune-mediated processes, genetic predisposition, infections, systemic diseases, and environmental factors, can contribute to the etiology of glomerular diseases. IgA nephropathy, lupus nephritis, and membranous nephropathy are examples of immune-mediated glomerular diseases caused by aberrant immune responses that target the mesangium or glomerular basement membrane. The glomerular basement membrane exhibits structural abnormalities in genetic disorders like Alport syndrome and thin basement membrane disease, which ultimately result in glomerular dysfunction.

The severity of kidney involvement and underlying pathology determine how glomerular diseases present clinically. Hematuria (blood in the urine), proteinuria (protein in the urine), edema, hypertension, and decreased urine production are typical symptoms. Systemic symptoms can also manifest as malaise, exhaustion, and weight loss, especially in cases of autoimmune or systemic kidney diseases.

The diagnosis of glomerular diseases is usually made by combining renal biopsy, imaging studies, laboratory testing, and clinical assessment. To assess kidney function and determine glomerular involvement, urinalysis, serum creatinine, and urine protein excretion assessment are crucial. The size and structure of the kidneys can be evaluated with imaging tests like an ultrasound or CT scan, while a renal biopsy confirms the histology and helps with treatment choices.

The goals of glomerular disease management are to lessen proteinuria, prevent kidney damage from getting worse, and maintain kidney function. Angiotensin-converting enzyme inhibitors (ACE inhibitors) or angiotensin receptor blockers (ARBs) to lower blood pressure and proteinuria, immunosuppressive therapy, and supportive measures like dietary and lifestyle adjustments are some possible treatment approaches. Dialysis or kidney transplantation might be required in extreme situations to restore lost kidney function and enhance patient outcomes.

Orientation and Directional Terms

Term	Definition	Illustration
Hematuria	Hematuria is blood in the urine. When the urine is red or pink this could be linked to blood in the urine and is called "gross" or "visible" hematuria.	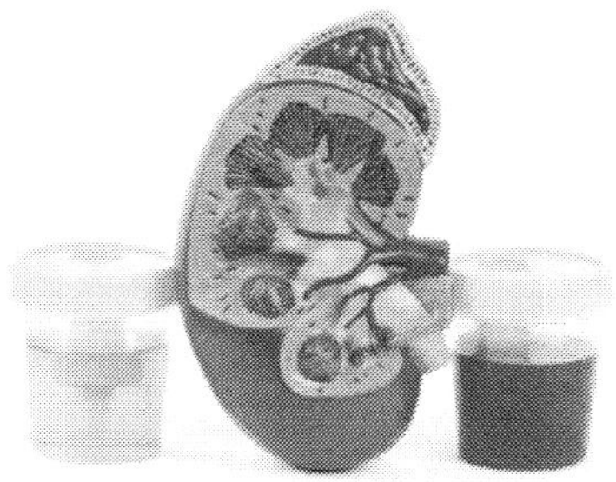
Podocytes	Podocytes are specialized cells in the kidney's glomerulus that wrap around capillaries and filter blood.	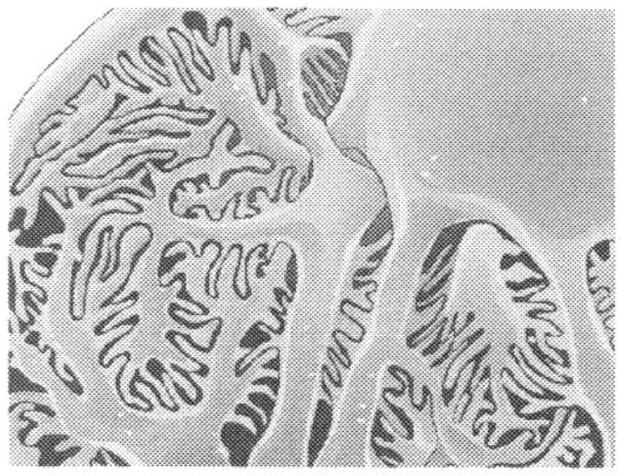
Nephritic	Nephritic refers to a clinical syndrome that includes signs of nephritis, which is inflammation of the kidneys. Nephritic syndrome is caused by inflammation of the glomerulus, which can be a kidney issue or a result of systemic disorders.	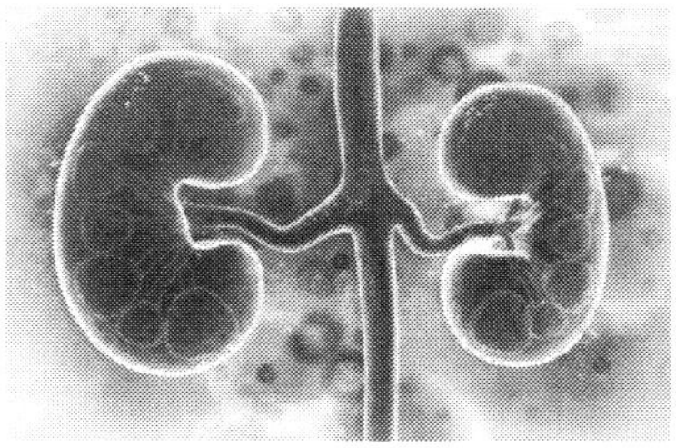
Nephrotic syndrome	Nephrotic syndrome is a kidney disorder that causes your body to pass too much protein in your urine.	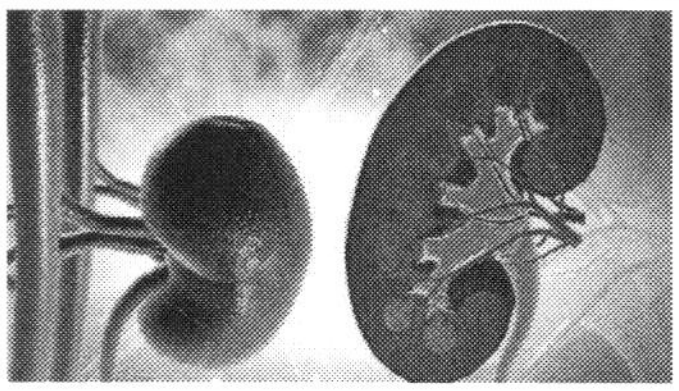
Glomerular filter	Glomerular filtration is a process by which blood plasma is filtered through the glomerular filtration membrane.	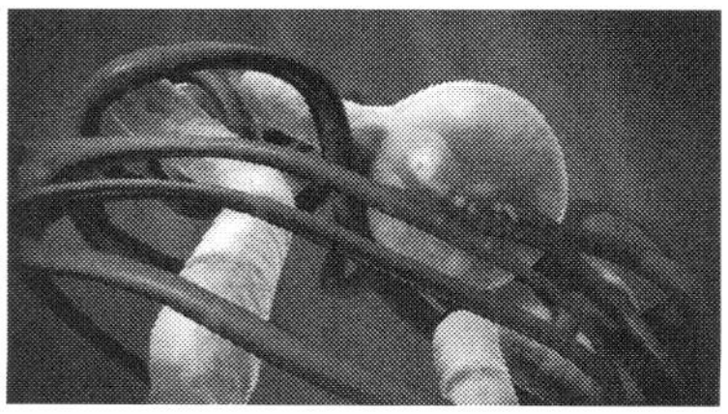

8.1. Overview of Glomerular Structure and Function

The kidneys perform many vital homeostatic tasks. These include the elimination of waste (NH3), the regulation of fluid and electrolyte balance, the metabolic blood acid-base balance, and the synthesis and modification of hormones related to blood pressure, calcium and potassium homeostasis, and the production of red blood cells. Most of these kidney functions are carried out by the renal tubules, which are responsible for reabsorption and excretion, and the renal corpuscle, which is the filtration unit of the kidney and includes the glomerulus and the surrounding glomerular or Bowman's capsule.

The kidney's distinctive blood flow, which features high perfusion autoregulation of flow across the glomerular capillaries over a range of pressures, contributes to its primary function of filtering blood. The kidneys are able to filter large amounts of blood because they receive a high percentage of blood—roughly 20% of cardiac output. Blood vessel arrangement causes blood flow to autoregulate across filtration capillaries (glomeruli). Unlike most other capillary beds, the glomerulus is positioned between two arterioles. Blood enters the glomerulus from the upstream afferent arteriole and exits via the downstream efferent arterioles (with an E for exit). Because of this configuration, the glomerular flow within the glomerulus and the rate of filtration can be precisely controlled through autoregulatory changes in the resistance arteriole diameters (vasodilation/vasoconstriction).

The kidney's main job is to filter blood and produce urine. Renal corpuscles, the kidney's filtering units, have histological structures that are essential to this function. Only the kidney cortex contains renal corpuscles, which number approximately 1 million per kidney, with racial variations. Three histological structures make up this particular filtration barrier: the glomeruli's capillary endothelium, podocytes, which are specialized cells, and the combined basement membranes of these two cells. Small molecules (less than 90 kDa) including water, ions, creatinine, glucose, and small proteins can all be filtered through this filtration barrier. Large blood proteins like albumin and immunoglobulins must not be filtered out by this structure.

Pathological conditions result from any deviation in this filtration barrier. Indeed, glomerular diseases account for about 90% of end-stage kidney disease. The main worry is that the kidneys' capacity for healing is restricted once they are injured. In fact, the majority of glomerular diseases progress gradually, with symptoms not showing up until a considerable percentage of the kidney's functional units have been compromised.

The glomerular filtration barrier is nearly always disrupted in glomerular diseases, which are diverse conditions with a wide range of etiologies and clinical manifestations. Based on the quantity of proteins entering the filtrate or glomerular filtration rate, these various kidney diseases can be broadly divided into two syndromes: nephrotic and nephritic. These syndromes are a collection of symptoms, indicators, and laboratory results that point to an underlying kidney disease, usually affecting the glomerulus, rather than diseases in and of themselves. Nephrotic and nephritic syndromes have a wide range of etiologies and pathologic alterations, but some helpful generalizations are achievable.

The primary cause of nephrotic syndrome is the degeneration of podocytes, which are essential components of the filtration barrier (think of the word "podocyte" as "O" for either protein or "podocyte"). Significant protein losses in the urine are a consequence of podocyte dysfunction.

On the other hand, kidney disorders linked to glomerular basement membrane disruption can result in nephritic syndrome. Hematuria, or blood in the urine, is a pathological change that is mainly caused by inflammation (nephrItic: think I for inflammation). This allows red blood cells to pass through the filtration membrane and gives the urine a cola color.

8.1.1. Structure

There are various histological structures that make up the renal corpuscle.

8.1.1.1. Glomerulus Capillaries

In the middle of the renal corpuscle, the glomerulus capillaries form a central tuft of looped capillaries. In addition to supplying blood, these capillaries provide a sizable surface area for renal filtration. The purpose of these capillaries is filtration. Because blood flow is controlled over wide pressure ranges, the glomerular filtration rate is largely maintained. The special positioning of the capillaries between the afferent and efferent resistance arterioles—think E for exit—allows for this regulation. They also offer a sizable porous surface area that is useful for filtration. About 20–50% of the endothelial surface of the glomerular capillary endothelium is made up of tiny transcellular pores, or fenestrations, or windows, with a diameter of about 60 nm. Despite the size of these pores, it is believed that molecules larger than 100 nm cannot pass through because of the negatively charged glycocalyx that covers the surface of the luminal endothelial cells. Finally, these capillaries are comparatively "free" inside the Bowman's capsule rather than embedded in an intracellular matrix that provides support. It makes sense, then, that the Greek word "filter" is where the term "glomerulus" originated."

8.1.1.2. Intraglomerular Mesangial Cells

Under the basement membrane, in the intercellular spaces, reside intraglomerular mesangial cells that support the glomerular capillaries. On the other side of the glomerulus from the podocytes, they are typically located. Because they are not encircled by interstitial tissue, glomerular capillaries need a special kind of support system. Very few stromal cells are found in the kidneys. These mesangial cells are indented, heterochromatic, and have a small, asymmetrical nucleus along with little cytoplasm. Mesangium is the collective term used to refer to both mesangial cells and their secreted extracellular matrix. Certain renal diseases cause the filtration area to decrease and glomerular capillaries to become occluded due to mesangial cell expansion (Haraldsson, 2008) (Figure 8.1).

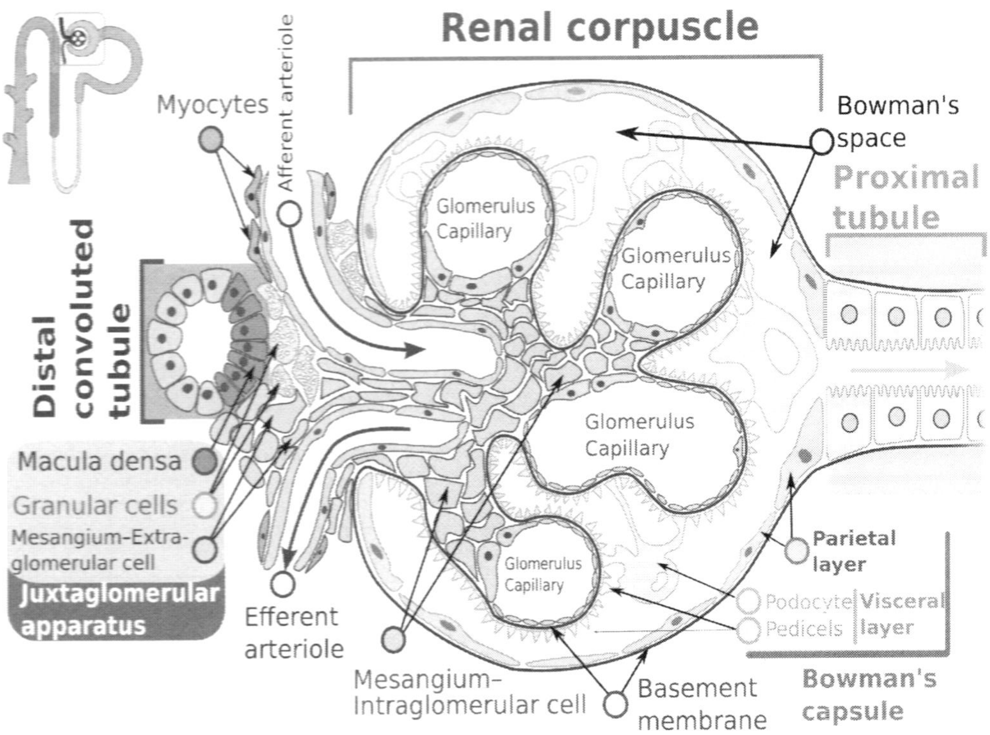

Figure 8.1. *Structure of glomerulus.*

Source. https://www.ncbi.nlm.nih.gov/books/NBK554544/bin/Renal_Corpuscle_Wikipedia.jpg.

In addition, mesangial cells perform phagocytic and contractile tasks. While there is some evidence that erythropoietin (EPO) can be secreted by mesangial cells, the more widely accepted theory is that peritubular cells produce EPO. In reaction to variations in blood pressure, the contractility modifies the glomerular capillary diameter, which fine-tunes glomerular filtration rates. Protein aggregates that become stuck in the glomerular filter, like immune complexes, are eliminated by the phagocytic function. Mesangial cells produce erythropoietin (EPO) in response to hypoxia, so the injury can also impact the production of red blood cells and hematocrit.

8.1.1.3. Bowman's Capsule

The layers of the parietal and visceral bodies make up Bowman's capsule. The glomerular capillaries are totally encircled by the inner visceral layer. Podocytes are specialized stellate epithelial cells that make up this structure. Bowman's capsule, on the other hand, has a single layer of simple squamous epithelium on its outer, or parietal, layer. Urine is filtered into the area that lies between these two layers.

8.1.1.4. Podocytes

Podocytes are a component of the glomerular filtration barrier as well as supporting glomerular capillaries. These are big cells with euchromatic nuclei that make up the Bowman's capsule's visceral layer, which is exposed to the urine space. A large portion of the surface of the glomerular capillaries is covered and encircled by the interdigitating secondary processes of the podocytes, also known as foot processes or pedicels. Actin is present in these foot processes, which may have some contractile activity to prevent the glomerular capillaries from distensing. These interdigitating pedicels create slit pores that are between 30 and 40 nanometers in width. Slit diaphragms, or thin membranes, cover these slits. Podocytes can regenerate foot processes (pedicels), but their capacity for repair is limited. Pedicel loss can also be called simplification, retraction, fusion, or effacement.

The slit diaphragms are specialized adherens junctions that form a structure resembling a zipper with tiny pores the size of an albumin molecule, along with nephron and other proteins. These tiny pores cause the filtrate to be sieved, which results in the protein barrier. A negatively charged glycocalyx, which also serves as a barrier by repelling negatively charged proteins like albumin, covers the podocytes and slit diaphragm in addition to the pores. It is noteworthy that electron microscopy is the only method by which the slight diaphragm can be seen. There is disagreement over whether the slit diaphragm plays a primary role in permeability selectivity.

8.1.1.5. The Glomerular Basement Membrane

Podocytes, capillary endothelium, and the glomerular basement membrane make up the filtration barrier's other two components. It is a composite basement membrane made up of podocytes and endothelial cells that also provides some glomerular capillary support. As a result, its thickness (240–270 nm) is greater than that of other capillary basement membranes (40–80 nm). It is a material that resembles gel and has a network of organized fibrous mesh that forms heterogeneous pores with a diameter of 10 nm. Type IV collagen makes up the majority of the material, but it also contains laminin, heparan sulfate, glycoproteins, and the proteoglycans agrin and perlecan. Negative charges combined with the mesh-like structure create a molecular sieve or barrier that keeps high molecular weight proteins like albumin and globulin (antibodies) from exiting the bloodstream. Although its exact function in selective permeability has recently been questioned, the glomerular basement membrane unquestionably limits fluid flow (Deen, 2001) (Figure 8.2).

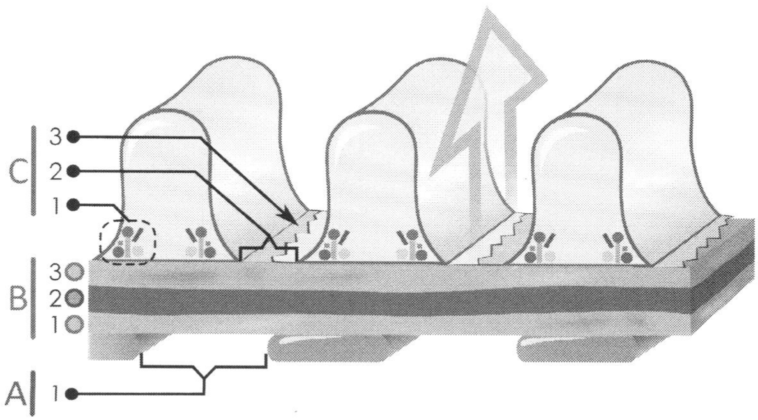

Figure 8.2. *Filtration barrier.*

Source: https://www.ncbi.nlm.nih.gov/books/NBK554544/bin/Filtration_Barrier_Wikipedia.jpg.

8.1.1.6. The Juxtaglomerular Apparatus

An essential collection of structures at the glomerulus's capillary entrance is called the juxtaglomerular apparatus. Two of these are specialized sensory structures with feedback mechanisms to control the rate of filtration and glomerular blood flow.

1. Macula Densa (thicker spot) is a thickened region of the distal convoluted tubule. It is characterized by apical nuclei and tightly packed columnar cells. It responds to the salt concentration in the tubule filtrate and is a tubuloglomerular feedback system that regulates the glomerular filtration rate. It is important to note that the macula Densa regulates the glomerulus that connects to the distal tubule, which detects the salt concentration.
2. Juxtaglomerular cells (also granular cells) are specialized smooth muscles in the walls of the afferent arteriole. These cells synthesize and secrete renin in response to decreased arteriolar blood pressure and activate the renin-angiotensin system to regulate blood pressure.
3. Lacis cells are extraglomerular mesangial cells and are in the stalk of the glomerular tuft of capillaries. They have similar functions as the intraglomerular mesangial cells.

8.1.2. Function

The filtration barrier's structure. A= Endothelial cells (pink) of glomerular capillaries with fenestrated walls; the fenestra, or pore, is represented by label 1. B is for the purple glomerular basement membrane. Three layers are discernible through electron microscopy. Labels for 1 are intracellular enzymes, 2 are slits, and 3 are slit diaphragms. C: Interdigitating podocytes end-feet with slits (blue) are labeled as 1 = lamina rara interna, 2 = lamina Densa, and 3 = lamina rara externa. The direction of the filtrate flow through the filtration barrier is indicated by the large orange arrow.

The glomerular capillary endothelium, podocytes, and the combined basement membranes of these two cell types make up this glomerular filtration barrier. The selective permeability by size and charge in the kidney's renal filtration of substances is caused by this filtration barrier. Salts and water are examples of small molecules (less than 10 kDa) that can be freely filtered because they are not attached to plasma carrier proteins. Filtration decreases with increasing molecular weights until proteins larger than approximately 90 kDa, at which point it stops.

It is important to remember that albumin only loses 0.1% of its molecular weight in plasma, despite having a negative charge and a molecular weight of about 66 kDa. This is because the filtration barrier also includes negative charges in addition to a barrier based on the sieving through pores. The glomerular basement membrane, podocytes, and endothelial lumen all have a net negative charge, which electrostatically repels negatively charged molecules like albumin.

The actual functional mechanism of glomerular filtration is a balance across the filtration barrier between hydrostatic and colloid osmotic pressures, also known as Starling forces. Water and salts from the blood are forced into the Bowman's urinary space by the glomerular capillary pressures. Albumin is mainly responsible for the colloid osmotic pressures because it retains water in the capillaries. Sodium's albumin binding essentially functions as a sponge, retaining and drawing excess bodily fluid into the blood. Glomerular capillary filtration occurs when hydrostatic pressures are higher than oncotic pressures.

The juxtaglomerular apparatus is another significant structure in the glomerulus. Its components react to both a drop in blood pressure and an increase in glomerular filtration rate (GFR). The distal tubule filtrate's elevated salt concentration is what the macula Densa interprets as an increase in the glomerular filtration rate (GFR). In response, the macula Densa releases chemicals that constrict blood vessels, the afferent arteriole, lowering blood pressure and flow, and restoring normal GFR. The granular (or juxtaglomerular) cells, so named because of the intracellular granules that store renin before release, control decreased glomerular blood pressure. Renin that has been stored in intracellular granules is released by these cells. To raise blood volume and restore normal blood pressure, renin triggers the renin-angiotensin system (via aldosterone mediating water reabsorption in the tubules).

8.1.3. Tissue Preparation

Clinical significance for glomerular histology evaluation is primarily seen in the context of renal biopsies for kidney disorders. Indications for renal biopsy are not well-established and somewhat controversial. Nephrotic syndrome is the most common medical reason for a renal biopsy worldwide. Renal biopsies changed the clinical strategy in 31 to 57% of patients with end-stage renal disease and/or chronic kidney disease. Furthermore, biopsies are essential for evaluating kidney tumors and monitoring for rejection in cases of renal transplantation, even though the glomerulus is not always the subject of these analyzes.

It is outside the purview of this review to describe in detail the pathologic assessment of the medical renal biopsy; nevertheless. It is crucial for medical students and physicians who are not pathologists to comprehend the complex relationship between the quality of the biopsy technique and the processing procedures used, and the significance of the information gleaned from the biopsy. To optimize the benefits of histologic evaluation, the highlights of renal biopsy processing will be briefly reviewed in the sections that follow.

In contrast to allografts, native kidney biopsies are typically carried out percutaneously on a prone patient using a 14–18 gauge needle. When no specific target can be identified, the lower pole of the kidney is usually biopsied to perform a general kidney assessment. Before inserting the needle, the skin is lanced and a local anesthetic is applied. Even though there is some risk associated with any procedure, contemporary renal biopsy practice is generally safe. Slightly more than one-third of patients will have hematuria, regardless of method, and 0.5% of patients will have gross hematuria. Less than 0.1% of cases involve severe complications that require transfusion.

Three assessment modalities are needed for a thorough pathologic evaluation of the biopsy: transmission electron microscopy, immunofluorescence/immunohistochemistry, and light microscopy. The pathologist's experience and the facilities at hand determine which immunofluorescence and immunohistochemistry to use. Whereas immunohistochemistry is used more frequently in Europe, immunofluorescence is more common in the United States. After the biopsy, the sample needs to be divided into three sections to be examined under a microscope. At this point, a pathologist or skilled technician should be present. One can use a dissecting microscope to see globuli. The biopsy core will be divided to guarantee that the glomerular tissue is positioned correctly in each of the three media.

8.1.4. Microscopy, Light

- **Light Microscopy:** The biopsy-bound portion can be transported at room temperature in a standard buffered formalin solution for light microscopy. To ensure that the tissue is not lost during processing, it should be wrapped in lens paper. If at all possible, avoid using net bags or sponges as they introduce artifacts that will impede interpretation. The tissue will be embedded in paraffin after fixation. Multiple sections per slide should be sectioned using serial sections measuring two to four micrometers. Regarding the number of slides created initially and the stains applied initially, each institution usually follows a set protocol. Hematoxylin and eosin (HandE), periodic acid-Schiff, trichrome, and a silver stain are examples of standard stains.
- **Immunofluorescent Microscopy:** The majority of immunofluorescent protocols require tissue to be frozen as opposed to fixed. Fixing tissue does not totally rule out the possibility of using immunofluorescence, but it is not the best option. Fixatives that cross-link, like glutaraldehyde and formalin, are great at maintaining morphologic integrity, but they also run the risk of cross-linking target antigens and adding excessive background autofluorescence. The tissue can be transported in ordinary saline if the biopsy is being done close to the lab performing the procedure. A Michel medium is a recommended medium if the sample needs to travel farther. A cryostat with sections of 2 to 4 μM can be used for sectioning. Once more, the standard workup varies by institution; however, IgG, IgM, and IgA, complement proteins (C3, C1q, and C4), fibrin, and kappa/gamma light chains are usually included in routine examinations, along with the relevant controls.

8.1.5. Microscopy, Electron

For electron microscopy, ice-cold glutaraldehyde (1 to 3%) is the most widely used fixative. While they can be used, other fixatives like formalin or paraformaldehyde are not as good. The institution's standard electron microscopy (EM) procedures are followed. Typically, a glomerulus in the given tissue is chosen by evaluating a relatively thick (1 micrometer) section, which is subsequently sectioned into extremely thin slices and positioned on a copper grid. Ultrastructure is inspected in several ways to evaluate every aspect of the glomerulus that was previously addressed.

8.1.6. Pathophysiology

Numerous indicators of glomerular dysfunction can be employed in the diagnostic process, as well as in the differentiation of diseases into nephrotic or nephritic syndromes.

- **Protein in the Urine (Proteinuria):** This is a hallmark measure of renal disease, and the primary measure used to differentiate between nephrotic and nephritic syndromes. Protein in the urine can be due to glomerular disease-causing proteins to leak into the urine, or a defect in protein reabsorption in the kidney tubules. Proteinuria may cause foamy urine. Generally, very high protein concentration in the urine or "nephrotic range" > 200 mg/l is associated with podocyte disruption, which results in non-selective protein loss. Loss of protein in the urine is typically associated with reduced proteins or albumin in the blood (proteinemia or hypoalbuminemia).

- **Blood in the Urine (Hematuria):** The presence of hemoglobin from leaked red blood cells gives the urine a pink or light brown (cola-colored). This presentation is a typical symptom of nephritic syndrome, along with lower proteinuria, and proteinuria is associated with nephritic attributable to a defect in the glomerular basement membrane.
- **Edema:** Protein losses from the blood result in a reduction of colloid oncotic pressure and increased filtration from the capillaries resulting in the excess, non-resorbed fluid accumulation within the intercellular spaces to cause swelling. This swelling due to edema is usually more noticeable in the hands, ankles, or periorbitally.
- **Uremia:** reduced glomerular filtration rate: Disruption of the barrier can also result in reduced filtration and thus the accumulation of waste products such as. Creatinine and urea nitrogen in the blood.
- **Acidosis:** This is beyond a discussion of the glomerulus, but still bears mentioning. Kidney tubules are involved in the metabolic acid-base homeostatic regulation of blood pH.

1. **Diseases with Nephritic Syndromes:** This syndrome is not a disease per se; rather, it is a collection of symptoms that are typically linked to inflammatory processes. Common symptoms include hypertension (salt retention), elevated blood urea nitrogen (BUN), creatine, oliguria, hematuria, and red blood cell casts. It is caused by disruption of the glomerular basement membrane. proteinuria with a daily value of less than 3.5 grams. (Watson S, et al., 2023) (Table 8.1).

Table 8.1. Diseases with Nephritic Syndromes

Disease	Notes	Histology
IgAnephropathy (Ban disease)	Most common cause of primary glomerulonephritis_ billammation_ blood in the mine_	LM: expanded mesangiunm, with increased matrix and/or hypercellularity_ IF: IgAmesangial deposits_

Acute post streptococcal glomerulonephritis	Most common in children > in boys_ -2-4 weeks after strep throat or, in rare cases after impetigo (skin infection)_	LM: diffuse enlargement of glomerular tufts and mesangial proliferation Hypercelhdlarity_ IF: ·starry sky· granular appearance IgG/Ight, and C3 along with GBM and mesangium EM: electron dense lumps in the subepithelial *space_*
Rapid progressive (crescentic) glomerulonephritis	Severe glomerulonepinitis with a rapidly progressive coarse, many etiologies	LM: Crescent formation (cellular aggregation in Bowman's space) in >50% of glomeruli, GMB rupture on saver stain IF: Fibrin deposition within crescents
Alport Syndrome	Genetic condition_ Mai - renal insufficiency@ 20s and total kidney failure by age 40	LM: Non-specific changes; foamy cells in interstitial spaces are common_ EMI· Thickened GBM with splitting and granulation of the lamina densa_

Source. Le et al. 2019 First Aid for the USMLE McGraw Hill pp 583–5. https://www.ncbi.nlm.nih.gov/books/NBK554544/bin/Table_1_StatPearls_Kidney_Path_Table_1.jpg.

GBM = glomerular basement membrane, LM= light microscopy, IF = immunofluorescence, EM = electron microscopy, IgG = immunoglobulin G, C3 = complement C3.

2. **Diseases with Nephrotic Syndromes:** This syndrome is a collection of symptoms rather than a standalone disease, and can be associated with various underlying conditions. Prevention strategies focus on managing the primary diseases that contribute to the syndrome. The condition is typically caused by disruption of podocytes, leading to a compromised charge barrier. Symptoms include significant protein loss in the urine (> 3.5g/day), low levels of albumin, high levels of lipids, and swelling. Adults with this syndrome are at an elevated risk of developing blood clots in the veins, particularly the renal vein. The swelling is a result of protein loss, while abnormal lipid levels may be related to altered cholesterol transport. Blood clotting issues are due to decreased levels of antithrombin III (Agrawal et al., 2018) (Table 8.2).

Table 8.2. Diseases with Nephrotic Syndromes

Disease	Notes	Histelogy
Diabetic nephropathy	Most common nephropathy: Increased permeability, hyper filtration due to hypertension. Common in persons of African, Native and Mexican descent	LM: Protein glycation — mesangial expansion_ Glomerular hypertrophy and seining (sclerosis). Glomerular basement membrane thickening.
Focal segmental glomerulosclerosis (FSGS)	Most common in people of African descent, Hispanics. Large number of etiologies_	Lit Focal v.-wring/sclerosis of glomeruli Permanent damage to capillaries. IF: Igm, C3 in lesions_ EM: Effacement of foot racemes/ foot *process* fusion.
Membranous nephropathy, also membranous glomeralopathy	Second most common nephrotic syndrome. Majority idiopathic, also systemic tapas erythernatosus, hepatitis WC	LM: Thickened Gat spaces_ Diffuse capillaries_ IF: Fine granular IIIG, C3 EM: Subepithelial deposits
Minimal change disease	Most common nephrotic syndrome in children_ Occurs in some adults Usually responsive to steroid treatment in children_	, LM: Normal_ Liquid drops may be present, but no waning_ IF: usually negative EM- Podocyte phenotypic switch_ effacement of foot processes foot process fusion_
Amyloidosis	Large, heterogeneous group of disorders characterized by deposition of amyloid fibrils	Highly dependent on amyloid type Key points: Identify wattle composition of amyloid and localization of amyloid (glomerular interstitial, vescular; etc).
Congenital Nephrotic Syndrome	Presort with nephrotic syndrome in first 3 months of life	Two basic types: Finish type: LM Ectasia (dilation) of proximal and distal tubules. Diffuse Mesangia A Sclerosis type: Lit Crowding of podocytes and sclerosis of mesangiun_

Source: Le et al. (2019). First Aid for the USMLE McGraw Hill pp 583–585, https://www.ncbi.nlm.nih.gov/books/NBK554544/bin/Table_2_StatPearls_Kidney_Path_Table_2.jpg.

GBM = glomerular basement membrane, LM= light microscopy, IF = immunofluorescence, EM = electron microscopy, IgG = immunoglobulin G, C3 = complement C3.

3. **Diseases with both Nephritic-Nephrotic Syndromes:** Severe glomerular basement membrane damage associated with severe nephritic syndrome, which alters the charge barrier. Proteinuria within the nephrotic range (>3.5 g/day) and nephrotic syndrome characteristics (Raza et al., 2023) (Table 8.3).

Table 8.3. Diseases with Both Nephritic-Nephrotic Syndromes

Disease	Notes	Histology
Mambranoproliferative glomerulonephiritis	Common in white adults, rare in children	**TYPE I** LM: Thickend GBM, proliferation IF:Granular IgG, C3 EM: Mesangial and subendothelial **TYPE II** LM:Lobulation. IF: C3 only EM= dense deposits, thickend GBM, granular immunollnorescence. Spike and dome, subepithelial immune complex deposition
Diffuse proliferative glomerulonephiritis	Systemic inflammatory disease affecting gromerulus. Mainly due to systemic lupus erythematosus (SLIT)>females	LM: wire looping of capillaries. Antoantibodies in the glomeruli, resulting in inflammation and scanning Hypercellularity

Source: Le et al. (2019). First Aid for the USMLE (pp 583–585). McGraw Hill. https://www.ncbi.nlm.nih.gov/books/NBK554544/bin/Table_3_StatPearls_Kidney_Path_Table_3.jpg.

GBM = glomerular basement membrane, LM= light microscopy, IF = immunofluorescence, EM = electron microscopy, IgG = immunoglobulin G, C3 = complement C3.

The pathologies that result from glomerular damage are listed below. With the use of blood and urine analysis, the pathologies are easily diagnosed. In addition, homeostatic control of red blood cell production (hematocrit), calcium and vitamin D homeostasis, blood pressure/volume, and acid-base balance should be considered in the case of kidney disease.

8.2. Common Glomerular Diseases Overview

A collection of illnesses collectively referred to as "glomerular disease" (also called "glomerulonephritides" or "glomerulopathies") harm the renal glomeruli. The location of filtration is represented by the glomeruli (i.e., where the kidneys' blood is filtered. Chronic kidney disease (CKD) and acute kidney injury (AKI) are both significantly influenced by glomerular diseases.

Glomerular diseases have historically been hard to understand. This is due to the large range of clinical presentations, the substantial overlap between conditions, and the confusing terminology that combines histopathological and clinical terms. The clinical manifestations of glomerular disease that are most frequently discussed are nephrotic syndrome and nephritic syndrome, which are covered in our previous notes.

Normal homeostasis depends on the kidneys. They perform a variety of tasks, such as blood pressure regulation, fluid balance, acid-base balance, calcium/phosphate balance, and waste product excretion.

8.2.1. The Nephron

The nephron is the microscopic name for the kidney's functional unit. The nephron is composed of various key structures that are involved in secretion, reabsorption, and filtering (Radhakrishnan, 2021) (Figure 8.3).

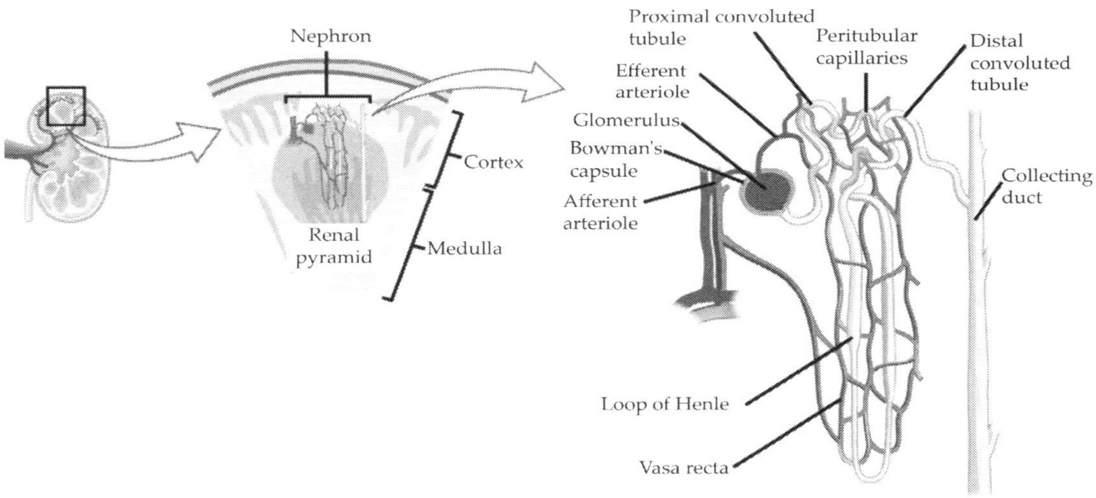

Figure 8.3. *The nephron.*

Source. https://courses.lumenlearning.com/suny-dutchess-ap1/chapter/nephrons-structure/.

8.2.2. Glomerulus

The process of extracting plasma free of proteins from the blood is known as filtration, and it is facilitated by the glomeruli. A tuft of capillaries encircled by a capsule (Bowman's capsule) is present in every glomerulus. The mesangium, a collection of cells and connective tissue, supports these capillaries (Radhakrishnan, 2021) (Figure 8.4).

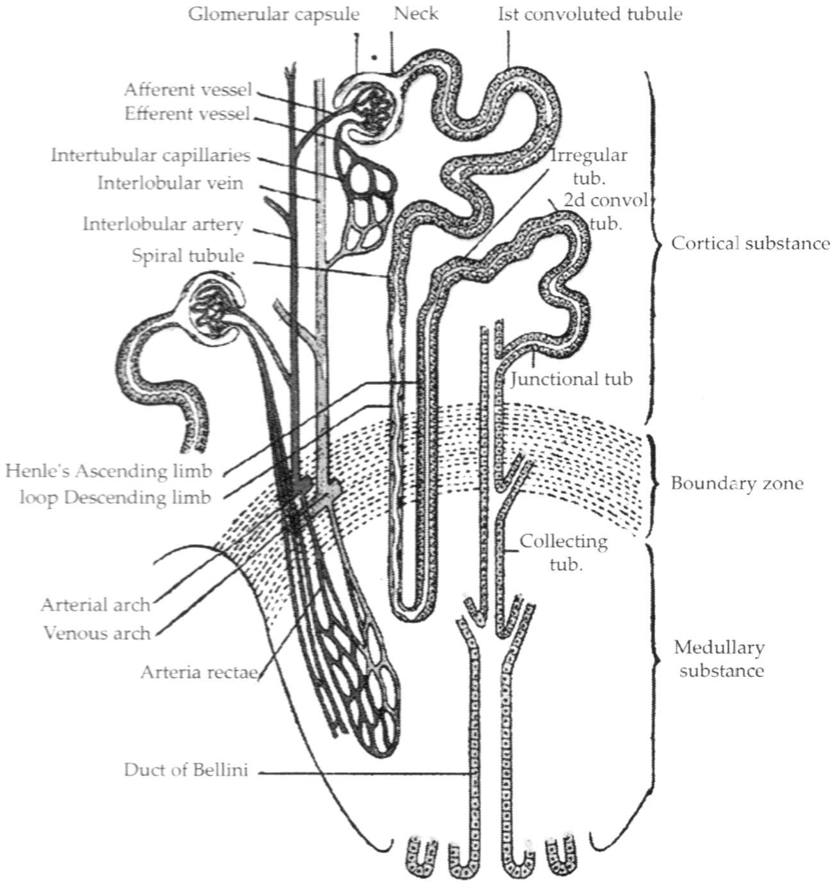

Figure 8.4. *The glomerulus.*

Source: By Henry Vandyke Carter – Henry Gray (1918) Anatomy of the Human Body (See "Book" section below)Bartleby.com: Gray's Anatomy, Plate 1128, Public Domain, https://commons.wikimedia.org/w/index.php?curid=567094.

The glomerulus's urinary space may receive substances and fluids from the capillaries. They then enter the proximal convoluted tubule of the kidney. The "filtration barrier" is composed of three layers that control the flow of fluid.

- Endothelium: capillary wall
- Basement membrane: provides a selective barrier to macromolecules based on size and charge
- Foot processes of podocytes: podocytes are specialized epithelial cells

The filtration barrier may be compromised by immune-mediated injury or structural alterations to the glomeruli. Red blood cell leakage may result from this (i.e., blood loss) and/or protein (i.e., proteinuria), which serves as the glomerular disease hallmark. (Radhakrishnan, 2021) (Figure 8.5).

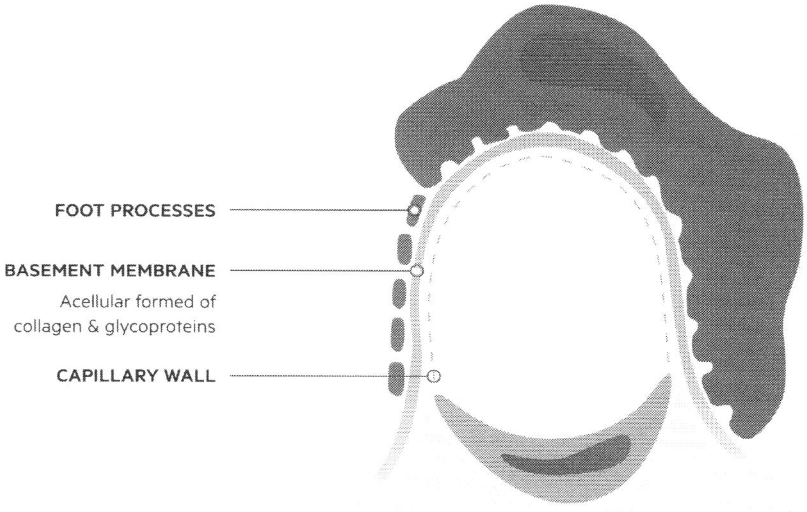

Figure 8.5. *Hematuria- filtration barrier.*

Source. https://d1z8zkw1yi6kd7.cloudfront.net/uploads/ckeditor/pictures/data/000/002/607//content/the_filtration_barrier.jpg.

Primary and secondary disorders can be used to broadly categorize glomerular disease. Glomerulopathies can be categorized and described in many ways. We go over some of the common terms here.

8.2.3. Primary Versus Secondary

Primary glomerular disease is defined as a glomerular injury resulting from a primary renal pathology, whereas secondary glomerular disease is a glomerular injury resulting from a systemic process.

- **Primary:** IgA nephropathy, minimal change disease, focal segmental glomerulosclerosis
- **Secondary:** Vasculitis (e.g., ANCA-associated vasculitis), amyloidosis, diabetes mellitus

Some conditions can be both a primary and secondary glomerulopathy if they occur alongside another systemic illness, such as focal segmental glomerulosclerosis.

8.2.4. Focal Versus Diffuse

A glomerulopathy can be diffuse, affecting all glomeruli, or focal, affecting only a portion of them. Typically, a broad cut-off of 50% is employed to distinguish between diffuse and focal. Renal biopsy and glomerulus sampling are used to determine whether a glomerulopathy is focal or diffuse.

8.2.5. Global Versus Segmental

A glomerulopathy can be classified as global or segmental, depending on the degree of involvement of each glomerulus. A threshold of 50% is commonly used to distinguish between the two categories based on histopathological evaluation.

8.2.6. Pathophysiology

Glomerular injury can be caused by a wide range of immune and non-immune mechanisms. Numerous pathways may result in glomerular injury, which in turn impacts the filtration barrier. The underlying mechanism responsible for glomerulopathy varies depending on its cause.

8.2.6.1. Mechanisms of Disease

The major pathological mechanisms can be divided into immune-mediated and non-immune mediated:

- **Immune-mediated:** deposition or *in situ* formation of immune complexes (collections of antibodies) that fix complement and activate a pro-inflammatory response. Alternatively, circulating antibodies may directly target key proteins on the basement membrane or endothelial cells precipitating an inflammatory reaction (e.g., ANCA-associated vasculitis).
- **Non-Immune Mediated:** the structure and/or function of podocytes may be affected that disrupts the filtration barrier (e.g., minimal change disease). This leads to larger macromolecules leaking through glomeruli. Alternatively, accumulation of non-immune material (e.g., proteins) can disrupt the glomeruli structure causing dysfunction (e.g., diabetes mellitus, amyloid).

8.2.6.2. Histopathological Changes

Every kind of glomerular injury frequently results in a distinct histological disease pattern that is visible under a microscope. A particular clinical presentation is frequently linked to these histological alterations.

The three major histological patterns include:

- **Proliferative:** increase in the number of cells in the glomerulus. May be located within the mesangium, capillary wall or outside the capillaries in Bowan's space. Typically associated with a marked inflammatory response due to deposition of immune complexes or antibody-binding. Causes glomerular inflammation with hematuria and/or nephritic syndrome.
- **Non-Proliferative (Structural):** glomerular damage characterized by structural changes and often sclerosis (scarring of the glomeruli). May show diffuse scarring or only subtle changes under the electron microscope. Typically associated with excess protein loss and nephrotic syndrome.
- **Crescents:** extra capillary lesions in Bowan's capsule due to accumulation of immune cells, fibroblasts, epithelial cells and fibrin. Crescents represent severe injury to the capillary wall that results in glomerular membrane rupture. Can be observed in any cause of inflammatory glomerular disease, but widespread crescents are typically seen in rapidly progressive glomerulonephritis (see Figure 8.6) (Radhakrishnan, 2021).

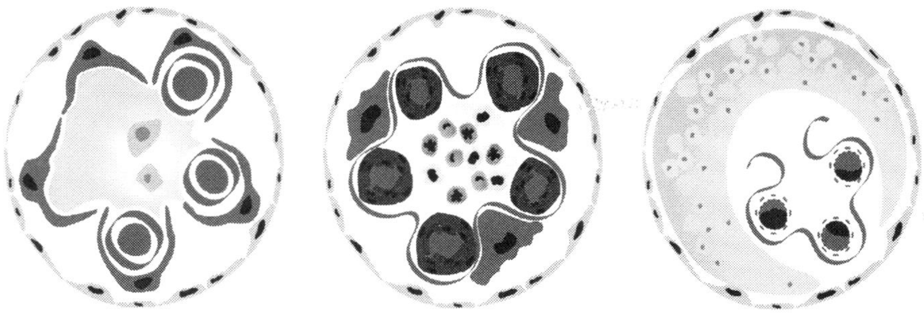

Figure 8.6. *Histopathology glomerular disease.*

Source: https://d1z8zkw1yi6kd7.cloudfront.net/uploads/ckeditor/pictures/data/000/002/608//content/histopathology_glomerular_disease.jpg.

Glomerular injury can be caused by a wide range of conditions. Glomerular disease has a variety of causes, which can be broadly categorized by the severity of renal impairment, presence of systemic features, and clinical presentation. These groups include:

- Isolated hematuria
- Isolated proteinuria
- Nephrotic syndrome
- Nephritic syndrome (i.e., glomerulonephritis)
- Rapidly progressive glomerulonephritis (RPGN)

Crucially, not every condition fits neatly into one of these groups. This is due to the fact that certain conditions can manifest in multiple ways (e.g., IgA nephropathy may result in nephritic syndrome, isolated hematuria, or infrequently, nephrotic syndrome.

8.2.7. Isolated Hematuria

Blood in the urine, which can be visible or invisible, is referred to as hematuria. Persistent hematuria without proteinuria and normal renal function is referred to as isolated hematuria. To ascertain whether hematuria is persistent, this needs to be reevaluated every one to four weeks.

Typical causes include:

- IgA nephropathy
- Alport syndrome
- Thin basement membrane disease: diffuse thinning of the basement membrane on electron microscopy. May be familial in up to 50% of cases

Crucially, blood can originate from any part of the urinary tract. Therefore, before confirming isolated hematuria, it's crucial to rule out other causes (e.g., MRI and cystoscopy. Features that are suggestive of blood from glomerular origin include:

- Dysmorphic red blood cells: red cell structure appears abnormal under the microscope
- Red blood cell casts: identification of red blood cells within urinary casts seen under the microscope. A cast is a microscopic cluster of particles wrapped in uromodulin (Tamm-Horsfall protein). Uromodulin is secreted by epithelial cells lining the loop of Henle, distal tubule & collecting duct.

8.2.8. Isolated Proteinuria

The term "proteinuria" describes the presence of protein in the urine, which can be overflowing (i.e., glomerular) or tubular. Either post-renal in origin (myeloma). Persistent proteinuria without any other urinary abnormalities is commonly referred to as isolated proteinuria e.g., hematuria, in conjunction with co-morbid conditions (diabetes and hypertension), and when renal function is normal.

The range of non-nephrotic proteinuria a 24-hour urine collection, a urine dipstick, or a spot urine protein: creatinine ratio can be used to detect levels below 3.5 g/day. A systemic disorder that requires more investigation or an underlying renal disease is typically indicated by persistent isolated non-nephrotic range proteinuria.

It is important to exclude more benign causes of proteinuria including:

- Transient proteinuria: common in young individuals. Absent on repeat testing and exercise is a common precipitant.
- Orthostatic proteinuria: the presence of proteinuria only in the upright position

8.2.9. Nephrotic Syndrome

The trio of heavy (nephrotic range) proteinuria > 3.5 g/day, hypoalbuminemia (< 35 g/L), and peripheral edema is commonly referred to as nephrotic syndrome. Hyperlipidemia and thrombotic disease (venous and arterial blood clots) may also coexist with the condition.

Patients experiencing severe fluid overload may experience pleural effusions and ascites. While it can happen, acute kidney injury is less common than glomerulonephritis. Nephrotic syndrome can be attributed to two main categories of disorders: primary renal disorders and secondary systemic conditions.

- Primary: minimal change disease, focal segmental glomerulosclerosis (FSGS), membranous nephropathy.
- Secondary: diabetes mellitus, amyloidosis, systemic lupus erythematosus, HIV infection

8.2.10. Nephritic Syndrome (i.e., Glomerulonephritis)

The traditional definition of the nephritic syndrome includes the following symptoms: hematuria, variable proteinuria (which can be a nephrotic range), oliguria (i.e., severe renal damage) and high blood pressure. When referring to inflammation within the glomeruli, the terms "nephritis" and "glomerulonephritis" are frequently used interchangeably.

Glomerulonephritis has quite a variable clinical presentation.

- Mild: presentation with minimal hematuria and proteinuria only
- Severe: typically presents with the classical 'nephritic syndrome'
- Self-limiting: development of an acute glomerulonephritis that gets better without treatment
- RPGN: severe glomerulonephritis that has a fulminant course with rapid deterioration in renal function over days to weeks to a few months.
- Chronic: slowly progressive renal disease presenting with features of CKD

There are three major causes of nephritic syndrome:

- Immune complex deposition: Poststreptococcal glomerulonephritis, autoimmune (e.g., lupus), IgA nephropathy
- Anti-GBM deposition: anti-glomerular basement membrane disease
- Small-vessel vasculitis: eosinophilic granulomatosis with polyangiitis, microscopic polyangiitis, polyangiitis with granulomatosis

8.2.11. Diagnosis & Investigations

Renal biopsy is the main test for a suspected glomerular disease. The pattern and clinical manifestation of renal injury (i.e., versus nephrotic), as well as serological indicators (e.g., specific antibodies) can all be utilized in conjunction with the findings of a renal biopsy to assist in determining the underlying diagnosis.

- **Urinary Tests:** Basic urinary tests are important to provide objective measurement of blood and/or protein in the urine
  - **Urine Dipstick:** most sensitive for detection of albumin
  - **Urinary Protein:** creatine ratio: a spot sample is collected to determine the protein content (level of protein divided by level of creatinine). Normal is < 30 mg/mmol
  - **24-hour Urinary Collection:** urine is collected over 24 hours to determine the protein content. Normal is < 0.2 g
- **Blood Tests:** A series of basic blood tests are required in any patient with suspected glomerular disease.
  - Full blood count
  - Urea & electrolytes
  - Bone profile
  - HbA1c
  - Blood gas
  - Lipid profile: hyperlipidemia seen in nephrotic syndrome
- **Renal Screen:** This is a reference to a battery of specialized blood tests meant to investigate the potential etiology of glomerular disease and acute renal impairment.

It is a comprehensive screen that can identify particular glomerular disease causes or, at the very least, offer crucial hints about a potential underlying cause.

  - Complement: typically low in vasculitis
  - Anti-nuclear antibody (ANA)
  - Anti-neutrophil cytoplasmic antibody (ANCA)
  - Anti-glomerular basement membrane antibody (GBM)
  - Anti-dsDNA: raised in systemic lupus erythematosus
  - Myeloma screen: serum-free light chains, protein electrophoresis
  - Anti-PLA2R autoantibody: raised in membranous nephropathy
  - Virology: Hepatitis B, Hepatitis C and Human immunodeficiency virus
  - Cryoglobulins: immunoglobulins that precipitate at low temperatures
  - Creatine kinase: may be raised in rhabdomyolysis

- **Imaging:** When diagnosing acute kidney injury and chronic kidney disease, imaging with a renal ultrasound or CT kidney, urinary, and bladder (CT KUB) is crucial for ruling out obstructive pathologies and evaluating the general anatomy of the kidneys (e.g., any polycystic features).
- **Renal Biopsy:** The primary test used to diagnose glomerular disease is a renal biopsy. The procedure entails obtaining a renal tissue sample via percutaneous biopsy guided by ultrasound. After that, the kidney tissue can be examined under a microscope to see the glomeruli and check for common disease patterns. Special stains can then be applied. The clinical history and these patterns worked together to support the diagnosis.

Sometimes a biopsy is not possible due to a strict or loose contraindication, or the diagnosis is safe based on the available clinical data (e.g., serological diagnosis) or there is a stereotypical presentation (e.g., pediatric nephrotic syndrome—probably a minimal change illness).

8.2.12. Management

The underlying cause of glomerular disease should be the focus of management. The underlying cause determines how any glomerular disease is managed, which is why a formal diagnosis is crucial.

The management of individual conditions is beyond the scope of these notes, but we should consider some key management principles for all glomerular diseases that includes:

- **Regular Monitoring:** rapid changes in renal function can occur with the development of complications
- **Treat Underlying Cause:** specific therapies may be available for some conditions. For example, corticosteroids are used in minimal change disease and potent immunosuppressive drugs may be utilized in ANCA-associated vasculitis
- **Determine Natural History:** for example, post-streptococcal glomerulonephropathy has a good

prognosis with only supportive treatment whereas anti-GBM disease is associated with rapid development of end-stage renal disease untreated

- **Treat Complications:** nephrotic syndrome is associated with hyperlipidemia and thrombotic complications that need addressing. Causes of nephritic syndrome may have extra-renal manifestations (e.g., pulmonary hemorrhage) that require urgent management.
- **Consider Renal Replacement Therapy:** early involvement of the renal physicians and/or intensive care team is vital in cases of severe AKI. It can lead to life-threatening complications including hyperkalemia, fluid overload, acidosis and uremia.

8.3. Glomerular Diseases Associated With Infection

More than two centuries have passed since the discovery of dark, scant urine during the convalescent stage of scarlet fever. The field of immune-mediated renal disease was first introduced by Clemens von Pirquet's groundbreaking theory at the turn of the 20th century, which held that the disease was caused by pathogenic antibodies rather than beneficial ones.

These days, infection-related glomerulonephritis (GN) is rare and typically linked to crippling illnesses like alcoholism, diabetes, malignant neoplasia, and acquired immunodeficiency syndrome (AIDS). Although a wide range of pathogens have been reported, streptococcus (27%) and staphylococcus (24%) account for the majority of infection-associated GN. Although other mechanisms may also occur, glomerular deposition of immune complexes containing bacterial antigens is typically the cause of GN. The upper respiratory tract (23%), skin (17%), lungs (17%), and heart valves (11.6%) are the most frequently infected sites. (Nasr, et al., 2008) (Figure 8.7).

Some Infectious Agents Associated with Renal Disease
Bacterial: *Streptococcus* (group A, *Streptococcus viridans*), *Staphylococcus (aureus, epidermidis)*, *Salmonella (typhi, paratyphi)*, *Escherichia coli*, *Leptospira*, *Treponema pallidum*, *Neisseria species*, *Mycobacterium leprae*, *Yersinia enterocolitica*, *Coxiella burnetii*, *Brucella abortus*, *Listeria monocytogenes*
Viral: Hepatitis A, B, and C; human immunodeficiency virus, varicella-zoster, parvovirus B19, cytomegalovirus, mumps, influenza, Epstein-Barr virus, coxsackievirus, and enteric cytopathic human orphan (ECHO) virus
Fungus: *Histoplasma capsulatum*, *Candida*
Protozoal: *Plasmodium* (*falciparum*, *malariae*, *vivax*, and *ovale*); *Trypanosoma*, *Toxoplasma*
Helminthic: *Schistosoma* (*mansoni*, *haematobium*), *Wuchereria bancrofti*, *Trichinella spiralis*, filaria (*Onchocerca volvulus*, *Loa loa*)

Figure 8.7. *Some infectious agents associated with renal disease.*

Source. https://www.ncbi.nlm.nih.gov/pmc/articles/PMC7151996/bin/f055-001-9780323058766.jpg.

8.3.1. Histologic Patterns and Pathogenesis

Generally speaking, mesangial proliferative GN is acute and self-limited. IgG, IgM, and C3 deposits are seen in conjunction with microscopic hematuria and non-nephrotic proteinuria. Serum complement might temporarily drop. Acute and self-limiting, diffuse proliferative GN occurs when the infection is eliminated. Electron-dense deposits are found in mesangial, subendothelial, and subepithelial locations; IgG, IgM, and C3 deposits are prominent in the mesangium and glomerular capillaries. Bacterial antigens and cryoglobulins may or may not be present in the immune complexes deposited in the glomeruli. Diffuse proliferative GN can be caused by staphylococcal infections, especially those that are resistant to methicillin. This is probably due to the presence of bacterial wall superantigens, which trigger a non-specific polyclonal immunoglobulin response that results in crescent formation and exclusive or predominant IgA deposition. Acute nephritic syndrome is the clinical manifestation. It is common to see membraneoproliferative GN (MPGN) in conjunction with persistent infections. The nephrotic syndrome typically manifests clinically as variable degrees of hypertension and microscopic hematuria. C3 deposits and immunoglobulins are present. When liver disease is present, such as when an infection with *Schistosoma mansoni* occurs, IgA may make up the majority of the immune deposits. Membranous nephropathy (MN), which manifests as nephrotic syndrome, is linked to recurrent infections. Lastly, bacterial (rarely streptococcus) or viral (particularly hepatitis B virus and human immunodeficiency virus) infections can cause vasculitis.

When clearing the infection or immune complexes is difficult, infection-related GN, especially when immune complex-associated, occurs more frequently and has a worse prognosis. These ailments include infection with the human immunodeficiency virus, infections contracted during the neonatal period (which frequently induces tolerance, as seen in the case of hepatitis B virus infection), diabetes, chronic alcoholism, and chronic liver disease.

Renal disease may also be linked to infections through non-immune complex-related mechanisms. HIV or parvovirus B19 infection can cause focal segmental glomerulosclerosis (FSGS) with glomerular collapse (collapsing glomerulopathy). Shigella or *Escherichia coli* species that produce verotoxins may be the cause of hemolytic-uremic syndrome. Chronic infections like schistosomiasis, leprosy, and tuberculosis can cause amyloidosis. Acute renal failure presenting as interstitial nephritis can be caused by a variety of bacterial (Legionella) or viral (Epstein-Barr virus) infections. Acute renal failure is caused by an infection of the interstitial capillaries and tubules, which is another hemorrhagic fever–renal failure syndrome that hantavirus can cause.

8.3.2. Bacterial Infections

8.3.2.1. Poststreptococcal Glomerulonephritis

8.3.2.1.1. Epidemiology

PSGN, or post-streptococcal glomerulonephritis, typically affects children between the ages of 2 and 14. It is more common in males (2:1). Only specific group A *Streptococcus pyogenes* nephritogenic strains have historically been linked to GN. PSGN typically follows streptococcal impetigo of M types 47, 49, 55, and 57 in the tropics and the southern United States. Nephritogenic streptococcus types 1, 2, 4, and 12 can also cause throat infections. Consumption of unpasteurized milk tainted with group C streptococcus (*Streptococcus zooepidemicus*) has been linked to at least one significant epidemic and clusters of cases more recently. In epidemics, the chance of developing nephritis can vary from 5% in cases of throat infections to up to 25% in cases of M type 49 pyoderma. Given the correlation between PSGN and HLA-DR4 and DR1, as well as the higher attack rates in siblings compared to the general population, a genetic predisposition is hypothesized. Early antibiotic treatment lowers the risk of PSGN.

PSGN is becoming less common in industrialized countries and is now more prevalent in elderly individuals, especially alcoholics, diabetics, and intravenous drug users. However, PSGN is still common in developing countries, affecting 9.3 to 9.8 cases per 100,000 population, particularly in communities with poor socioeconomic conditions. The decline in PSGN incidence is likely due to increased use of antibiotics, while fluorination of water may also help reduce the expression of virulence factors in cultures of *S. pyogenes*.

8.3.2.1.2. Pathogenesis

Nephritis-associated plasmin receptor (NAPLr), also known as glyceraldehyde-3-phosphate dehydrogenase (GAPDH), and streptococcal proteinase exotoxin B (SPEB) along with its more immunogenic precursor, zymogen, have been identified as the two nephritogenic streptococcal antigens. Renal biopsy specimens from acute PSGN have been found to contain GAPDH and SPEB, and the majority of convalescent sera have elevated antibody titers to both of these antigens. Although GAPDH is not co-localized with complement or immunoglobulin, it has been localized in glomeruli with plasmin-like activity, suggesting a local direct mechanism of glomerular inflammatory damage. Conversely, SPEB exhibits co-localization with complement and IgG, indicating its involvement in immune-mediated glomerular damage. Moreover, the most common histologic lesion of acute PSGN, subepithelial electron-dense deposits known as humps, have only been shown to harbor SPEB, the putative streptococcal nephritogenic antigen. Renal biopsy specimens from PSGN patients typically show the presence of SPEB but not GAPDH, according to studies conducted in Central Europe and Latin America. In contrast, a study involving Japanese patients found that PSGN had GAPDH. These divergent findings give rise to the intriguing hypothesis that distinct streptococcal antigens may cause acute nephritis in various ethnic populations. In fact, an analysis of the C S group. The absence of the gene linked to SPEB in the zooepidemicus strain that caused the epidemic outbreak in Brazil indicates that this antigen was not involved in that epidemic. (Beres et al., 2008) (Figure 8.8).

The pathogenesis of PSGN is believed to be the development of circulating immune complexes and antigenemia brought on by persistent streptococcal infection. These complexes primarily settle in the subendothelial and mesangial locations and set off an inflammatory cascade that includes local complement activation, neutrophil recruitment, and monocyte-macrophage recruitment. The development of subepithelial immune deposits, or humps, is caused by cationic antigens (e.g., SPEB) or immune complex dissociation in the subendothelial space with transit and re-formation on the glomerular basement membrane's exterior surface. Helper (CD4) T lymphocytes are essential for cell-mediated immunity. Additionally, cytokines are involved in localized injury and inflammation. During the acute phase of PSGN, the level of proteinuria is correlated with urinary monocyte chemoattractant protein 1.

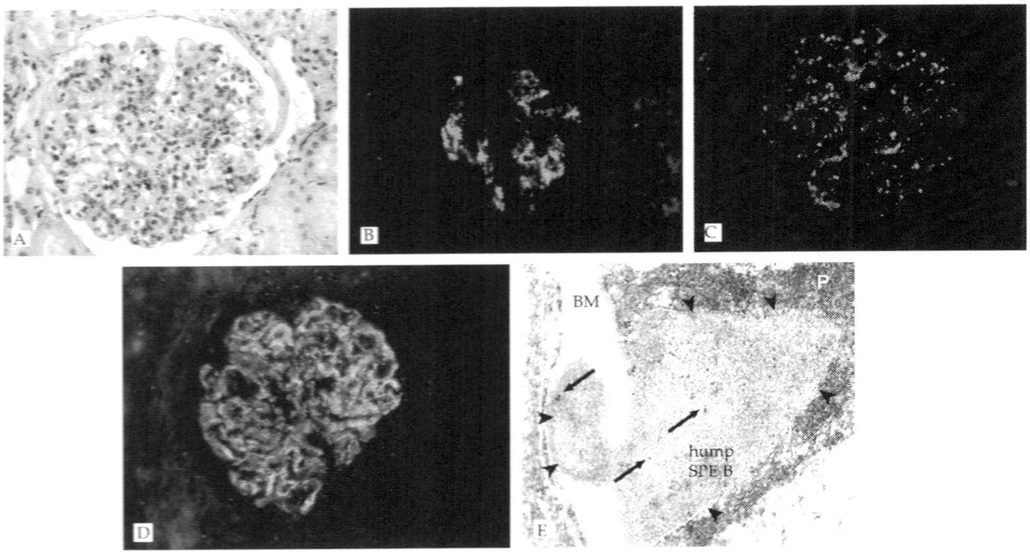

Figure 8.8. *Poststreptococcal glomerulonephritis.*

Note: A diffuse proliferative and exudative glomerulonephritis can be seen by light microscopy. B-D, Immunofluorescence showing the mesangial (B), starry sky (C), and garland (D) patterns. E, Immune electron microscopy showing the characteristic subepithelial electron-dense deposits (humps) (arrowheads), inside which streptococcal proteinase exotoxin B (SPEB) is demonstrated (arrows) (immunogold staining). BM, basement membrane; P, podocyte.

Source. Batsford SR, Mezzano S, & Mihatsch M. (2005). Is the nephritogenic antigen in poststreptococcal glomerulonephritis pyrogenic exotoxin B (SPE B) or GAPDH? Kidney Int., 68, 1120–1129.

Many problems are still unsolved. For instance, immune complex disease typically activates the classical complement pathway; however, only C3 is typically detected in the deposits, and C4 levels are typically normal. Antigens (like GAPDH) that activate the alternative pathway may be the cause of this. It has been shown that C3Nef IgG antibodies in sera can activate the alternative complement pathway in certain patients. Although it has been suggested that bacterial antigens activate the lectin complement pathway, PSGN can still occur in people who are genetically incapable of doing so.

Lastly, it's still unclear how autoimmune processes function. One-third of patients have serum levels of cryoglobulins and rheumatoid factors, particularly IgG rheumatoid factor, during the first week of the illness. An antibody to IgG known as rheumatoid factors has been detected in one-third of renal biopsy specimens and in the kidney's eluate in a fatal case. The loss of sialic acid from autologous IgG as a result of streptococcal neuraminidase (sialidase) or the binding of the IgG Fc fragment to type II Fc receptors in the streptococcal wall can both lead to anti-IgG reactivity. Anti-C1q antibodies are additional manifestations of autoimmune reactivity, especially in severe cases. Anti-DNA reactivity, antineutrophil cytoplasmic antibody (ANCA), and autoimmune hemolytic anemia are less common manifestations.

8.3.2.1.3. Pathology

A diffuse endocapillary GN with mesangial and endothelial cell proliferation is seen in the renal biopsy. Monocytes and lymphocytes are infiltrating the glomerulus and interstitial space. Neutrophil globular accumulation, or exudative GN, is a common occurrence. The mesangium and glomerular capillary loops contain glomerular immune deposits of C3 (which accounts for 100% of cases), IgG (62%), IgM (76%), properdin, and the terminal membrane attack complex C5b-C9 (which accounts for 85% of cases and is typically codeposited with C3). Sorger and Colleagaues' seminal work described three patterns of immunofluorescence in the glomeruli, along with their clinical correlates: the garland pattern formed by gross deposits in the capillary loops; the starry sky pattern formed by deposits scattered in mesangium and capillary walls; and the mesangial pattern of irregular and heavy immune deposits. The garland pattern is linked to numerous electron-dense subepithelial immune deposits and heavy proteinuria, making it clinically significant. Ultrastructural studies show the subepithelial humps, which are characteristic but not pathognomonic of PSGN because they can also be seen in cryoglobulinemia, lupus nephritis, and postinfectious GN of other causes (classically endocarditis-associated GN secondary to Staphylococcus infection).

The excess cells undergo apoptosis to end GN. Even in the absence of clinical illness, biopsy specimens obtained years later reveal varying degrees of focal glomerulosclerosis and mesangial expansion. Residual renal injury is a common occurrence. It is unknown what these changes mean clinically.

8.3.2.1.4. Clinical Manifestations

The majority of patients report having had a prior streptococcal infection, even though it was frequently healed at the time of presentation. After skin infections, the incubation period lasts for several weeks as opposed to two weeks for throat infections.

The acute nephritic syndrome is the classic presentation. In 80% of cases, hypertension is present. Ascites is extremely uncommon; edema occurs in 80–90% of cases and is the primary complaint in 60% of cases. Edema, hypertension, and increased intravascular volume are all related to primary sodium retention. Aldosterone and plasma renin activity are decreased. Hematuria is a common condition that manifests as macroscopic in 30% of cases.

20% of adults and 2% of children may develop nephrotic syndrome at some point in their lives. Less than 1% of patients experience rapidly progressing renal failure due to extracapillary crescent formation. Up to 83% of adults and 25 to 40% of children have impaired renal function.

10 to 70% of cases during epidemics and 20 to 25% of sporadic cases have positive cultures for streptococcus. More than two-thirds of patients with PSGN following throat infections have elevated antistreptolysin O (ASO) titers, and 73% of post-impetigo cases have elevated anti-DNAse B titers. More than 80% of subjects tested positive for the more sensitive streptozyme panel, which measures antibodies to four antigens: anti-DNAse B, antihyaluronidase, ASO, and antistreptokinase. Despite being more specific and sensitive, antibody titers to GAPDH and SPEB/zymogen are not commercially accessible.

In the first week of the illness, serum C3 levels drop in over 90% of patients and then return to normal in less than two months. C4, a gauge of the activation of the classical complement pathway, might be normal. 80% of the cases have elevated serum IgG and IgM, while IgA is normal, in contrast to another post-streptococcal disease called rheumatic fever. Up to one-third of patients have cryoglobulins, elevated rheumatoid factor, and anti-C1q antibodies; a small percentage of patients may have low titers of anti-DNA and ANCA.

Subclinical disease, which can be seen through microscopic hematuria and a decrease in serum complement levels, is four to five times more common than clinically obvious disease. It often affects siblings of individuals diagnosed with the illness. Occasionally, entire families show different symptoms of PSGN. Therefore, it is crucial to ask about a history of streptococcal infections and signs of nephritic syndrome among all family members.

8.3.2.1.5. Management

Renal biopsy is not usually necessary for PSGN, but it might be needed if the condition exhibits peculiar symptoms, such as nephrotic proteinuria, decreased C3 levels that have persisted for more than a month (which suggests lupus or hypocomplementemic MPGN), or progressive renal dysfunction (which suggests crescentic GN).

Treatment for any leftover streptococcal infection and culture are included in management. Prompt antibiotic administration is probably going to stop PSGN. Penicillin (1.22 million units of benzathine penicillin in adults, or half this dose in small children), orally administered phenoxymethyl or phenoxyethyl penicillin G 250 mg [adults] or 125 mg [children], every 6 hours for 7 to 10 days) is the recommended course of treatment. Alternatively, erythromycin (250 mg every 6 hours in adults and 40 mg/kg in children) is administered to individuals allergic to penicillin. Cephalosporins can be applied with comparable or even superior outcomes. In populations that are at risk during epidemics and in siblings of index cases, preventive antibiotic treatment is warranted.

Restricting sodium and fluid intake as well as treating circulatory congestion with loop diuretics are two treatments for acute nephritic syndrome. For the most part, an oral long-acting calcium antagonist is adequate to manage hypertension. Under exceptional circumstances, nitroprusside is used to treat hypertensive encephalopathy. About 25–30% of adults require dialysis, either hemodialysis or peritoneal dialysis, but children hardly ever need it.

Cerebral vasculitis, cerebral vasogenic edema, and posterior reversible leukoencephalopathy are uncommon consequences of acute PSGN. The final one can be mistaken for hypertensive encephalopathy and presents with headaches, convulsions, visual hallucinations, and mental disturbances. Studies using magnetic resonance imaging are necessary for the diagnosis.

Pulse methylprednisolone therapy may be beneficial for rare patients with crescentic GN associated with PSGN, according to anecdotal reports. If spontaneous improvement is not seen after two weeks, this therapy may be tried. Although a full recovery may be anticipated in less than half of the cases, the prognosis for crescentic PSGN is noticeably better than that of crescentic GN owing to other causes.

8.3.2.1.6. Prognosis

The majority of PSGN kids get better. Higher rates of acute complications, such as mortality (25%), congestive heart failure (40%), nephrotic proteinuria (20%), and renal impairment (60 to 70%), are seen in older subjects.

Following recovery, microscopic hematuria and mild proteinuria (<500 mg/day) may continue for up to a year without adversely affecting the prognosis in the long run. However, some subjects—especially adults—may experience persistently high blood pressure, proteinuria, or impaired renal function. However, fewer than 1% of the children seen for a period of one to two decades following the acute attack develop end-stage renal disease (ESRD).

A high incidence of chronicity has been reported in certain epidemics, possibly due to the population's predominance of adults. Older age and the co-existence of diabetic nephropathy are risk factors for the development of chronic kidney disease. Nephrotic-range proteinuria is one such risk factor. Additionally, some groups—like the Australian aborigines—have a poorer prognosis in the long run.

8.3.2.2. Endocarditis-Associated Glomerulonephritis

According to population-based surveys, the incidence of community-acquired native valve endocarditis in the United States and Western Europe is 1.7 to 6.2 cases per 100,000 person-years, and it has not changed over the past three decades. Every year, 15,000 new cases of infective endocarditis are reported in the US. The bacteria that cause infections most frequently are *Streptococcus viridans*, *S. aureus*, and *Staphylococcus epidermidis*. *Enterococcus faecalis*, *E. pyogenes*, and less frequently *E. coli*, Proteus, and bacteria from the species Candida and Bartonella. The reduction in the percentage of cases linked to rheumatic heart disease and the rise in cases linked to health care are the two most notable changes in epidemiology that have been noticed. Chronic hemodialysis patients are the most significant subgroup, with an incidence 20–60 times higher than the general population. Synthetic grafts and long-term venous dialysis catheter use are major risk factors in this population. Impaired renal function affects one-third of patients with bacterial endocarditis, and the risk rises with age, history of hypertension, thrombocytopenia, and prosthetic valve infection.

GN was found in 26% of the 62 patients with infective endocarditis in a recent survey where renal tissue was available for analysis. Many of these cases were pauci-immune renal vasculitis. Additional pathologic alterations included 10% of interstitial nephritis, which was primarily caused by antibiotics, and localized infarcts (31%), of which 50% were septic. In 10% of the cases, cortical necrosis was discovered.

Diffuse proliferative GN is the most prevalent pathologic alteration of the glomerulus. Spocular GN, MN, and MPGN type I are less common. About half of the proliferative GN forms have crescent formation. Typically, there is widespread IgM, IgG, and C3 deposition as well as electron-dense subendothelial, mesangial, and subepithelial deposits that resemble poststreptococcal humps. Mesangial immune deposits and focal segmental proliferative lesions with fibrinoid necrosis or capillary thrombi may be seen in subacute endocarditis. Variable degrees of atrophy and fibrosis as well as tubulointerstitial cellular infiltration may be observed. A different diagnosis, such as acute interstitial nephritis brought on by antibiotics, should be considered in case of intense eosinophilic infiltration.

Immune complexes containing bacterial antigens are deposited in glomeruli during the pathogenesis of endocarditis-associated GN; this mechanism is similar to that suggested for PSGN. 50% of subjects have cryoglobulins (polyclonal or type III type), which can be found in glomeruli. Certain microorganisms (typically methicillin-resistant S. aureus) produce superantigens that can directly activate T cells, resulting in the development of immune complex GN and polyclonal gammopathy.

8.3.2.2.1. Clinical Manifestations and Diagnosis

Patients frequently arrive with purpura, anemia, arthralgias, and fever. Rarely, infectious endocarditis can occur as a primary renal disease without exhibiting typical systemic symptoms. Seldom are classic endocarditis findings like splinter hemorrhages, Janeway lesions, and Osler's nodes observed. The typical renal manifestations include microscopic hematuria, mild proteinuria (except membranous GN, which can cause nephrotic range proteinuria), and mild impairment of renal function (except renal vasculitis, which frequently results in renal failure). Nephrotic syndrome or a fast-moving clinical course are uncommon. Reduced C3 and C4 levels (corresponding with activation of the classical complement pathway), high titers of rheumatoid factor, circulating immune complexes, and type III cryoglobulins are examples of abnormal serologic test results. Although complement levels may be normal in superantigen-mediated GN, these serologic findings are seen in a greater percentage of patients with endocarditis-associated GN and in 50% of subjects with subacute bacterial endocarditis. Rare cases of GN and subacute endocarditis have been linked to cytoplasmic ANCA.

Embolism, interstitial nephritis, and antibiotic-associated nephrotoxicity are among the differential diagnoses. If the foramen ovale is patent, embolism may come from the right or left side of the heart. Small or large emboli can block small or large vessels; fungal or hemophilus endocarditis has been linked to the latter. Large emboli can cause hematuria, pyuria, and flank pain; microemboli cause microabscesses and localized infarcts that give the kidney the traditional "flea-bitten" look. Frequent symptoms of interstitial nephritis include fever, eosinophilia, and eosinophiluria. Regretfully, fever can also be a symptom of endocarditis-associated GN, and eosinophiluria can exacerbate crescentic nephritis of any cause.

Treatment with antibiotics for 4 to 6 weeks typically eliminates endocarditis and corrects abnormal serologic levels, but some kidney issues like hematuria, proteinuria, and elevated serum creatinine may persist for months. Improvement in C3 levels during treatment is associated with a positive outcome. In cases of crescentic glomerulonephritis, corticosteroid therapy and plasma exchange may be considered alongside antibiotics, though their effectiveness is uncertain. The mortality rate for bacterial endocarditis is 20%, rising to 36% in patients who experience renal failure.

8.3.2.3. Staphylococcal Infections with Glomerular IgA Deposition

In 1995, Koyama and colleagues identified a new severe form of glomerulonephritis linked to methicillin-resistant staphylococcal infections. This condition was characterized by kidney damage, high levels of protein in the urine, and varying degrees of crescent formation. Patients exhibited IgA dominant or codominant deposits along with other immunoglobulins and complement deposits, with increased levels of serum IgA and specific T-cell receptor Vβ + subsets observed. The researchers suggested that staphylococcal superantigens played a role in the development of the disease. The prevalence of this condition is uncertain, but it accounts for 1.6% of kidney biopsies in one medical facility. (Satoskar et al., 2006) (Figure 8.9).

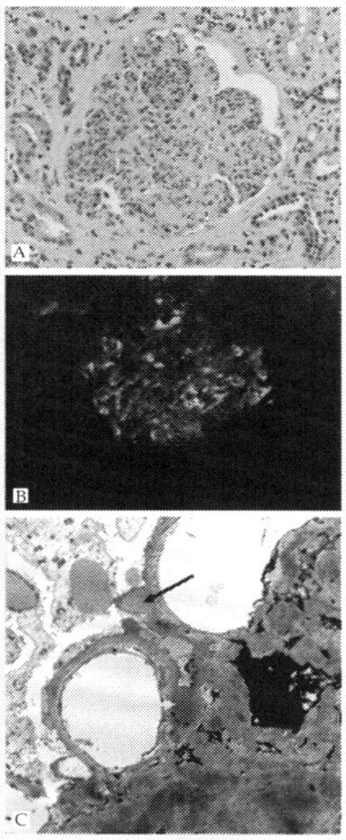

Figure 8.9. *Glomerulonephritis in a diabetic subject with methicillin-sensitive S. aureus infection.*

Note: A diffuse exudative GN is present with neutrophil infiltration. B, Immunofluorescence shows IgA-dominant mesangial deposits. C, Electron microscopy shows domeshaped subepithelial deposits (black arrow) and mesangial deposits (yellow arrow).

Source: https://www.ncbi.nlm.nih.gov/pmc/articles/PMC7151996/bin/f055-004c-9780323058766.jpg.

8.3.2.3.1. Clinical and Pathologic Characteristics

The first cases primarily showed severe glomerulonephritis with acute kidney injury, high levels of protein in the urine, and blood in the urine. However, the condition can also have a less severe clinical presentation. While many cases are linked to infections from methicillin-resistant Staphylococcus bacteria, they can also arise from infections with methicillin-sensitive bacteria. Diabetic glomerulosclerosis is often present alongside this condition. Complement levels may be either low or within the normal range.

Mesangial and intracapillary hypercellularity, either with or without crescent formation, are seen in varying degrees in renal biopsies. Tubular atrophy and interstitial fibrosis can be mild or severe. Electron microscopy reveals electron-dense deposits in subendothelial regions and the mesangium of the glomerular basement membrane. Some series report large subepithelial electron-dense deposits. IgA deposition can be dominant or codominant with other Ig deposits, and it can be mild, moderate, or intense. Deposits of C3 are typically found.

8.3.2.3.2. Pathogenesis

The exact cause of IgA glomerulonephritis related to staphylococcal infection is not fully understood. Koyama and his colleagues have suggested that staphylococcal superantigens may directly bind to antigen-presenting cellular major histocompatibility complex class II molecules, leading to the activation of T cells via the Vβ T-cell receptor region. This results in intense T cell activation and cytokine production, which in turn stimulates B cells to produce both IgG and IgA antibodies. They have also found that a cell envelope antigen from *Staphylococcus aureus* is localized in the same area as the IgA deposits in the glomeruli. Further research is needed to determine if staphylococcus antigens play a role in the development of IgA nephropathy.

8.3.2.3.3. Differential Diagnosis and Treatment

Treatment with antibiotics is recommended for GN related to IgA-dominant staphylococcus because renal function may recover. Since corticosteroid therapy is contraindicated, it is crucial to differentiate it from IgA nephropathy, for which corticosteroids may be necessary in severe cases. The association with a staphylococcal infection (as opposed to upper respiratory infection in IgA nephropathy), the frequent occurrence of massive proteinuria (which is uncommon in IgA nephropathy), and the acute renal failure (which is uncommon in IgA nephropathy) are clinical characteristics that may be useful in the differential diagnosis.

8.3.2.3.4. Shunt Nephritis

About 30% of cases with atrioventricular shunts may result in an infection. 0–7% to 2% of patients with infected atrioventricular shunts may develop GN; this can happen two months to several years after implantation. Usually, S are the infectious organisms. *S. epidermidis* and *S. aureus*, and less commonly Serratia, Phtheroids, Pseudomonas, or *Propionibacterium acnes*. Ventriculoperitoneal shunts, in contrast to atrioventricular shunts, are rarely complicated by GN.

Symptoms of patients include a slow onset of mild fever, joint pain, weight loss, anemia, skin rash, enlarged liver and spleen, high blood pressure, and signs of pressure in the brain. Nearly all patients have trace amounts of blood in their urine, and protein levels are often very high, indicating kidney problems. Blood tests show positive results for rheumatoid factor, cryoglobulinemia, and low levels of certain proteins. Elevated levels of c-ANCA may also be present.

Nearly 60% of cases with renal histology show MPGN type I, and the remaining cases show non-IgA mesangial proliferative GN. There are deposits of IgM, IgG, and C3 in the mesangium and glomerular capillary.

Antibiotic therapy and the quick removal of the infected atrioventricular shunt—which is typically replaced by a ventriculoperitoneal shunt—are necessary for treatment. The prognosis for the renal lesion deteriorates with time following the diagnosis and shunt removal. If dialysis is necessary, hemodialysis is the recommended method since patients with a ventriculoperitoneal shunt are at risk of meningitis from peritonitis that complicates chronic peritoneal dialysis. Over half of the patients experience full recovery; of these, 22% have persistent urinary abnormalities and 6% have end-stage renal disease (ESRD).

8.3.2.3.5. Glomerulonephritis Associated with Other Bacterial Infections

Glomerulonephritis (GN) is often associated with osteomyelitis and abscesses in various areas of the body such as the abdomen, pelvis, pleura, and teeth. Infections can go undiagnosed for months before symptoms appear. Renal disease can range from mild urinary issues to rapidly progressive GN, with nephrotic syndrome being the most common presentation. Unlike other infection-related GN, complement levels are typically normal in these cases. Renal tissue samples may show membranoproliferative GN, diffuse proliferative GN, or mesangial proliferative GN, with possible presence of crescents. Early antibiotic treatment can lead to recovery of renal function.

GN may be linked to both congenital and secondary (or early latent) syphilis. Patients with congenital syphilis typically exhibit anasarca 4–12 weeks postpartum. 8% of patients have nephrotic syndrome, which may be the main clinical symptom (as opposed to the more traditional triad of rhinitis, osteochondritis, and rash). Renal involvement affects 0.3% of patients with acquired syphilis. Adults sometimes exhibit an acute nephritic picture or the nephrotic syndrome.

The results of the rapid plasmin reagin, VDRL, and fluorescent treponemal antibody absorption test serologic tests for syphilis are positive.

Although diffuse proliferative GN with or without crescents, mesangial proliferative GN, and MPGN have also been observed, MN remains the most common renal pathologic process. It has been determined that the immune deposits contain treponemal antigens. Antibiotic therapy is effective in treating syphilitic GN, though remission might take 4 to 18 months.

Acute typhoid fever caused by Salmonella typhi is identified by symptoms such as fever, splenomegaly, and gastrointestinal issues. In severe cases, shock and acute renal failure may develop due to conditions like disseminated intravascular coagulation or hemolytic-uremic syndrome, although these occurrences are rare.

About 2% of cases may involve overt mesangial proliferative GN, while around 25% may exhibit mild proteinuria and microscopic hematuria. Diagnosis typically involves identifying the organism through blood or stool cultures or through rising antibody levels in the Widal test. In some cases, GN may also be seen in individuals with schistosomiasis and a coexisting Salmonella infection of the urinary tract (Chugh, 1990) (Figure 8.10).

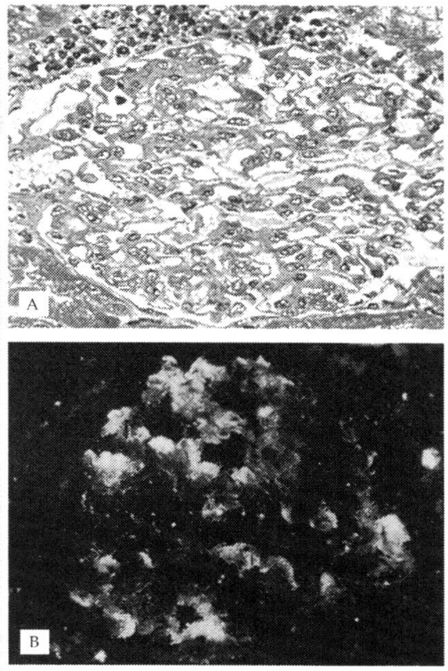

Figure 8.10. *Glomerulonephritis in typhoid fever.*

Note: A, Mesangial proliferative GN. B, Immunofluorescent staining demonstrates granular deposition of Salmonella typhi Vi antigens in the mesangium.

Source. https://www.ncbi.nlm.nih.gov/pmc/articles/PMC7151996/bin/f055-005b-9780323058766.jpg.

Autopsy studies have shown that leprosy, caused by *Mycobacterium leprae* infection, can be linked to various renal complications such as glomerulonephritis (5% to 14% of cases), interstitial nephritis (4% to 54%), and amyloidosis (4% to 31%). Clinical manifestations of glomerulonephritis are rare, affecting less than 2% of patients, and there is debate about whether it is more common in lepromatous leprosy compared to tuberculoid leprosy. Urinary abnormalities consistent with glomerulonephritis often occur during episodes of erythema nodosum leprosum. Nephrotic syndrome is the most common presentation, followed by acute nephritic syndrome and rarely rapidly progressive glomerulonephritis. Biopsy results may show MPGN or diffuse proliferative glomerulonephritis with various deposits. Treatment response for renal complications in leprosy is variable, with prednisolone (40 to 50 mg/day) being used in short courses for erythema nodosum leprosum associated with glomerulonephritis. Amyloidosis with nephrotic syndrome is another rare complication, particularly in lepromatous leprosy, along with interstitial nephritis.

Rarely, especially if treatment is postponed, microhematuria and proteinuria may be linked to pneumococcal pneumonia. There have been reports of diffuse proliferative GN as well as mesangial proliferative GN, and the immune deposits contain pneumococcal antigens. Pneumococcal neuraminidase obscures the Thomsen-Friedenreich antigen in glomeruli, allowing preformed antibodies to attach and trigger an immune response. This is the rare way in which pneumococcal pneumonia can also be linked to hemolytic-uremic syndrome.

Campylobacter jejuni-induced gastroenteritis has been linked to diffuse proliferative or mesangioproliferative GN. Other bacterial infections, including those caused by *E. coli* can also result in, Meningococcus, Yersinia, and Mycoplasma pneumoniae.

8.3.3. Viral Infections

Interstitial nephritis (HANTAV, influenza virus, dengue, BK virus, coronavirus, cytomegalovirus, hepatitis A virus) and chronic GN (hepatitis B virus [HBV], hepatitis C virus [HCV], human immunodeficiency virus [HIV], parvovirus B19) are among the conditions that can result from viral infections. The most prevalent infections are linked to HIV, HBV, and HCV. The formation of autoantibodies against endogenous antigens altered by viral damage, the deposition or in situ formation of exogenous (viral) immune complexes, the release of proinflammatory cytokines, chemokines, adhesion molecules, and growth factors by the virus, and the direct cytopathic effects of viral proteins are some of the pathogenetic mechanisms.

8.3.3.1. Hepatitis A Virus–Associated Renal Disease

Severe hepatitis A virus infection can lead to renal failure, which may be caused by interstitial nephritis or acute tubular necrosis. In rare cases, immune complex-related diffuse proliferative glomerulonephritis with immunoglobulin and C3 deposits can develop, presenting as nephritic or nephrotic syndrome with impaired renal function. Typically, recovery from glomerulonephritis occurs as hepatitis improves.

8.3.3.2. Hepatitis B Virus–Associated Renal Disease

The only known natural host of the DNA virus HBV, which belongs to the Hepadnaviridae family, is the human. Immune response against hepatocytes that are infected causes hepatitis.

Symptoms of acute HBV infection can include nausea, vomiting, fever, enlarged liver, and a short-term serum sickness-like syndrome with symptoms such as rash, neuropathy, joint pain, and urinary issues. A renal biopsy may reveal mesangial proliferative glomerulonephritis. The clinical presentation typically improves on its own as the hepatitis resolves.

While acute HBV infection may go away without any problems, chronic infection (defined as persistence of HBsAg-positive serology but negative for IgM antibodies to HBV core antigen) affects over 90% of infected infants, 25% to 50% of children infected between the ages of 1 and 5 years, and 6% to 10% of older children and adults. Maternal-infant transmission at birth, or vertical transmission, is typically found in endemic regions like Southeast Asia and China. Direct contact with mucous membranes or blood contamination are the two ways that horizontal transmission happens. The infection is more commonly acquired by carriers as adults or adolescents through horizontal transmission following drug abuse, blood transfusions, or sexual interactions; the prevalence is higher in Europe and the US. HBV carriers may present with a variety of renal syndromes.

8.3.3.2.1. HBV-Associated Membranous Nephropathy

Membranous nephropathy (MN) can be found in individuals with chronic HBV infection. In children, there is a higher prevalence in males and they often exhibit asymptomatic proteinuria or nephrotic syndrome, along with microscopic hematuria and normal kidney function. Their liver disease is usually minimal and the prognosis is typically positive, with spontaneous remission often occurring when anti-HBe antibodies are detected in the blood. On the other hand, adults with MN may have impaired kidney function, and evident liver disease, and are at a higher risk of progressing to renal failure. C3 and C4 levels are decreased in a significant percentage of cases. MN is confirmed via biopsy, which may show mesangial immune deposits in addition to the typical MN features. Virus-like particles have been observed in the glomeruli, and HBeAg can be detected in the immune deposits using immunohistochemistry.

8.3.3.2.2. HBV-Associated Membranoproliferative Glomerulonephritis

The most prevalent glomerular lesion among adult HBV carriers is MPGN. There may be cryoglobulinemia, particularly if there is an HCV infection going on at the same time. Even though chronic liver disease is typically present, it may not show any symptoms at all. Proteinuria, whether nephrotic or non-nephrotic, is frequently accompanied by microhematuria. Typical type I MPGN is seen in the biopsy, and immune deposits occasionally contain HBsAg.

8.3.3.2.3. Mesangial Proliferative Glomerulonephritis with IgA Deposits

A renal lesion that resembles IgA nephropathy in cases of HBV infection has been reported multiple times. This could be the result of hepatic IgA nephropathy brought on by chronic liver disease with decreased clearance of IgA circulating immune complexes.

8.3.3.2.4. Treatment of HBV-Associated Glomerulonephritis

The goal of treatment is to eradicate the HBV virus. Pegylated interferon alfa or interferon alfa at a dose of 5 million units per day for six months may induce remission, particularly in MN linked to HBV. In HBV-associated MN, lamivudine (100 mg taken orally once a day for 52 weeks) has also been shown to eradicate the HBV virus and cause remission. When the glomerular filtration rate (GFR) falls below 50 ml/min per 1.73 m^2, a dose reduction is required. The initial dose is 100 mg, and if the GFR is 30 to 49 ml/min per 1.73 m^2, this is followed by 50 mg taken orally every day; if the GFR is 15 to 29 ml/min per 1.73 m^2, the initial dose is the same, and subsequent doses are decreased to 25 mg daily. The starting dose for ESRD patients is 35 mg, and then there is a daily 10 mg dose. With continued use, strains resistant to lambivudine may develop. An alternative may be offered by entecavir and adefovir dipivoxil, but adefovir's nephrotoxicity is a turnoff, even though the risk is minimal at standard dosage if renal function is normal. Because corticosteroid treatment is ineffective, it may speed up the progression of liver disease and delay or prevent seroconversion. Therefore, it is contraindicated.

The general consensus has been that since most children with HBV-associated MN experience spontaneous remission, treatment is not necessary. In controlled studies, however, approximately half of the children had clearance of HBV DNA and HBeAg, and the treated group had a higher incidence of proteinuria resolution. It is reasonable to treat when proteinuria is severe or renal disease progresses because HBV-associated MN in children rarely progresses to ESRD.

As evidenced by the 10-fold decrease in incidence in Taiwan and the 67% reduction in the United States 10 years after universal vaccination was enacted in 1991, active immunization is the most effective preventive measure.

8.3.3.2.5. Polyarteritis Nodosa

HBV-related vasculitis, also known as HBV-related polyarteritis nodosa [PAN], is a rare condition that primarily affects adult men who use drugs or receive blood transfusions and who become infected with HBV less than a year after a mild hepatitis attack. In regions of the world where HBV infection is contracted at birth or during childhood, like Asia, it is uncommon and hardly ever seen in children. Unlike HBV-associated serum sickness, which goes away on its own when the HBsAg is cleared, the typical patient with HBV-related PAN exhibits signs of serum sickness both before and during a mild or asymptomatic attack of hepatitis. The disease advances in these patients to the point where it affects multiple organs. Medium-sized arteries are usually involved, and it can manifest in many ways, such as cerebral ischemia, mesenteric angina, myocardial ischemia, and mononeuritis multiplex. Microhematuria, nephrotic or non-nephrotic proteinuria, and renin-dependent hypertension are signs of renal vasculitis. While pulmonary and cutaneous manifestations are uncommon, patients with HBV-associated PAN more commonly have orchitis and gastrointestinal and renal vessel involvement. Overall, symptoms are similar to those seen in noninfectious PAN. In HBV-related PAN, rapidly progressing GN, as observed in microscopic polyangiitis, is rare.

The pathophysiology of PAN linked to HBV is believed to be the deposition of immune complexes HBsAg-antiHBs in the arterial wall, which triggers an inflammatory response and complement activation. IgM and HBsAg are frequently predominant in the vessels, indicating that HBsAg-IgM complexes are mediating the injury. Antibodies against HBc and HBsAg are detected by serologic tests. ANCA are not present, and serum complement is typically normal.

The identification of circulating HBsAg in conjunction with biopsy or angiographic evidence of vasculitis is necessary for the diagnosis. Vascular lesions, which are usually panmural and vary in stage of development, are shown by biopsy studies. Leukocyte infiltration, fibrin deposition, and fibrinoid necrosis are all present in varying degrees. The vessel wall is where HBsAg, IgM, and occasionally IgG are deposited. Compared to biopsies, angiographic studies that show saccular or fusiform aneurysms as well as narrow segments in the renal or celiac arteries have a higher diagnostic yield.

A liver biopsy may reveal acute hepatitis in rare cases or chronic active or persistent hepatitis. Along with the arteriolar lesions, the renal biopsy may reveal largely intact glomeruli in the glomerular tuft, with varying degrees of collapse most likely due to ischemic changes. Necrotizing lesions with crescent formation are uncommon in idiopathic microscopic polyangiitis. There have been reports of diffuse proliferative GN, MPGN, MN, and mesangial proliferative GN.

Interferon alfa therapy or lamivudine are administered after a brief course of corticosteroids (prednisone 1 mg/kg per day for 2 weeks) and plasma exchange (9 to 12 exchanges over 3 weeks).

8.3.3.3. Hepatitis C Virus–Associated Renal Disease

The RNA virus known as HCV, which belongs to the Flaviviridae family, is frequently responsible for hepatoma, cirrhosis, and chronic hepatitis. Numerous forms of glomerular disease can also be linked to the development of chronic HCV infection. MPGN, with or without cryoglobulinemia, is the most prevalent. MN may also be linked to HCV, particularly in individuals who have had renal transplants. Except the presence of HCV RNA and anti-HCV antibodies in the blood, the clinical and histologic findings are comparable to those seen in idiopathic MN. Additional correlations that have been reported include thrombotic microangiopathy with anticardiolipin antibodies, focal glomerulosclerosis (particularly in African Americans), and fibrillary GN (particularly following renal transplantation).

8.3.3.4. Human Immunodeficiency Virus–Associated Renal Disease

HIV infection is linked to a variety of renal complications, the most prevalent of which is HIV-associated nephropathy. HIV infection is associated with human immunodeficiency virus-associated renal disease.

8.3.3.5. Other Virus-Associated Renal Disease

Reduced renal function may result from polyomavirus nephropathy caused by the BK virus, which is becoming more widely recognized in the context of renal transplantation.

Renal transplant recipients are frequently affected by cytomegalovirus (CMV) infection. In these patients, the virus can infect tubular cells and macrophages in the interstitium, leading to the characteristic intracytoplasmic "owl-like" inclusions. There is no proof that this causes glomerular injury, but there is some evidence that it might be the cause of tubular dysfunction. On rare occasions, nontransplant subjects have experienced a diffuse proliferative GN with immune deposits containing CMV antigens due to CMV. Furthermore, in individuals who are not HIV-positive, a rare report has connected CMV infection to collapsing glomerulopathy and end-stage renal disease.

Parvovirus B19 is a single-stranded DNA virus that has a strong preference for erythroid precursor cells. In certain conditions where there is an increase in the destruction or decrease in the production of red blood cells, infection with parvovirus may lead to aplastic anemia, such as in cases of renal transplantation and sickle cell disease. In individuals with sickle cell disease, parvovirus-induced aplastic crises can sometimes be followed by nephritic or nephrotic syndrome, which is believed to be caused by immune complex deposition. Various kidney conditions, including diffuse proliferative GN, MPGN, and collapsing focal glomerulosclerosis (similar to those seen in heroin- and HIV-associated nephropathy), have been linked to parvovirus B19 infection. Some studies have found viral DNA in kidney biopsy samples, along with the presence of C3 and IgG in capillary walls and subendothelial deposits. Additionally, there is evidence suggesting a connection between renal parvovirus infection and chronic allograft nephropathy.

Acute interstitial nephritis and hemorrhagic fever are caused by the hantavirus. Acute renal failure is the presenting symptom in severe cases, which are more common in endemic areas. Fever, hepatitis, and mild renal dysfunction are symptoms of milder forms. If severe acute respiratory distress syndrome (SARS) is present, it is likely linked to multiorgan failure; acute renal failure itself may result in tubulointerstitial nephritis.

Varicella, mumps, adenovirus, coxsackievirus, influenza, and diffuse proliferative GN, in which viral antigens are detected in the mesangium, are among the numerous viral infections that can cause transient microscopic hematuria and non-nephrotic proteinuria. Although measles is more well-known for its rare capacity to induce remission in patients with minimal change disease and nephrotic syndrome, it can also result in a diffuse proliferative GN.

The family Flaviviridae comprises four serotypes that can cause dengue hemorrhagic fever. Clinical signs of increased vascular permeability include cramping in the muscles, gastrointestinal distress, and, in more extreme situations, shock and bleeding symptoms. Severe cases may be accompanied by acute renal failure; in certain patients who are not as sick, acute endocapillary GN with mesangial proliferation may occur and show up as proteinuria and microhematuria. IgG, IgM, and C3 are typically found in concentrated granular deposits in mesangial regions and to a lesser extent in capillary walls.

Acute Epstein-Barr virus (EBV) infection can also cause mild renal abnormalities; in 10 to 15% of cases, proteinuria and microhematuria are observed. The most frequent renal complication is most likely acute interstitial nephritis, but MPGN and diffuse proliferative GN can also happen. Replicating EBV was found in proximal tubular cells, which were demonstrated to express the EBV CD21 receptor, in addition to infiltrating macrophages. One theory suggested that EBV may be a primary cause of long-term interstitial nephritis (Carton, 2006).

A Closer Look

Podocyte Dysfunction

Podocytes are specialized cells located within the Bowman's capsule of the kidney's nephron, playing a critical role in maintaining the integrity and function of the glomerular filtration barrier. Dysfunction of podocytes can lead to disruption of this barrier, resulting in proteinuria and impaired kidney function. Podocyte dysfunction can occur due to various factors, including genetic mutations, immune-mediated mechanisms, metabolic disorders, and environmental insults.

Genetic mutations affecting podocyte structure and function are implicated in several inherited kidney diseases, collectively known as podocytopathies. Mutations in genes encoding proteins crucial for podocyte structure, such as nephrin, podocin, and α-actinin-4, can disrupt the intricate architecture of podocyte foot processes, compromising their ability to maintain the glomerular filtration barrier. These genetic defects underlie conditions such as focal segmental glomerulosclerosis (FSGS), minimal change disease (MCD), and Alport syndrome.

Immune-mediated mechanisms, particularly in autoimmune diseases like lupus nephritis and membranous nephropathy, can lead to podocyte injury and dysfunction. Autoantibodies targeting podocyte antigens, immune complex deposition, and inflammatory cytokines can trigger podocyte apoptosis, podocyte foot process effacement, and disruption of the glomerular filtration barrier. This immune dysregulation contributes to proteinuria and progressive kidney damage in affected individuals.

Metabolic disorders such as diabetes mellitus and obesity are also associated with podocyte dysfunction. High blood glucose levels in diabetes can induce podocyte injury through various mechanisms, including oxidative stress, advanced glycation end-products (AGEs) formation, and activation of inflammatory pathways. Similarly, dyslipidemia and adipokine dysregulation in obesity can impair podocyte function, promoting proteinuria and glomerulosclerosis.

Environmental insults, including exposure to toxins, drugs, and infections, can adversely affect podocyte health and function. Certain medications, such as nonsteroidal anti-inflammatory drugs (NSAIDs), calcineurin inhibitors, and chemotherapeutic agents, have been implicated in podocyte toxicity and nephrotoxicity. Viral infections, particularly HIV and parvovirus B19, can directly infect podocytes or trigger immune responses leading to podocyte injury and proteinuria.

Summary

- Glomerular diseases encompass a group of conditions affecting the glomeruli, the tiny filtration units in the kidneys responsible for removing waste products and excess fluid from the bloodstream.
- The kidneys have several essential homeostatic functions. These functions include waste removal (NH_3), fluid/electrolyte balance, metabolic blood acid-base balance, as well as producing/modifying hormones for blood pressure, calcium/potassium homeostasis, and red blood cell production.
- Glomerulus capillaries form a central tuft of looped capillaries located in the center of the renal corpuscle. These capillaries deliver blood and create a large surface area for renal filtration.
- Bowman's capsule consists of the visceral and parietal layers. The inner visceral layer completely encircles the glomerular capillaries. It is comprised of specialized stellate epithelial cells termed podocytes.
- The glomerular basement membrane is the third component of the filtration barrier, along with the capillary endothelium and podocytes.
- This glomerular filtration barrier is comprised of three structures: the glomerular capillary endothelium, podocytes, and the fused basement membranes of both of these cells.
- The glomeruli are important for filtration, which describes the process of removing protein-free plasma from the blood.
- A glomerulopathy may be focal (only some glomeruli are involved) or diffuse (all glomeruli are affected).
- Hematuria refers to blood in the urine that may be visible or non-visible. Isolated hematuria is broadly defined as persistent hematuria in the absence of proteinuria and normal renal function.
- Nephrotic syndrome is broadly defined as a triad of heavy (nephrotic range) proteinuria > 3.5 g/day, hypoalbuminemia (< 35 g/L) and peripheral edema.
- Today, infection-related glomerulonephritis (GN) is uncommon and usually associated with debilitating conditions such as diabetes, malignant neoplasia, acquired immunodeficiency syndrome (AIDS), and alcoholism.

References

1. Agrawal, S., Zaritsky, J. J., Fornoni, A., & Smoyer, W. E. (2018). Dyslipidaemia in nephrotic syndrome: Mechanisms and treatment. *Nature Reviews Nephrology, 14*(1), 57–70. doi: 10.1038/nrneph.2017.161.
2. Alpers, C. E., & Kowalewska, J. (2007). Emerging paradigms in renal pathology of viral diseases. *Clinical Journal of the American Society of Nephrology, 2*(Suppl 1), S6–S12. doi: 10.2215/CJN.01980507.

3. Badour, L. M., Wilson, W. R., & Bayer, A. S. (2005). Infective endocarditis: Diagnosis, antimicrobial therapy, and management of complications. *Circulation, 111*, 3167–3184. doi: 10.1161/CIRCULATIONAHA.105.539568.
4. Balter, S., Benin, A., & Pinto, S. W. (2000). Epidemic nephritis in Nova Serrana, Brazil. *Lancet, 355*, 1776–1780. doi: 10.1016/S0140-6736(00)02295-0.
5. Barsoum, R. S. (1998). Malarial nephropathies. *Nephrology Dialysis Transplantation, 13*(7), 1588–1597. doi: 10.1093/ndt/13.7.1588.
6. Barsoum, R. S. (2006). Parasitic infections in transplant recipients. *Nature Clinical Practice Nephrology, 2*(9), 490–503. doi: 10.1038/ncpneph0290.
7. Barzon, L., Murer, L., & Pacenti, M. (2009). Investigation of intrarenal viral infections in kidney transplant recipients unveils an association between parvovirus B19 and chronic allograft injury. *Journal of Infectious Diseases, 199*(3), 372–380. doi: 10.1086/597635.
8. Batsford, S. R., Mezzano, S., & Mihatsch, M. (2005). Is the nephritogenic antigen in poststreptococcal glomerulonephritis pyrogenic exotoxin B (SPE B) or GAPDH? *Kidney International, 68*(3), 1120–1129. doi: 10.1111/j.1523-1755.2005.00482.x.
9. Beres, S. B., Sesso, R., & Pinto, S. W. (2008). Genome sequence of a Lancefield group C Streptococcus zooepidemicus strain causing epidemic nephritis: New information about an old disease. *PLoS ONE, 3*(12), e3026. doi: 10.1371/journal.pone.0003026.
10. Carton, J., et al. (2006). *Clinical Pathology*. Oxford Core Texts.
11. Casey, J. R., & Pichichero, M. E. (2004). Meta-analysis of cephalosporin versus penicillin treatment of group A streptococcal tonsillopharyngitis in children. *Pediatrics, 113*(4), 866–882. doi: 10.1542/peds.113.4.866.
12. Chugh, K. S., & Sakhuja, V. (1990). Glomerular disease in the tropics. *American Journal of Nephrology, 10*(6), 437–450. doi: 10.1159/000139064.
13. Davies, M. (1994). The mesangial cell: A tissue culture view. *Kidney International, 45*(2), 320–327. doi: 10.1038/ki.1994.45.
14. Deen, W. M., Lazzara, M. J., & Myers, B. D. (2001). Structural determinants of glomerular permeability. *American Journal of Physiology Renal Physiology, 281*(4), F579–596. doi: 10.1152/ajprenal.2001.281.4.F579.
15. Doe, J. Y., Funk, M., & Mengel, M. (2006). Nephrotic syndrome in African children: Lack of evidence for "tropical nephrotic syndrome"? *Nephrology Dialysis Transplantation, 21*(3), 672–676. doi: 10.1093/ndt/gfk010.
16. Eckardt, K. U. (1996). Erythropoietin production in liver and kidneys. *Current Opinion in Nephrology and Hypertension, 5*(1), 28–34. doi: 10.1097/00041552-199601000-00007.
17. Ehrich, J. H., & Eke, F. U. (2007). Malaria-induced renal damage: Facts and myths. *Pediatric Nephrology, 22*(5), 626–637. doi: 10.1007/s00467-007-0457-4.
18. Faul, C., Asanuma, K., Yanagida-Asanuma, E., Kim, K., & Mundel, P. (2007). Actin up: Regulation of podocyte structure and function by components of the actin cytoskeleton. *Trends in Cell Biology, 17*(9), 428–437. doi: 10.1016/j.tcb.2007.07.002.
19. Fiorentino, M., Bolignano, D., Tesar, V., Pisano, A., Van Biesen, W., D'Arrigo, G., Tripepi, G., & Gesualdo, L. (2016). Renal biopsy in 2015–From epidemiology to evidence-based indications. *American Journal of Nephrology, 43*(1), 1–19. doi: 10.1159/000441352.

20. Fisher, J. W. (2003). Erythropoietin: Physiology and pharmacology update. *Experimental Biology and Medicine (Maywood), 228*(1), 1–14. doi: 10.1177/153537020322800101.

21. Fukuda, M., Motokawa, M., & Usami, T. (2006). PR3-ANCA–positive crescentic necrotizing glomerulonephritis accompanied by isolated pulmonic valve infective endocarditis, with reference to previous reports of renal pathology. *Clinical Nephrology, 66*, 202–209. doi: 10.5414/CNP66202.

22. Gerl, K., Miquerol, L., Todorov, V. T., Hugo, C. P., Adams, R. H., Kurtz, A., & Kurt, B. (2015). Inducible glomerular erythropoietin production in the adult kidney. *Kidney International, 88*(6), 1345–1355. doi: 10.1038/ki.2015.296.

23. Greka, A., & Mundel, P. (2012). Cell biology and pathology of podocytes. *Annual Review of Physiology, 74*, 299–323. doi: 10.1146/annurev-physiol-020911-153327.

24. Guruswamy Sangameswaran, K. D., Hashmi, M. F., & Baradhi, K. M. (2023). *Focal Segmental Glomerulosclerosis*. StatPearls Publishing. Retrieved from: https://www.statpearls.com (accessed on 31 July 2024).

25. Haraldsson, B., Nyström, J., & Deen, W. M. (2008). Properties of the glomerular barrier and mechanisms of proteinuria. *Physiological Reviews, 88*(2), 451–487. doi: 10.1152/physrev.00050.2006.

26. Hebert, L. A., Parikh, S., Prosek, J., Nadasdy, T., & Rovin, B. H. (2013). Differential diagnosis of glomerular disease: A systematic and inclusive approach. *American Journal of Nephrology, 38*(3), 253–266. doi: 10.1159/000351902.

27. Iwata, Y., Ohta, S., & Kawai, K. (2004). Shunt nephritis with positive titers for ANCA specific for proteinase 3. *American Journal of Kidney Diseases, 43*(1), e11–e16. doi: 10.1053/j.ajkd.2003.11.024.

28. Johnson, R. J., & Couser, W. G. (1990). Hepatitis B infection and renal disease: Clinical, immunopathogenetic, and therapeutic considerations [Editorial review]. *Kidney International, 37*(3), 663–676. doi: 10.1038/ki.1990.90.

29. Johnston, F., Carapetis, J., & Patel, M. S. (1999). Evaluating the use of penicillin to control outbreaks of acute poststreptococcal glomerulonephritis. *Pediatric Infectious Disease Journal, 18*(4), 327–332. doi: 10.1097/00006454-199904000-00014.

30. Kitterer, D., Gürzing, K., Segerer, S., Alscher, M. D., Amann, K., Braun, N., & Latus, J. (2015). Diagnostic impact of percutaneous renal biopsy. *Clinical Nephrology, 84*(6), 311–322. doi: 10.5414/CN107883.

31. Koyama, A., Kobayashi, M., & Yamaguchi, N. (1995). Glomerulonephritis associated with MRSA infection: A possible role of bacterial superantigen. *Kidney International, 47*(1), 207–216. doi: 10.1038/ki.1995.20.

32. Koyama, A., Sharmin, S., & Sakurai, H. (2004). Staphylococcus aureus cell envelope antigen is a new candidate for the induction of IgA nephropathy. *Kidney International, 66*(1), 121–132. doi: 10.1111/j.1523-1755.2004.00759.x.

33. Lai, A. S. H., & Lai, K. N. (2006). Viral nephropathy. *Nature Clinical Practice Nephrology, 2*(5), 254–262. doi: 10.1038/ncpneph0183.

34. Lai, K. N., Li, P. K., & Lui, S. F. (1991). Membranous nephropathy related to hepatitis B virus in adults. *New England Journal of Medicine, 324*(21), 1457–1463. doi: 10.1056/NEJM199105233242104.

35. Lau, G. K., Piratvisuth, T., & Luo, K. X. (2005). Peginterferon Alfa-2a HBeAg-Positive Chronic Hepatitis B Study Group: Peginterferon alfa-2a, lamivudine, and the combination for HBeAg-positive chronic hepatitis B. *New England Journal of Medicine, 352*(26), 2682–2695. doi: 10.1056/NEJMoa043386.

36. Lomonte, C., Chiarulli, G., & Cazzato, F. (2004). End-stage renal disease in leprosy. *Journal of Nephrology, 17*(2), 302–305. doi: 10.1007/s40620-017-0330-8.

37. Majumdar, A., Chowdhary, S., & Ferreira, M. A. A. S. (2000). Renal pathological findings in infective endocarditis. *Nephrology Dialysis Transplantation, 15*(11), 1782–1787. doi: 10.1093/ndt/15.11.1782.

38. Menè, P., & Cinotti, G. A. (1989). Paracrine and autocrine functions of glomerular mesangial cells. *Journal of Endocrinological Investigation, 12*(7), 497–509. doi: 10.1007/BF03349238.

39. Nasr, S. H., Markowitz, G. S., & Stokes, M. B. (2008). Acute postinfectious glomerulonephritis in the modern era: Experience with 86 adults and review of the literature. *Medicine (Baltimore), 87*(1), 21–32. doi: 10.1097/MD.0b013e318160fe77.

40. Nasr, S. H., Markowitz, G. S., & Whelan, J. D. (2003). IgA-dominant acute poststaphylococcal glomerulonephritis complicating diabetic nephropathy. *Human Pathology, 34*(12), 1235–1241. doi: 10.1016/j.humpath.2003.07.010.

41. Ngu, J. L., Chatelanat, F., & Leke, R. (1985). Nephropathy in Cameroon: Evidence for filarial derived immune complex pathogenesis in some cases. *Clinical Nephrology, 24*, 128–132. doi: 10.5414/CNP24128.

42. Oda, T., Yamakami, K., & Omasu, F. (2005). Glomerular plasmin-like activity in relation to nephritis-associated plasmin receptor in acute poststreptococcal glomerulonephritis. *Journal of the American Society of Nephrology, 16*(1), 247–254. doi: 10.1681/ASN.2004070556.

43. Okocha, E. C., Ibeh, C. C., Ele, P. U., & Ibeh, N. C. (2005). The prevalence of malaria parasitaemia in blood donors in a Nigerian teaching hospital. *Journal of Vector Borne Diseases, 42*(1), 21–24. doi: 10.4103/0972-9062.16348.

44. Pagnoux, C., Cohen, P., & Guillevin, L. (2006). Vasculitides secondary to infections. *Clinical and Experimental Rheumatology, 24*(Suppl 41), S71–S81.

45. Parra, G., Rodríguez-Iturbe, B., & Batsford, S. (1998). Antibody to streptococcal zymogen in the serum of patients with acute glomerulonephritis: A multicentric study. *Kidney International, 54*(2), 509–517. doi: 10.1038/ki.1998.317.

46. Pavenstädt, H., Kriz, W., & Kretzler, M. (2003). Cell biology of the glomerular podocyte. *Physiological Reviews, 83*(1), 253–307. doi: 10.1152/physrev.00024.2002.

47. Quaggin, S. E., & Kreidberg, J. A. (2008). Development of the renal glomerulus: Good neighbors and good fences. *Development, 135*(4), 609–620. doi: 10.1242/dev.005953.

48. Radhakrishnan, J. (2021). Glomerular disease: Evaluation and differential diagnosis in adults. *UpToDate*. Retrieved from: https://www.uptodate.com (accessed on 31 July 2024).

49. Rajapurkar, M. M. (1994). Renal involvement in malaria. *Tropical Nephrology, 40*, 132–134.

50. Rawla, P., Padala, S. A., & Ludhwani, D. (2022). *Poststreptococcal Glomerulonephritis*. StatPearls Publishing. Retrieved from: https://www.statpearls.com (accessed on 31 July 2024).
51. Raza, A., & Aggarwal, S. (2023). *Membranous Glomerulonephritis*. StatPearls Publishing. Retrieved from: https://www.statpearls.com (accessed on 31 July 2024).
52. Reiser, J., Kriz, W., Kretzler, M., & Mundel, P. (2000). The glomerular slit diaphragm is a modified adherens junction. *Journal of the American Society of Nephrology, 11*(1), 1–8. doi: 10.1681/ASN.V1111.
53. Roccatello, D., Fornasieri, A., & Giachino, O. (2007). Multicentric study on hepatitis C virus–related cryoglobulinemic glomerulonephritis. *American Journal of Kidney Diseases, 49*(1), 69–82. doi: 10.1053/j.ajkd.2006.10.017.
54. Rodríguez-Iturbe, B. (1984). Epidemic poststreptococcal glomerulonephritis. *Kidney International, 25*(1), 129–136. doi: 10.1038/ki.1984.17.
55. Rodríguez-Iturbe, B., & Batsford, S. (2007). Pathogenesis of poststreptococcal glomerulonephritis a century after Clemens von Pirquet. *Kidney International, 71*(10), 1094–1104. doi: 10.1038/sj.ki.5002174.
56. Rodríguez-Iturbe, B., & Musser, J. M. (2008). The current state of poststreptococcal nephritis. *Journal of the American Society of Nephrology, 19*(9), 1855–1864. doi: 10.1681/ASN.2008010012.
57. Satoskar, A. A., Nadasdy, G., & Plaza, J. A. (2006). Staphylococcus infection–associated glomerulonephritis mimicking IgA nephropathy. *Clinical Journal of the American Society of Nephrology, 1*(6), 1179–1186. doi: 10.2215/CJN.01690706.
58. Schoener, B., & Borger, J. (2023). *Erythropoietin Stimulating Agents*. StatPearls Publishing. Retrieved from: https://www.statpearls.com (accessed on 31 July 2024).
59. Scott, R. P., & Quaggin, S. E. (2015). Review series: The cell biology of renal filtration. *Journal of Cell Biology, 209*(2), 199–210. doi: 10.1083/jcb.201411085.
60. Sesso, R., & Pinto, S. W. L. (2005). Five-year follow-up of patients with epidemic glomerulonephritis due to *Streptococcus zooepidemicus*. *Nephrology Dialysis Transplantation, 20*(9), 1808–1813. doi: 10.1093/ndt/gfh010.
61. Sorger, K., Gessler, M., & Hübner, F. K. (1987). Follow-up studies of three subtypes of acute postinfectious glomerulonephritis ascertained by renal biopsy. *Clinical Nephrology, 27*, 111–124.
62. Tapia, C., & Bashir, K. (2023). Nephrotic syndrome. In *StatPearls* [Internet]. StatPearls Publishing. Treasure Island, FL.
63. Tlevjeh, I. M., Steckelberg, J. M., & Murad, H. S. (2005). Temporal trends in infective endocarditis: A population-based study in Olmsted County, Minnesota. *JAMA, 293*, 3022–3028.
64. Tomlinson, L., Borskin, Y., & McPhee, I. (2003). Acute cytomegalovirus infection complicated by collapsing glomerulopathy. *Nephrology Dialysis Transplantation, 18*, 187–189.
65. Varghese, R. T., & Jialal, I. (2023). Diabetic nephropathy. In *StatPearls* [Internet]. StatPearls Publishing. Treasure Island, FL.
66. Vaziri, N. D. (2016). Disorders of lipid metabolism in nephrotic syndrome: Mechanisms and consequences. *Kidney International, 90*(1), 41–52.

67. Vivarelli, M., Massella, L., Ruggiero, B., & Emma, F. (2017). Minimal change disease. *Clinical Journal of the American Society of Nephrology, 12*(2), 332–345.

68. Waldman, M., & Kopp, B. J. (2007). Parvovirus B19 and the kidney. *Clinical Journal of the American Society of Nephrology, 2*(Supplement 1), S47–S56.

69. Walker, P. D. (2009). The renal biopsy. *Archives of Pathology & Laboratory Medicine, 133*(2), 181–188.

70. Wang, G. L., & Semenza, G. L. (1996). Molecular basis of hypoxia-induced erythropoietin expression. *Current Opinion in Hematology, 3*(2), 156–162.

71. Watson, S., Padala, S. A., Hashmi, M. F., & Bush, J. S. (2023). Alport syndrome. In *StatPearls* [Internet]. StatPearls Publishing. Treasure Island, FL.

72. White, A. V., Hoy, W. E., & McCredie, D. A. (2001). Childhood post-streptococcal glomerulonephritis as a risk for chronic renal disease in later life. *Medical Journal of Australia, 174*, 492–496.

73. White, K. E. (2012). Research into the structure of the kidney glomerulus–making it count. *Micron, 43*(10), 1001–1009.

74. Wiggins, R. C. (2007). The spectrum of podocytopathies: A unifying view of glomerular diseases. *Kidney International, 71*(12), 1205–1214.

75. Yoshizawa, N., Yamakami, K., & Fujino, M. (2004). Nephritis-associated plasmin receptor and acute poststreptococcal glomerulonephritis: Characterization of the antigen and associated immune response. *Journal of the American Society of Nephrology, 15*, 1785–1793.

Chapter 9

CYSTIC DISEASES OF THE KIDNEY

Contents

Introduction

Kidney cystic diseases encompass a wide spectrum of conditions that manifest in infants, children, and adults with multiple phenotypic manifestations. These represent approximately 10% of end-stage renal disease (ESRD) patients and are common across all racial, ethnic, and gender groups globally. Typically, the age at which they present, clinical characteristics, renal imaging studies that show the location and distribution of cysts, and extra-renal manifestations all help with the clinical diagnosis. Kidney cyst diseases rank among the most important monogenic causes of renal morbidity and mortality in adult and pediatric populations. Over the last 10 years, significant progress has been made in determining and describing the genes causing these illnesses. This chapter will focus on the genetic components, molecular pathogenesis, clinical manifestations, and management of these disorders. While there are acquired forms of cystic renal disease, this chapter will primarily address the inherited forms.

Orientation and Directional Terms

Term	Definition	Illustration
Bardet-Biedl syndrome	Bardet-Biedl syndrome is a rare autosomal recessive ciliopathy with multisystemic compromise, affecting vision, kidneys, and eventually heart, liver and digestive system. Obesity, mental retardation, hypogonadism and polydactilia are common findings.	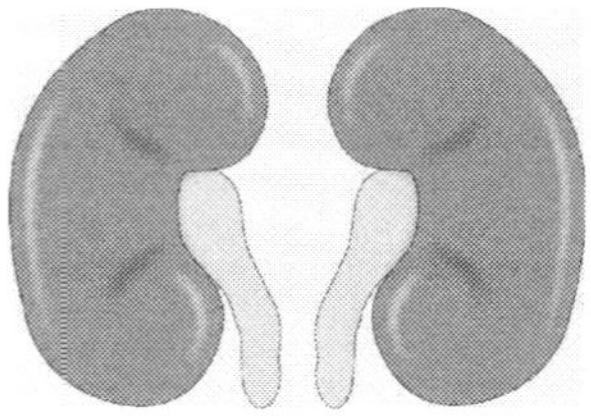
Medullary sponge kidney	Medullary sponge kidney (MSK) is a rare congenital disorder that causes cysts to form in the kidney's tubules, giving the kidney a sponge-like appearance. The cysts can be 1–8 millimeters in diameter.	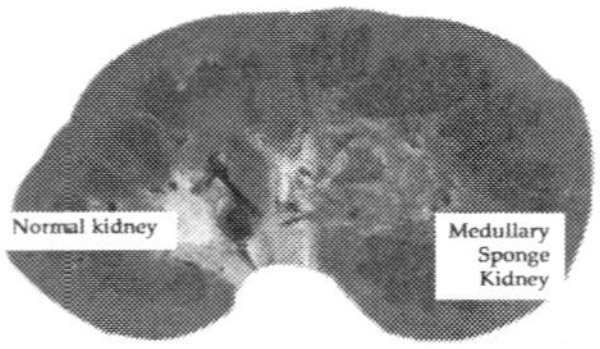
Nephronophthisis	Nephronophthisis (NPHP) is a cystic kidney disease that's caused by mutations in 11 genes that encode proteins involved in the function of primary cilia. It's the most common genetic cause of renal failure in children and young adults, and the most frequent genetic cause of end-stage renal disease up to the third decade of life.	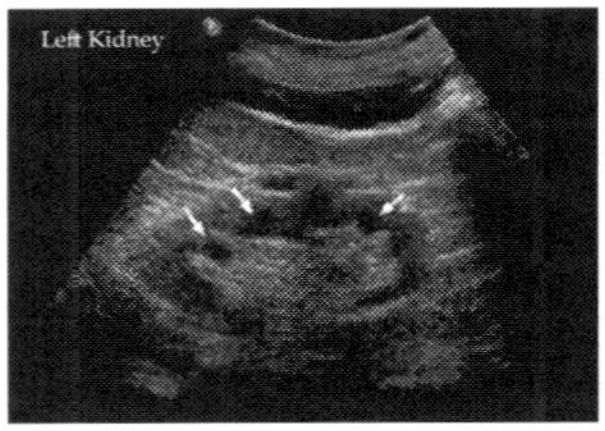
Simple renal cysts	A simple renal cyst is a fluid-filled sac that forms on the surface of the kidney. They are the most common type of kidney cyst and can form in one or both kidneys.	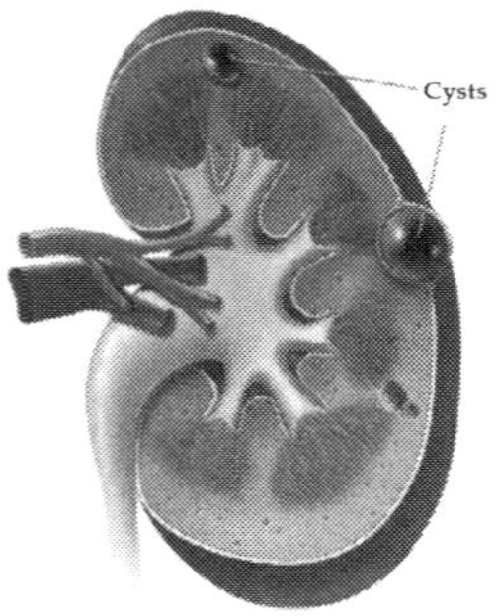
von Hippel-Lindau syndrome	Von Hippel-Lindau syndrome is a rare genetic disorder that causes tumors and cysts to grow in various parts of the body.	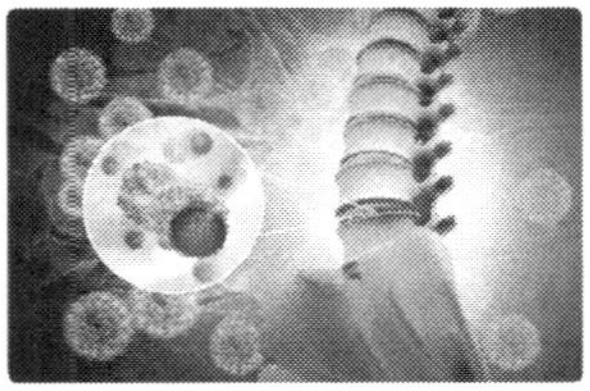

9.1. Classification of Cystic Kidney Diseases

A cyst is essentially defined as a cavity filled with liquid or semisolid material that is surrounded by epithelium. One or both kidneys may contain one or more cysts. They could be big, dangerous, and enlarging, or they could be tiny, non-enlarging, and clinically insignificant. Table 9.1 presents the classification of diseases affecting the cystic kidney. As shown in Table 9.2, kidney cyst disease can also be categorized according to the pattern of inheritance.

Table 9.1. Classification of Cystic Kidney Disorders

Autosomal dominant polycystic kidney disease (ADPKD)
Autosomal recessive polycystic kidney disease (ARPKD)
• Tuberous sclerosis complex
• von Hippel-Lindau syndrome
Autosomal dominant medullary cystic kidney disease
Hereditary recessive ciliopathies with interstitial nephritis, cysts or both
• Nephronophthisis
• Bardet-Biedl syndrome
Renal cystic dysplasias
• Multicystic kidney dysplasia
Other cystic kidney disorders
• Simple cysts
• Medullary sponge kidney
• Acquired cystic kidney disease
Renal cystic neoplasms
• Cystic renal cell carcinoma
Cysts of nontubular origin
• Cystic disease of the renal sinus
• Perirenal lymphangiomas
Pyelocalyceal cysts

Source: OP Kalra and Deepak Jain. Cystic Diseases of the Kidney. In book: Essentials of Nephrology, Edition 3, Volume 1, pp 265–72 (pp.265–72). https://www.researchgate.net/publication/333872295_Cystic_Diseases_of_Kidney.

Table 9.2. Classification of Cystic Diseases of the Kidney Based on Inheritance

Genetic	*Nongenetic*
1. Autosomal dominant polycystic kidney disease (ADPKD)	1. Multicystic kidney
2. Autosomal recessive polycystic kidney disease (ARPKD)	2. Multilocular cyst
3. Juvenile nephronophthisis—medullary cystic complex	3. Simple cysts—solitary or multiple
4. Cysts associated with multiple malformation syndromes: Tuberous sclerosis, von Hippel-Lindau's disease, Meckel's syndrome, Orofacial syndrome and chromosome disorders like trisomy 21,13,18 and trisomy C	4. Multiple parapelvic cysts
	5. Medullary sponge kidney
	6. Acquired renal cystic disease

Source: OP Kalra and Deepak Jain. Cystic diseases of the kidney. In book: Essentials of Nephrology, Edition 3, Volume 1, pp 265–72. https://www.researchgate.net/publication/333872295_Cystic_Diseases_of_Kidney.

Of these, this chapter primarily discusses four types of cysts that are frequently seen in adults. A genetic condition known as autosomal dominant polycystic kidney disease (ADPKD) can cause progressive renal failure. Acquired cystic kidney disease (AKCD) may be linked to chronic renal failure of unclear etiology. In the absence of particular kidney pathology, sporadic presence of simple cysts may be reported; these cysts have modestly negative clinical consequences. Lastly, another common cystic kidney disease seen in routine clinical practice is the medullary sponge kidney. Retinal cysts in their remaining forms are comparatively uncommon.

9.2. Autosomal Dominant Polycystic Kidney Disease

With an incidence of 1 in 400–1,000 births, ADPKD is one of the most prevalent genetic disorders affecting all ethnic groups worldwide. In North America and Europe, it represents over 5% of ESRD cases. Two different genetic mutations have been connected to ADPKD. ADPKD can result from mutations in the PKD1 gene, which is found on chromosome 16 and encodes polycystin-1, or the PKD2 gene, which is found on chromosome 4 and encodes polycystin-2. PKD1 mutations are the cause of about 85% of cases. The localization of the primary cilia of the renal epithelium and intracellular calcium signaling are both controlled by polycystin-1 and polycystin-2.

9.2.1. Mechanisms of Cyst Formation

To date, no single mechanism put forth to account for the formation of cysts has been able to provide solid evidence for the development of cysts. Furthermore, the fact that normal renal cells cannot form cysts when grown in culture, only human PKD cells can, implies the existence of a genetic defect that directly causes cyst formation. The anomalies in tubular sodium reabsorption may be caused by the translocation of the basolateral membrane Na-K ATPase pump to the luminal membrane. This would therefore encourage the cyst's early phases of development and growth to secrete sodium and water. This happens early and could be a result of the cyst-lining cells dedifferentiating later on. The apical membrane of ADPKD cells contains the cystic fibrosis transmembrane conductance regulator (CFTR). This channel promotes cyst growth by acting as a chloride channel that is dependent on cyclic AMP (cAMP). Cyst growth in ADPKD has been linked to activation of the mammalian target of rapamycin (mTOR) pathway. Renal cyst formation and changes in blood glucose metabolism have been related. Cyst formation results from the renal cellular preferential switch to aerobic glycolysis. Finally, angiogenesis may contribute to the development of cysts and the advancement of ADPKD.

9.2.2. Clinical Features

Adults with ADPKD typically experience symptoms in their third or fourth decade of life. By the time they are 55 years old, nearly two-thirds of the patients have a diagnosis. Initial manifestations can range from a state of no symptoms to hematuria, mild proteinuria, hypertension, or renal insufficiency. Although palpable kidneys are present in about half of younger patients, the incidence of palpable kidneys is significantly higher in older patients. Cysts of varying sizes may be dispersed throughout the renal tissue in the patient (Figures 9.1 and 9.2). One of the most prevalent signs of ADPKD is flank pain, which is primarily brought on by renal calculi, hemorrhage, or urinary tract infection. Increased erythropoietin production by the kidney's ischemic parenchyma may be the cause of polycythemia. Anemia is rare in ADPKD, even in cases where ESRD develops. Fever, loin pain, and discoloration of the cyst contents can all be signs of cyst infection. Hematuria may result from bleeding into a cyst that is in communication with the drainage system. About 20% of patients develop renal stones, primarily as a result of urine stasis brought on by distorted renal anatomy. Malignancy developing within a cyst is uncommon. As the cysts grow larger and compress the remaining renal parenchyma, renal failure may occur. Renal failure frequently develops gradually and advances to end-stage renal disease (ESRD). The related tubulointerstitial damage may also lead to the development of polyuria, polydipsia, and a salt-losing state.

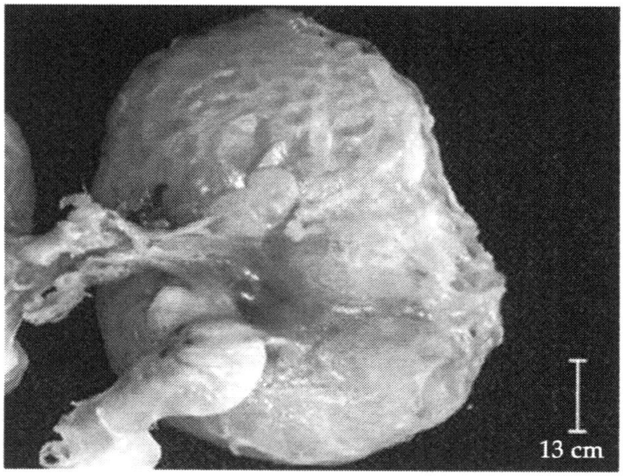

Figure 9.1. *Autosomal dominant polycystic kidney disease—external surface showing multiple cysts with variable sizes.*

Source: *OP Kalra and Deepak Jain. Cystic Diseases of the Kidney. In book: Essentials of Nephrology, Edition 3, Volume 1, pp 265–72 (pp.265–72). https://www.researchgate.net/publication/333872295_Cystic_Diseases_of_Kidney.*

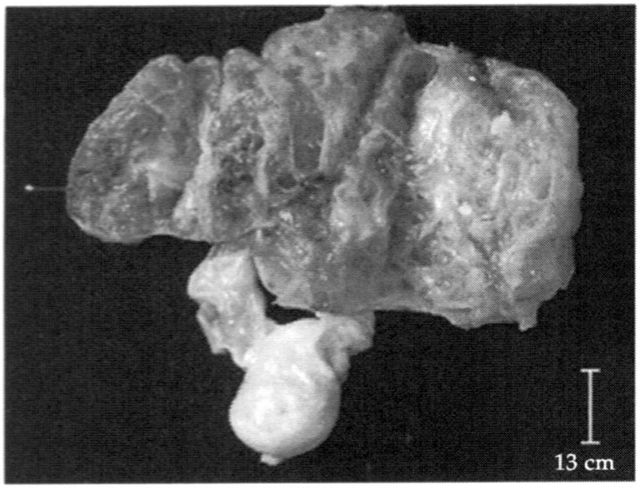

Figure 9.2. *Autosomal dominant polycystic kidney disease—cut surface showing multiple cysts with variable sizes.*

Source: *OP Kalra and Deepak Jain. Cystic Diseases of the Kidney. In book: Essentials of Nephrology, Edition 3, Volume 1, pp 265–72 (pp.265–72). https://www.researchgate.net/publication/333872295_Cystic_Diseases_of_Kidney.*

One of the most prevalent extrarenal manifestations of ADPKD is polycystic liver disease. When there are four or more cysts in the hepatic parenchyma, it should be suspected. The majority of the time, there are no symptoms, but cystic or massive hepatic enlargement may cause them. About 8% of patients with ADPKD develop intracranial aneurysms. The aneurysm's size determines the rupture risk, which is typically very low in these patients. The most prevalent valvular abnormality detected by echocardiography in about 25% of ADPKD patients is mitral valve prolapse. The other significant associated features are cardiac valvular incompetence and primary dilatation of the aortic root. There have also been reports of cyst formation in the ovary, thyroid, spleen, pancreas, arachnoid membrane, etc. The other associations are with immotile sperms, corneal dystrophy, horseshoe kidney, and colonic diverticulosis.

9.2.3. Laboratory, Imaging, and Histopathologic Findings

Studies on serum electrolytes are normal unless ESRD is present. About 40–45% of urine tests show microscopic or gross hematuria, particularly when there is cyst hemorrhage. 30% of patients have microalbuminuria and 20% have dipstick proteinuria. Even in cases of severe cystic disease, liver transaminases, alkaline phosphatase, and indicators of hepatic synthetic function like prothrombin time and partial thromboplastin time are typically normal. Hepatic cyst burden is correlated with γ-glutamyltransferase levels.

Diagnosing ADPKD is best done with abdominal ultrasonography. The Ravine criteria are very specific—nearly 100%—but their sensitivity varies with age, that is to say. e. The chance of illness decreases with the length of time a person stays negative. Due to the later age of onset, 67% of PKD2 patients are younger than 30 years old. As a result, if a person is at risk for PKD2, they should continue to receive ultrasonography surveillance or undergo molecular diagnostic testing after the age of 30. There are numerous anechoic cysts of different sizes distributed throughout the cortex of the enlarged kidneys, which distort the normal pelvicalyceal architecture. Echogenic debris within a cyst may be indicative of hemorrhage or infection. Ultrasound can also be used to see cysts in the spleen, pancreas, and liver. When higher resolution imaging is needed, magnetic resonance imaging (MRI) or computed tomography (CT) with intravenous contrast can be used to diagnose ADPKD.

Patients with ADPKD should not have renal biopsies due to the possibility of bleeding. Cysts covering the surface of the kidney enlarge gross renal specimens. Cut specimens show cysts throughout the kidney's thickness that are filled with a brown, serosanguinous, or straw-colored fluid. Purulent material fills the infected cysts. In the parenchyma in between cysts, interstitial fibrosis and intact nephrons are visible under a microscope. Renal epithelium, which primarily originates from the collecting duct and proximal convoluted tubule, lines the cysts. Biliary duct epithelium lines the inside of hepatic cysts.

9.2.4. Diagnosis

Imaging methods are necessary for the diagnosis of ADPKD in patients with a positive family history. The kidneys' large size is frequently visible on a plain X-ray of the KUB region. An excretory urogram demonstrates the recognizable "spider leg" deformity. Ultrasonography is the most widely used imaging modality for ADPKD diagnosis, as it can confirm kidney enlargement. Table 9.3 contains the revised criteria that have been suggested to increase the diagnostic accuracy of ultrasonography in ADPKD. A renal cyst or normal kidneys found on ultrasonography in a person 40 years of age or older has a 100% negative predictive value. The "gold standard" for diagnosis, particularly in less evident cases involving children and young adults, is a CT scan. Additionally, if cysts are present, it can identify malignant changes and other abdominal organ cysts.

Table 9.3. Sonographic Criteria for Diagnosis or Exclusion of ADPKD

Age (yr)	*Criteria for positive diagnosis*	*PPV(%)*	*Sensitivity (%)*
15–29	≥3 cysts, unilateral or bilateral	100	81.7
30–39	≥3 cysts, unilateral or bilateral	100	95.5
40–59	≥2 cysts in each kidney	100	90.0
≥60	≥4 cysts in each kidney	100	100
	Revised criteria for diagnosis exclusion	*NPV (%)*	*Specificity (%)*
15–29	≥1 cyst	90.8	97.1
30–39	≥1 cyst	98.3	94.8
40–59	≥2 cysts	100	98.2

PPV: Positive predictive value; NPV: Negative predictive value

Source: OP Kalra and Deepak Jain. Cystic Diseases of the Kidney. In book: Essentials of Nephrology, Edition 3, Volume 1, pp 265–72 (pp.265–72). https://www.researchgate.net/publication/333872295_Cystic_Diseases_of_Kidney.

9.2.4.1. Molecular and Prenatal Diagnosis

The preferred diagnostic procedure is abdominal ultrasonography, particularly for those who may be at risk for PKD1. If higher-resolution studies are needed and ultrasound is inconclusive, CT or MRI may be used as an adjunct. Molecular diagnostic testing is offered for sale for PKD1 and PKD2.

For PKD1, sequence analysis has a mutation detection rate of about 90%. Multiplex ligation-dependent probe amplification can identify gross rearrangements in an additional 4% of patients. Direct sequence analysis for PKD2 identifies more than 90% of the mutations. Molecular testing is not without its limitations, though. There are very few recurrent PKD1 and PKD2 mutations; the majority are "private mutations." As a result, it's important to interpret sequencing results carefully because some sequence variations might correspond to benign polymorphisms. It is actually known that each person carries more than 10 polymorphic variants in the PKD1 gene. Furthermore, mutations in the noncoding sections of the genes cannot be found by exon sequencing.

Analysis of cells from amniocentesis or chorionic villus sampling can be used for prenatal diagnosis if linkage to a particular haplotype or disease-causing mutation has already been established. However, unless there is a family history of a severely affected infant, prenatal diagnosis is typically not done due to the availability of treatment, lack of cognitive impairment, and adult onset of disease.

9.2.5. Prognosis

Up until their fourth decade of life, the majority of ADPKD patients have normal renal function. After that, the glomerular filtration rate starts to decrease annually at a rate of 4–4–5 ml/minute. Risk factors for poor prognosis and progression to ESRD in individuals with ADPKD include genetic factors (PKD1 has a comparatively poorer prognosis than PKD2), hypertension, early onset of symptoms such as proteinuria and hematuria, male gender, larger kidneys (PKD1 mutations result in larger kidneys), increased left ventricular mass index, and low birth weight.

9.2.6. Treatment and Management

In ADPKD, there is no particular treatment to stop or slow the progression of renal structural disease. Nonspecific treatments for ADPKD include regulating dietary protein, eating a low-salt diet, drinking more water, closely controlling hypertension—ideally with the use of angiotensin receptor blockers (ARBs) or ACEIs—and taking statins, which may slow the disease's progression and lower cardiovascular death. Over the past 10 years, mTOR inhibitors, somatostatin analogs, vasopressin receptor antagonists (tolvaptans), and maximal inhibition of the renin-angiotensin-aldosterone system have all been proposed as novel, promising treatments. The final three crucial components of treating ADPKD are supportive therapy for pain management, total bed rest during gross hematuria, and cyst infection treatment.

When ADPKD patients reach ESRD, they need renal replacement therapy, such as dialysis or kidney transplantation. Because it is more challenging to infuse large volumes of peritoneal dialysate fluid when the kidneys are severely enlarged, hemodialysis is preferred over peritoneal dialysis. Additionally, it is linked to a higher risk of peritonitis brought on by a cyst infection or diverticular disease complications. In ADPKD, nephrectomy should be avoided whenever possible. On rare occasions, patients may need a nephrectomy of one or both cystic kidney(s) to make more room for the allograft, or they may need it for persistent pain, renal cell carcinoma, recurrent UTIs, or chronic hematuria necessitating frequent blood transfusions. For patients with ADPKD who have ESRD, renal transplantation is the recommended course of treatment.

Despite its great significance, genetic counseling is frequently overlooked when treating patients with ADPKD. It is important to inform recently diagnosed patients about the etiology and pattern of inheritance. Initial screening is necessary for asymptomatic family members, as is ongoing blood pressure monitoring and recurring ultrasound evaluation. Individuals who are at risk for ADPKD must undergo screening before engaging in physically demanding activities or sports.

The management of ADPKD is restricted to monitoring for and managing the disease's complications because there is currently no conclusive treatment for the underlying genetic defect. On the other hand, several innovative treatments are presently being tested in clinical trials and may eventually be employed in the treatment of these patients.

9.2.6.1. Hypertension

Given that the RAA system is the primary mechanism underlying hypertension in ADPKD and that both hypertension and proteinuria are predictive of an earlier onset of ESRD, the treatment of choice would seem to be angiotensin-converting enzyme inhibitors (ACE-i), which target the RAA system and lower blood pressure and proteinuria. According to epidemiologic and nonrandomized research, ACE-i can lessen proteinuria and delay the development of renal insufficiency. The few prospective, randomized studies on ACE-i, however, have shown different results. Treatment with a low-protein diet or ACE-i did not slow the loss of glomerular filtration rate (GFR), according to the Modification of Diet in Renal Disease (MDRD) Study Group, a randomized, prospective trial that included 200 patients with ADPKD (Schrier et al., 2003). The ACEi in Progressive Renal Insufficiency Study, which involved 64 ADPKD patients, discovered that benazepril treatment had no effect on the proportion of patients who needed to start dialysis or experienced a doubling of their serum creatinine. Lastly, there was no discernible difference in the decline in GFR among hypertensive ADPKD patients receiving enalapril or atenolol, a ß-blocker. There was also no discernible drop in microalbuminuria. Enalapril-treated normotensive ADPKD patients did not significantly slow down the decline in GFR when compared to non-treated patients. Antihypertensive medication does not appear to lower the risk of cardiac illness or intracranial hemorrhage in ADPKD patients, according to available data. A randomized study, however, found that patients receiving strict control of their hypertension (blood pressure less than 135–140/85–90 mmHg as opposed to 120/80 mmHg) had a significantly lower left ventricular mass index, which is a risk factor for cardiovascular disease. Although the results of this study suggest that antihypertensive medication is likely helpful in ADPKD, cardiac end-points like myocardial infarction, cardiomyopathy, or congestive heart failure were not investigated. Angiotensin receptor blockers (ARBs), which function similarly to ACE-i, are an additional treatment option. Therapy with ACE inhibitors and/or ARBs is advised because hypertension is a separate factor that raises the morbidity of ESRD patients.

9.2.6.2. Dialysis and Renal Transplantation

Renal replacement therapy with dialysis should be started as soon as end-stage renal disease (ESRD) manifests, or patients should be assessed for preemptive kidney transplantation if living donors are available. Before considering the implantation of a peritoneal catheter, a ventral hernia should be evaluated because they can cause problems with peritoneal dialysis. The 5-year and 10-year graft survival rates are 73% and 67%, respectively, for renal transplant patients who are not diabetics, and the 5-year and 10-year patient survival rates are 84% and 73%, respectively, for renal transplant recipients. The most frequent reason for graft failure and patient death is malignancy brought on by persistent immunosuppression (Errasti et al., 2003). Patients with ADPKD make excellent transplant candidates; however, due to the high risk of disease in relatives and the late onset of cysts in some, transplantation from living related donors needs to be carefully considered. Due to these worries, prospective living relatives should be thoroughly screened for signs of ADPKD or undergo genetic testing before making a live donation.

9.2.6.3. Polycystic Liver Disease

Since the majority of patients with polycystic liver disease do not exhibit symptoms, there is no recommended course of treatment and no effective medical therapies exist. It was suggested to avoid estrogen because postmenopausal women with ADPKD receiving hormone replacement therapy had a higher burden of hepatic cysts; however, no studies have shown that estrogen avoidance or estrogen receptor blockade is beneficial. CT-guided aspiration/sclerosis or laparoscopic cyst fenestration may be appropriate for patients with symptomatic liver disease and a few dominant cysts; however, most symptomatic patients have too many cysts for these procedures to be helpful. These procedures carry a risk of bleeding, bile leak, ascites, or recurrent symptoms; some patients may need to have an open laparotomy. Patients with hepatomegaly and severe symptoms have been tried with partial liver resection; however, there is a significant risk of perioperative morbidity. Patients with ESRD and severe refractory liver disease, as well as those with symptomatic portal hypertension, Budd-Chiari syndrome, or intrahepatic biliary obstruction, are candidates for orthotopic liver transplantation (OLT) or combined liver and kidney transplantation. For OLT alone, the five-year survival rate is 69%; for OLT plus renal transplantation, it is 76% (Everson et al., 2004).

9.2.6.4. Abdominal Pain

Given the prevalence of nephrolithiasis, renal cyst bleeding, diverticulitis, lower UTI, and cyst (hepatic or renal) infection, abdominal pain in patients with ADPKD should not be disregarded. Bed rest, hydration, and analgesics are the recommended treatments for nephrolithiasis. Renal cyst hemorrhage is typically self-limiting and can be managed similarly to nephrolithiasis; however, if pain intensifies, cautious measures should be taken because severe blood loss and hypovolemia have been reported in conjunction with retroperitoneal hemorrhage. Patients with end-stage ADPKD need to be treated for diverticulitis with antibiotics and bowel rest as soon as possible. The typical presentation of a lower UTI is dysuria, urgency, and frequency. For the recommended amount of time, oral antibiotics that treat gram-negative Enterobacteriaceae should be given.

On the other hand, cyst infections are more challenging to diagnose and cure. The observation that 92% of cyst infections occur in females suggests that ascending infection is most likely the cause of renal cyst infections. Hepatic cyst infections typically show up with fever and tenderness in the right upper quadrant, while renal cyst infections typically show up with fever and focal pain overlying the affected kidney. Some patients do, however, exhibit more subdued clinical symptoms. Positive urine cultures and pyuria are not always present in patients with renal cyst infections. The best diagnostic test for renal and hepatic cyst infection has been demonstrated to be a blood culture, although leukocytosis and elevated erythrocyte sedimentation rate can help in the diagnosis process. Although it can be costly, 18F-fluorodeoxyglucose positron emission tomography has emerged as a potentially useful tool for identifying infected cysts. For patients who have a suspected cyst infection, empirical therapy with an enteric-coating antibiotic (ciprofloxacin, trimethoprim-sulfisoxazole, or vancomycin) should be started. The common pathogens are Enterobacteriaceae. To ensure proper cyst penetration, if an organism is found, the patient should undergo an extended course of treatment that lasts at least four weeks. If the cyst infection does not improve, CT-guided drainage might be required.

9.2.6.5. Cardiac Disease

To check for valvular disease, left ventricular hypertrophy, and aortic root dilatation, periodic echocardiography should be carried out. If there is hemodynamically significant valvular insufficiency, subacute bacterial endocarditis prophylaxis should be administered before dental and gastrointestinal procedures. When regurgitation is severe and symptomatic, valve replacement is recommended.

If the aortic root diameter reaches 4 cm, monitoring of the aortic root should be done every month or every two months. If the aortic root diameter exceeds 5 cm, aortic root replacement is recommended. However, the data used to make this recommendation comes from patients who have Marfan syndrome. Studies on ADPKD patients that monitor the rate of aortic root dilatation or evaluate the association between aortic root diameter and the risk of aortic dissection do not currently exist. Furthermore, it is unknown if ß-blockade can effectively slow the rate of dilatation, as in Marfan syndrome, in ADPKD patients with aortic root dilatation.

9.2.6.6. Screening of Intracranial Aneurysm

It was not advised to routinely screen all ADPKD patients before the development of MRI and magnetic resonance angiography (MRA) due to the high risk of complications associated with the screening test, intraarterial angiography, which included the possibility of permanent neurologic deficit. The preferred method for screening for aneurysms is now high-resolution time-of-flight magnetic resonance imaging. The method is very sensitive and specific for aneurysms larger than 5 mm in diameter, but its sensitivity decreases significantly for smaller aneurysms. While CT angiography has been demonstrated to have higher sensitivity, patients with end-stage renal disease (ESRD) or chronic renal insufficiency (CRI) may not be able to participate in this study due to the intravenous contrast requirement.

The benefits of preventing SAH were outweighed by the operative complications, postoperative morbidity, and long-term loss of function that followed the successful identification of small, asymptomatic aneurysms through screening relatives of patients with the condition. It is imperative to exercise caution when extrapolating the data to patients with ADPKD, as only theoretical cost-benefit analyzes have been conducted.

Starting at age 20, the current recommendation is to screen only ADPKD patients with a family history of SAH or aneurysm, or with a history of SAH in the past. Other groups have recommended screening those planning major elective surgery because aneurysm rupture has been reported after renal transplantation. It has also been determined that those in "high-risk" occupations, like airline pilots, should undergo screening.

In a 10-year longitudinal study, very few people (2.4%), who had no aneurysm detected at initial screening, developed one. Research on patients whose screening aneurysm was discovered has demonstrated that aneurysmal enlargement or the formation of new aneurysms happens gradually. In one study, out of 18 patients whose aneurysm was discovered during screening, one had an enlargement of the preexisting aneurysm and the other developed a new one. The group of 10 patients who were imaged over an average of 10 years and who had previously been reported in a different study experienced both events. After being monitored for 10 years or longer, none of the patients experienced another aneurysm. In a different study, during an average follow-up period of 15 years, 25% (5 of 20) of people with previously diagnosed aneurysms developed new aneurysms. None of the five had recurrent intercranial bleeding; instead, four of them had intracranial aneurysms that were first discovered when they suffered an intercranial bleed. These results are consistent with other studies that have demonstrated a higher risk of aneurysm rupture in individuals who have had SAH, and they also indicate that these individuals have a high incidence of developing new aneurysms. These data suggest that individuals who screened negative should have the longest interval for reimaging (5–10 years), those with asymptomatic aneurysms an intermediate interval (3–5 years), and those with a prior history of SAH the shortest (1–3 years), even though there are no specific recommendations for imaging intervals. When an aneurysm is larger than 10 mm or symptomatic, patients should have intra-arterial coiling or clipping of the aneurysm performed.

9.2.6.7. Novel Therapies

Numerous promising medications that are undergoing clinical trials have been found as a result of improved pathophysiology knowledge and the accessibility of animal models. It has been demonstrated that inhibiting cAMP slows the growth of cysts. Vasopressin V2 receptor antagonists (VPV2R) inhibit the development of cysts in animal models by lowering renal levels of cAMP. Phase II clinical trials for the VPV2R tolvaptan have been completed, and a phase III trial is currently underway (NCT00428948). In the liver and kidney, cAMP is inhibited by somatostatin. For PKD and cystic liver disease, octreotide and lanreotide are being used in clinical trials (NCT00309283, NCT00426153, NCT00565097). Additionally, research on animals has demonstrated that the mTOR pathway plays a role in coordinating cell division and growth, an activity whose unchecked activation has been linked to the etiology of ADPKD. The mTOR inhibitors sirolimus and/or everolimus considerably impede cyst growth and safeguard renal function in animal models. These medications are being studied in prospective, randomized clinical trials (NCT00346918, NCT00286156, NCT00414440) (Torres et al., 2009).

9.3. Autosomal Recessive Polycystic Kidney Disease

The cystic kidney disease known as autosomal recessive polycystic kidney disease (ARPKD) typically affects children. Since this is a disorder that is recessively inherited, siblings may experience it while parents do not. Previously referred to as "infantile polycystic kidney disease," it is typified by renal collecting duct cystic dilations and hepatobiliary system developmental abnormalities, which lead to varied degrees of congenital hepatic fibrosis. About one case of ARPKD occurs for every 20,000 live births.

9.3.1. Pathogenesis

The PKHD1 gene on chromosome 6p21, which codes for the gene fibrocystin, is the cause of this disorder. Fibrocystin is present in the cortical and medullary collecting ducts, the thick ascending limb of the loop of Henle, and the hepatic bile duct's epithelial cells. In this disorder, abnormal renal cilia function is disrupted due to defective fibrocystin, which forms cysts. Patients with ARPKD typically have kidneys full of microcysts, which are typically smaller than 2 mm. These are observable as pinpoints on the surface of the kidney and radiate from the medullary junction to the cortex. The collecting ducts exhibit bilateral cystic dilatations on histopathologic examination of renal biopsies; however, there is no obstruction to the urine flow within these ducts. The proportion of nephrons with cysts directly affects the severity of renal manifestations. Renal cysts up to 1 cm in diameter and interstitial fibrosis can occur over time. Children who survive the neonatal period experience a progressive deterioration of their renal function as a result.

Almost invariably, developmental abnormalities of the biliary system are linked to ARPKD. This frequently manifests as massive dilatation and biliary dysgenesis, which can cause hepatomegaly and portal hypertension. It can also lead to varying degrees of congenital hepatic fibrosis and intrahepatic bile duct dilatation (Caroli disease).

9.3.2. Clinical Features and Natural History

The age at which ARPKD first manifests affects its clinical profile. Most often, patients show up with either hepatic or renal involvement. Individuals who are diagnosed with congenital hepatic fibrosis, whether as adolescents or adults, usually exhibit symptoms such as hepatomegaly and portal hypertension. ARPKD has been classified into the following forms based on their presenting features:

1. **Prenatal Form**: ARPKD is often detected prenatally during routine ultrasonography. Usually, it is considered in the presence of characteristic findings of markedly enlarged echogenic kidneys accompanied by oligohydramnios and the absence of urine in the fetal bladder.
2. **Neonatal Form**: Neonatal ARPKD presents with respiratory distress in a newborn due to pulmonary insufficiency resulting from pulmonary hypoplasia. A subset of patients may also have features of skeletal deformities. Renal insufficiency or hypertension may develop during the first few weeks of life.
3. **Infantile and Childhood Form**: This is the least severe form of ARPKD and over time there is gradual deterioration of renal function, eventually culminating in ESRD. A subset of older patients may present with signs and symptoms due to liver disease, with little evidence of renal involvement.

Without regard to ethnic variation, ARPKD affects roughly 1 in 10,000–40,000 live births. Since patients with mild disease may not receive a diagnosis until later in life and severely affected infants may pass away as newborns without a diagnosis, the true incidence may be higher. According to reports, the causative gene's carrier frequency is 1:70. Formerly thought to be a fatal condition that struck children, more recent case series show that the phenotypic severity and age of onset of ARPKD can vary widely. Roughly half of the cases are detected during pregnancy through ultrasound technology or at birth. ARPKD is strongly suggested by oligohydramnios, nephromegaly, echogenic kidney parenchyma, small cysts less than 2 cm in diameter, and loss of corticomedullary differentiation. Nevertheless, not all afflicted fetuses, especially those with milder involvement, exhibit these signs, making ultrasound an unreliable prenatal diagnostic tool.

Pneumothorax or pneumomediastinum due to pulmonary hypoplasia, talipes equinovarus from extrinsic compression, and Potter facies (hypertelorism, prominent infraorbital creases, flattened nasal bridge and tip, low-set, flattened, fleshy pinnae, and micrognathia) are all consequences of oligohydramnios. Neonatal mortality is attributed to critical respiratory insufficiency rather than renal or liver disease, with estimates ranging from 20 to 50% depending on the case series.

Research indicates that infants who make it through the first month of life are likely to survive the first year as well; survival rates at one year and five years are 78–87% and 50–87%, respectively. The estimated 10-year survival rate is 87%, while the 15-year survival rate varies between 67 and 79%. Significant morbidities await survivors and those in need of neonatal mechanical ventilation experience earlier onset of symptoms. 40% of patients have chronic renal failure, with a median onset of one day and one year in ventilated and nonventilated patients, respectively; approximately 20 to 25% of patients have growth retardation; and 65% have systemic hypertension. This disparity is most likely the result of children who were not diagnosed with ARPKD until later in infancy or childhood due to milder symptomatology and lack of respiratory insufficiency. 10 to 30% of patients have ESRD, which usually manifests in the first 10 years of life. Renal size does not grow as renal insufficiency worsens, in contrast to ADPKD.

The reliability of clinical signs and imaging results is lower in children who present beyond the neonatal period. Hepatic disease appears to be the more constant characteristic in these kids. A condition known as Caroli's disease, liver disease is characterized by aberrant intrahepatic biliary duct hyperproliferation and dilatation, which leads to hepatocellular damage, inflammation, and fibrosis. The function of hepatic synthesis is unaffected. Subsequent complications of ARPKD include portal hypertension, hepatosplenomegaly, recurrent cholangitis, and associated esophageal varices and upper gastrointestinal bleeding. According to the North American case series, 15–34% of patients had portal hypertension, with a median age of onset of 7 months for ventilated patients and 4.6 years for nonventilated patients. A small proportion of patients (2.4–7%) needed liver transplantation or portocaval shunting due to severe portal hypertension. There was no correlation found between the severity of hepatic disease and the presence of systemic hypertension or renal disease.

9.3.3. Gene Mapping, Structure, Function, and Genotype–Phenotype Correlations

Allelism of ARPKD to the PKD1 locus was not found in the early studies. The ARPKD locus, known as PKHD1 (polycystic kidney and hepatic disease 1), was discovered at 6p21-cen by the initial linkage studies. It was later refined to a 3.8 centiMorgan (cM) segment from 6p21.1–12 in the absence of evidence for a second locus. Seven years later, the gene was independently found within a month of each other by two groups, one using a rat model system to trace back to the human gene and the other looking through a cDNA transcription map of the PKHD1 region.

One of the biggest disease genes in the human genome, PKHD1 has at least 86 exons with different slice forms, the longest of which is 472 kb long. It is translated into a 447 kDa protein containing 4074 amino acids after encoding a 16.2 kb mRNA. The gene, which is termed polyductin by one group and fibrocystin by another, consists of a single transmembrane domain, a large, highly glycosylated N-terminal segment that contains multiple plexin and immunoglobulin-like domains, and a short cytoplasmic tail at the C-terminal. Fibrocytin's exact role is unknown, but domain analysis points to potential roles for the protein in the control of cellular adhesion, repulsion, and proliferation as well as the maintenance and control of the hepatic bile ducts and renal collecting tubules. In renal tubular epithelial cells, the PKHD1 protein product localizes to primary cilia and is concentrated in the basal body area.

There have been reported to be 702 distinct PKHD1 mutations to date, 378 of which are considered pathogenic. 36 (10%) splice site mutations, 56 (15%) nonsense mutations, 78 (21%) frameshift mutations, and 202 (53%) missense mutations are among them. Large PKHD1 deletions have also been reported, although they account for a much smaller percentage of cases. There is no sign of clustering among the mutations; they are dispersed throughout the gene. Similar to PKD1 and PKD2, every family has a different set of mutations that lead to a shortened protein product. One mutation, 107C>T (T36M), is probably a "hot spot" for mutations because it has been seen in unrelated patients from various ethnic backgrounds. In the Finnish population, there are two founder mutations: R496X and V3471G.

Although the correlation between genotype and phenotype is not entirely reliable due to intrafamilial phenotypic heterogeneity and high rates of compound heterozygosity, certain trends were evident in the results of the mutation analysis. Regardless of where the truncation occurred, all patients with a truncating mutation on both parental alleles passed away soon after birth. A study conducted on families categorized as "severe"—meaning that at least one child had to present with perinatal disease and neonatal death—found that 57% of the mutations found were truncating. 70% of families with "moderate" status (survival or diagnosis longer than one month) had missense mutations. On the other hand, perinatal death was associated with seven missense mutations. When only one mutant allele was found in a patient, it may indicate that there are more extensive genomic rearrangements, regulatory elements, or intron-specific mutations that are too small to be detected by gene sequencing. There is no distinct pattern of mutation in those with significant hepatic involvement.

9.3.4. Laboratory, Imaging, and Histopathologic Findings

Among these patients, decreased urinary concentrating ability is consistently observed. Serum chemistries and urinalysis reveal 25% hyponatremia, 60–67% elevated blood urea nitrogen (BUN) and serum creatinine, and 10–55% proteinuria. Nephromegaly, increased echogenicity, loss of corticomedullary differentiation, and numerous small cysts are all visible on renal ultrasonography. When a patient exhibits the typical signs of renal ultrasonography and is found to have hepatic fibrosis, parental consanguinity, no renal cysts in the parents, or a previous sibling with renal/hepatic pathology-diagnosed ARPKD, ARPKD can be diagnosed.

Dilation and elongation of the channels radiating from the medulla to the cortex at right angles to the cortical surface give kidney specimens a sponge-like appearance. Histopathologically, the cysts originate from the collecting ducts and distal convoluted tubules, in contrast to ADPKD cysts that can originate from any part of the nephron. Hepatic fibrosis and the usual ductal plate abnormality with biliary duct proliferation and dilatation are visible in the histopathology of the liver.

9.3.5. Diagnosis

The majority of the time, distinctive renal and hepatic findings on ultrasonography are used to diagnose ARPKD. Other imaging modalities, such as MRI or genetic testing, may be helpful in making the diagnosis in cases where it is unclear.

9.3.5.1. Molecular and Prenatal Diagnosis

Clinically available molecular testing for ARPKD can be carried out via linkage analysis or direct sequencing of the PKHD1 gene. Similar to PKD1 and PKD2, the abundance of private mutations and the ambiguous nature of variants may make it challenging to interpret sequence results. The mutation detection rate for the whole spectrum of ARPKD is now close to 85% thanks to the growing number of mutations registered in databases and new algorithms to assess the pathogenicity of variations. In certain instances, screening for significant deletions or gross rearrangements in PKHD1 may improve the diagnostic yield. Given that 35.7% of 14 children with isolated congenital hepatic fibrosis had PKHD1 mutations, molecular testing for the gene has been recommended for children with isolated Caroli's disease.

It is impossible to conduct routine ARPKD screening for all pregnant women because prenatal ultrasonography is specific but not sensitive. Because of this, families who seek a prenatal diagnosis of ARPKD frequently have a child or family member who is affected. This puts the expectant parents in a challenging and extremely emotional situation, necessitating a high level of sensitivity on the part of the prenatal counselor to their psychosocial needs. If the mutation(s) are known, then direct mutation detection is feasible. If not, cultured amniocytes or cytotrophoblasts can be used for linkage analysis or PKHD1 sequencing. A variant with unclear clinical significance or a mutation on only one allele, however, presents another challenging counseling scenario because the absence of a mutation in one allele does not imply the absence of disease. Preimplantation genetic diagnosis may become accessible as more facilities start providing prenatal diagnostic testing.

9.3.6. Management and Outcome

As of right now, there is no known cure for ARPKD. Supportive intervention for newborns' respiratory symptoms and renal replacement therapy—including hemodialysis and kidney transplantation—are the mainstays of care for patients who develop ESRD. Prenatal genetic testing is another component of counseling for siblings and family members of affected patients who might be carriers of a PKHD1 mutation. The age at presentation, the severity of renal and hepatic fibrosis, and the degree of pulmonary hypoplasia all influence the course of ARPKD.

9.4. Medullary Cystic Kidney Disease/Nephronophthisis

Small to normal-sized cysts at the corticomedullary junction are a defining feature of a group of genetic disorders known as nephronophthisis (NPH)/medullary cystic kidney disease (MCKD). Autosomal dominant MCKD and autosomal recessive NPH are the modes of inheritance. The type of extrarenal organ involvement and the age at which ESRD first manifested are additional characteristics.

10 to 20% of pediatric cases of renal failure are caused by NPH. It is linked to congenital hepatic fibrosis, cerebellar involvement, and retinitis pigmentosa in about 15% of the families. The majority of NPH cases are caused by NPHP1 gene defects. Depending on when ESRD first manifested, three different types of NPHP have been identified: infantile, juvenile, and adolescent.

MCKD is a chronic, progressive kidney disease that can reduce or preserve the kidney size. It is characterized by tubulointerstitial nephropathy and bilateral, multiple medullary cysts. MCKD comes in two varieties: type 1 and type 2.

Mutations in the MCKD1 gene, found on chromosome 1q21, cause type 1 MCKD, while mutations in the MCKD2 gene, found on chromosome 16p12, cause type 2 MCKD. Polyuria, polydipsia, hyperuricemia, and gradually worsening renal parenchymal disease that eventually leads to ESRD are characteristics of MCKD. The cornerstones of the diagnosis are the clinical features, hyperuricemia, gout, and adjuvant imaging studies. The imaging results show multiple cysts at the bilateral medulla/corticomedullary junction along with either preserved or reduced renal size. Renal replacement therapy combined with kidney transplantation is the only proven treatment for NPH/MCKD patients. The recurrence of MCKD in kidney transplant recipients is unknown.

9.4.1. Nephronophthisis

The four previously mentioned criteria collectively refer to a class of autosomal-recessive inherited renal disorders known as NPH. NPH usually manifests in childhood and is frequently linked to involvement of the extrarenal system. Although it is less common in the US population, it is the most common genetic cause of kidney failure in children and adolescents in Europe (>15%). Three common genetic mutations are known:

1. **NPH1**: Associated with juvenile NPH
   a. Associated with up to 85% of NPH cases
   b. Encodes for a protein called nephrocystin-1 that has an important function in cell–matrix interactions.
2. **NPH2**: Associated with infantile NPH
   a. Encodes for the protein inversin
   b. Age at onset of kidney failure is typically less than 30 months and always less than 5 years.
3. **NPH3**: Associated with adolescent NPH
   a. Specific protein has yet to be revealed
   b. The median age of kidney failure is approximately 19 years.

Renal cysts in NPH patients are limited to the medulla or the corticomedullary junction, and both kidneys are small. Clinical signs that are common include anemia, polyuria, growth retardation, salt wasting, and progressive kidney failure. In late childhood (mean age, 13 years), kidney failure and death occur without treatment, with dialysis or transplantation being the only options.

9.4.1.1. Clinical Features and Natural History

The most frequent genetic cause of renal failure during the first 30 years of life is nephronophthisis (Wolf et al., 2011). Nephronophthisis was first identified by Fanconi in 1950. Due to their similar renal histopathologic appearance and presenting symptoms, the two conditions were previously categorized together as medullary cystic kidney disease (MCKD). However, due to its autosomal dominant inheritance and later onset age compared to familial nephronophthisis, MCKD was later classified into a separate category.

Nephronophthisis is an autosomal recessive disorder with variable presentation and considerable locus heterogeneity (Caridi et al., 2000). Based on the age of onset, three distinct variants have been identified and categorized. Between the first and second decades of life, juvenile nephronophthisis typically manifests by the age of six, and end-stage renal disease (ESRD) develops by the median age of 13. When moms notice that their infants are changing their diapers too often, they may have infantile nephronophthisis. The adolescent variant presents with ESRD at a median age of 19 years. In all types, progressive CRI is invariable, and anemia develops out of proportion to the degree of renal insufficiency. CRI progresses to ESRD, and if untreated, death occurs by uremia.

9.4.1.1.1. Juvenile Nephronophthisis

Out of the three variations, juvenile nephronophthisis is the most prevalent. Patients show up with decreased urinary concentrating ability and polyuria due to tubular dysfunction. These kids have low urine osmolality despite being dehydrated, and vasopressin does not raise it, simulating nephrogenic diabetes insipidus. Because of sodium waste, hypertension is uncommon.

9.4.1.1.2. Infantile Nephronophthisis

The unusually early onset of infantile nephronophthisis and many phenotypic variations led to its recognition as a unique form of nephronophthisis. Premature birth is associated with oligohydramnios, Potter facies, and severe respiratory insufficiency without hepatic fibrosis, phenotypes similar to ARPKD. Individuals with hypertension and hyperkalemia instead of the usual polyuria and polydipsia are seen in infants and early childhood illnesses.

There may be cardiac abnormalities and situs inversus totalis. While tubular cell atrophy, interstitial cell infiltration, and fibrosis are typical of nephronophthisis, the renal histological phenotype is different from that of juvenile nephronophthisis in that it exhibits features of ARPKD (e.g., nephromegaly, microcystic cortical dilatation).

Infantile nephronophthisis is primarily caused by mutations in the NPHP2 gene. There is locus heterogeneity for infantile nephronophthisis, as evidenced by the recent reports of mutations in NPHP3 and NPHP9 in patients with very early-onset nephronophthisis.

9.4.1.1.3. Adolescent Nephronophthisis

With a reported median age of 19 years (range 4–37 years), ESRD is observed in late adolescence and early adulthood in cases of adolescent nephronophthisis. The first gene found to be responsible for adolescent nephronophthisis was NPHP3. RTPV-4 mutations cause retinitis pigmentosa in roughly 10% of families with affected children. Nonetheless, retinitis pigmentosa affects every patient who carries an NPHP5 mutation.

9.4.1.2. Syndromic Forms of Nephronophthisis

The condition's correlation with extrarenal malformations is another feature of nephronophthisis that sets it apart from MCKD. Separate kindsreds have reported cases of liver fibrosis, optic nerve colobomas, and cone-shaped epiphyses. This article discusses other types of nephronophthisis that have syndromic nomenclature and particular extrarenal malformations.

9.4.1.2.1. Joubert Syndrome

Congenital hypotonia, psychomotor retardation, tachypnea alternating with apnea, cerebellar ataxia, oculomotor apraxia, and, most significantly, aplasia or hypoplasia of the cerebellar vermis, which results in the well-known "molar tooth sign" on brain neuroimaging, are the characteristics of Joubert syndrome, an autosomal recessive condition. 25% of patients with Joubert syndrome have renal disease, which most frequently takes the form of nephronophthisis. Children usually exhibit polyuria and polydipsia in their first 10 years of life, which is followed by CRI and, by the time they reach their second decade of life, renal failure. While nephronophthisis with an infantile or adolescent onset is possible, juvenile nephronophthisis is the most frequently found type linked to Joubert syndrome.

Joubert syndrome is known to be caused by at least 10 distinct genes; additional loci are still unknown. AHI1, NPHP6, MKS3, and CC2D2A mutations each account for about 10% of cases. 1 to 2% of patients have an NPHP1 deletion that is homozygous (Parisi et al., 2006).

9.4.1.2.2. Senior–Løken Syndrome

This condition, which also goes by the names Senior syndrome and renal-retinal syndrome, is characterized by a mix of nephronophthisis and retinal pigment epithelium degeneration. It makes up roughly 10–15% of all cases of nephronophthisis. The histopathology and renal symptoms, including the age range of onset, are the same as in isolated nephronophthisis. Comparably, ocular pathology can begin at any time between birth and childhood. When a baby has Leber's congenital amaurosis, they exhibit near-absent pupillary reaction, nystagmus, blindness, or severe visual impairment. Elderly kids first exhibit nyctalopia, or night blindness, before gradually losing both of their peripheral vision. There is one report of an adult patient who has some preservation of visual fields and acuity, but color perception and central visual acuity are lost until end-stage disease, which usually happens in adolescence. A fundoscopic examination reveals the optic disk's pallor and attenuated blood vessels, but not the typical "bone spicule" retinal pigmentary abnormalities associated with retinitis pigmentosa.

Senior-Løken syndrome is primarily caused by mutations in NPHP5, although there have also been reports of mutations in NPHP1, NPHP2, NPHP3, and NPHP4 in addition to the classic 290 kb deletion. Furthermore, 20% of cases of Leber congenital amaurosis—a condition marked by an early onset of severe vision impairment from retinitis pigmentosa—are caused by mutations in NPHP6 and do not involve renal disease. Depending on the gene involved, retinitis pigmentosa in Senior-Løken syndrome can occur at different frequencies: 6% in cases of NPHP1 and 100% in cases of NPHP5 and NPHP6.

9.4.1.2.3. Meckel–Gruber Syndrome

With an estimated incidence ranging from 1:140,000 to 1:13,250 births, Meckel-Gruber syndrome is a severe and potentially fatal multiple congenital anomaly syndrome during fetal development. Similar to those with ARPKD, the infants have bilaterally enlarged, cystic kidneys as well as hepatic ductal plate dysplasia, biliary proliferation, and fibrosis. Both the medulla and the cortex are affected by renal cysts. Medullary cysts are larger, up to several millimeters in diameter, and separated by thick fibromuscular walls, whereas cortical cysts are typically small, thin-walled, and surrounded by normal glomeruli. Malformations of the central nervous system are severe. The most prevalent deformity is posterior encephalocele, but other patients have aplasia or hypoplasia of different central nervous system (CNS) structures, including the corpus callosum, cerebellum, cerebrum, optic or olfactory tracts. Another essential characteristic of the syndrome is preaxial or postaxial polydactyly. Transvaginal ultrasonography can detect Meckel-Gruber syndrome in fetuses as early as 10–12 weeks of gestation.

There is a well-established locus of heterogeneity and autosomal recessive inheritance. Meckel-Gruber syndrome has been linked to mutations in MKS1, TMEM216, MKS3/TMEM67, NPHP6/CEP290, NPHP8/RGRIP1L, NPHP3, and CC2D2A. Numerous of these genes are also associated with Joubert syndrome, indicating that these conditions are not distinct from one another but rather represent a spectrum of phenotypic variation.

9.4.1.2.4. Cogan-Type Oculomotor Apraxia

Individuals who have Cogan-type oculomotor apraxia are unable to initiate horizontal saccades and make voluntary, smooth movements of their eyes. They have to make abrupt, jerky movements of their heads to bring objects into view. There is no impairment to involuntary horizontal eye movements, suggesting normal firing of the oculomotor nerves. This disorder has been reported to be associated with nephrophilia; however, in contrast to Joubert syndrome, these patients do not exhibit retinitis pigmentosa or the molar tooth sign.

Patients with nephronophthisis and Cogan-type oculomotor apraxia have been found to have mutations in NPHP1 and NPHP4. One patient has been found to have the classic deletion of one allele and an inactivating splice junction point mutation of the other, while another patient has been reported to have homozygosity of the classic NPHP1 deletion. There is also evidence of homozygosity for the frameshifting 3272delT mutation in NPHP4.

9.4.1.2.5. Mainzer–Saldino Syndrome

It has been reported that cone-shaped epiphyses and nephronophthisis are related. Patients with this syndrome may also experience cerebral ataxia and retinal degeneration.

9.4.1.3. Gene Mapping, Structure, Function, and Genotype–Phenotype Correlations

In addition to the genes causing the syndromic forms of nephronophthisis, at least nine additional genes have been linked to the condition. A homozygous deletion of NPHP1 is the most frequent mutation in patients with nephronophthisis, accounting for 21% of cases. In 3% of cases, the remaining genes are involved, and in 70% of cases, the mutation is not known.

9.4.1.3.1. NPHP1

Nephronophthisis's initial gene locus was located at 2p through linkage analysis of 22 multiplex families. Using fine mapping techniques, the locus was first refined to 2q13 and then to a 2Mb critical region. In 80% of familial cases of nephronophthisis, a deletion of about 250 kb was found to map to the 2q13 locus. Within the deleted region, two ORFs were found; one encoded a small protein of 148 amino acids that was involved in cellular trafficking, and the other encoded a protein that was unknown at the time but was later found to be mutated in nephronophthisis patients.

The NPHP1 protein, also known as nephrocystin-1, encodes a 4.5kb mRNA and has 20 exons that cover 83 kb of the genome. The predicted protein has a length of 732 amino acids and a mass of 83 kDa. Protein-protein interaction motifs, coiled-coil domains and Src-homology 3 domain (SH3) are both present in it. Generally, "adapter" proteins—which link other proteins—have SH3 domains.

Nephrocystin-1 was demonstrated to bind the focal adhesion complex protein p130cas using the yeast 2-hybrid system. Nephrocystin-1 and p130cas have been shown by immunofluorescence to co-localize in vivo at basolateral cell membrane focal adhesions. The focal adhesion complex, which mediates signal transduction from the extracellular matrix to the nucleus, contains the cytosolic protein p130cas. Nephrocystin-1 was also discovered to co-localize at the transition zone of renal cell primary cilia with ß-tubulin and E-cadherin at adherens junctions. Furthermore, it forms a multiprotein complex through interactions with Jouberin and other nephrocystin proteins. These findings highlight the significance of cilia and cell–cell and cell–matrix interactions in inherited kidney disease, as do related findings from PKD1, PKD2, and PKHD1 localization.

As mentioned earlier, homozygous 290 kb deletion of NPHP1 is present in over 80% of patients with juvenile nephronophthisis. With two adjacent 45 kb repeats and two 330 kb inverted repeats surrounding the gene, the segment is vulnerable to intrachromosomal loop excision and unequal homologous recombination, which could result in an interstitial deletion.

There have also been reported nonsense, frameshift, and splice site mutations in NPHP1, all of which probably cause nephrocystin-1 to stop working. There is only one missense mutation known to exist, 1,024G>A, which results in a nonconservative amino acid alteration in a residue that is conserved in NPHP1 in dogs and mice.

It is unclear why some patients with the classic NPHP1 deletion only exhibit renal symptoms, while others have Cogan-type oculomotor apraxia, Senior-Løken syndrome, or Joubert syndrome. Extrarenal disease may be caused by additional genes that are located within the deleted region or near the deletion boundaries. Triallelic inheritance is a plausible explanation whereby multisystemic disease is caused by a mutation in a different gene in addition to NPHP deletion. Alternative hypotheses encompass minute reorganizations of breakpoints that remain imperceptible through haplotype analysis, or interference with enhancer sequences that modify the expression of genes beyond the deletion area.

9.4.1.3.2. NPHP2

The gene locus was identified by linkage analysis in an inbred Bedouin family with infantile nephronophthisis at 12.9cM, or 9q22–q31. The location of human inversin within the NPHP2 critical region and the finding of inversin mutations in the inv/inv mouse, which has enlarged, cystic kidneys, situs inversus, and histopathologic findings similar to nephronophthisis, strongly suggested that inversin was the candidate gene. The gene, later dubbed NPHP2 or INVS, was found to have recessive mutations in seven families with infantile nephronophthisis, providing confirmation.

NPHP2, a 100 kb genomic DNA gene with 17 exons, codes for the 1065 amino acid protein nephrocystin-2/inversin, which is conserved in both mice and zebrafish. A protein involved in the anaphase-promoting complex is bound by two “destruction” or D boxes, which also contain a split nuclear localization signal, two calmodulin-binding IQ domains, a highly conserved N-terminal domain with 16 tandem ankyrin repeats, and a cell-cycle regulatory ubiquitin ligase that controls the transition of cells from metaphase to anaphase and mitosis to G1. Inversin links with other proteins involved in cilia formation, maintenance, and intraflagellar transport by co-localizing with nephrocystin-1 in the renal tubular epithelium's primary cilia. Additionally, the idea that nephrocystin-2/inversin is involved in the preservation of normal planar cell polarity is supported by the cell-cycle-dependent expression of NPHP2 and its function in the Wnt signaling pathway.

In NPHP2, frameshift, missense, and splice site mutations have all been documented; the majority of these mutations cause truncation of the protein. In unrelated families, five recurrent mutations have been identified: Q485fsX509, Q671X, R899X, R907X, and E970fsX971. There are no discernible relationships between genotype and phenotype. One patient with homozygous missense mutations in a cohort of seven families with NPHP2 mutations did not experience ESRD until the age of five, and children of a family with compound heterozygous truncating mutations did not either. The only patient with mutations in both alleles that eliminated all domains C-terminal to the ankyrin repeats, including the nuclear localization domains, was the one with situs inversus totalis. This patient also had homozygous truncating R603X mutations.

9.4.1.3.3. NPHP3

Nephronophthisis in a large inbred Venezuelan family was found to be different from juvenile and infantile nephronophthisis at the time due to the later age of onset and the different gene locus. After a complete genome scan and higher resolution haplotype analysis, the family locus was located at 3q22, within a 3.3Mb interval. During this time, eight expressed sequence tags (ESTs) and seven genes with known functions were discovered.

Five ESTs were identified as potential genes after multiple families with Senior-Løken syndrome were mapped to the same region. Subsequent sequencing identified mutations in NPHP3, a 40.5 kb gene. Nephrocystin-3 is a 1,330 amino acid cytosolic protein product that is translated from a 3,990 nucleotide mRNA encoded by the 27 exons that make up NPHP3. The protein interacts with nephrocystin-1 and nephrocystin-2/inversin and has a tubulin tyrosine ligase domain and a coiled-coil region at the N-terminus. mRNA is expressed in the brain, retina, liver and biliary tract, renal tubules, respiratory epithelium, and node during gastrulation in embryonic mice. The pcy mouse mutant, which has cystic kidney disease because of a hypomorphic Nphp3 allele, is the result of mutations in the murine ortholog Nphp3. It's interesting to note that administering a vasopressin-2 receptor antagonist to PCY mice has been demonstrated to improve their condition by reducing renal cAMP levels. This finding could result in additional therapeutic initiatives.

As more cases are gathered, the phenotypic spectrum linked to NPHP3 mutations has expanded and now encompasses nephronophthisis in infants and adolescents, nephronophthisis with liver fibrosis, nephronophthisis with retinitis pigmentosa, and defects in embryonic patterning. In terms of genotype–phenotype correlations, missense and other non-truncating mutations are linked to a milder and later-onset disease, whereas truncating and splice site mutations in NPHP3 result in a more severe phenotype akin to Meckel–Gruber syndrome.

9.4.1.3.4. NPHP4

Even with the identification of NPHP1, NPHP2, and NPHP3, some kindreds were still not mapped to any of these loci. After those families were collected, a 2Mb region inside 1p36.31 was identified by linkage analysis. Six genes were found within a 700 kb interval after the region was narrowed by higher resolution haplotype mapping. Two teams designated the same gene, NPHP4, after discovering mutations in it.

Encoding nephrocystin-4/nephroretinin, a 1,426 amino acid protein product lacking known homologs in the human genome, is NPHP4, a large, 30-exon gene spanning 130 kb. With orthologs in the mouse, cow, pig, zebrafish, Xenopus, Ascaris, and Caenorhabditis elegans, it is a highly conserved protein. The ortholog from C. elegans has only 24% sequence identity with the human sequence, compared to 78% with the ortholog from mice. A putative nuclear localization signal, an acidic domain, and an SH3 domain are revealed by domain analysis; the latter two are also characteristics of nephrocystin-1. Nephrocystin-1, p130Cas, Pyk2, and other proteins combine to form a complex with nephrocystin-4. Its localization to centrosomes, basal bodies, and primary cilia is in line with the pathogenic mechanism of cystogenesis that has been linked to other nephrocystin proteins. Furthermore, Leber congenital amaurosis is caused by a deficiency in RPGRIP1 (retinitis pigmentosa GTPase regulator interacting protein 1), which is localized to the connecting cilia of photoreceptor cells where nephrocystin-4 interacts with it.

In 250 patients with nephronophthisis, NPHP4 underwent a recent mutational analysis. Of those patients, 26 (10%) had 23 novel sequence variants. Five out of eight (63%) of the six patients with homozygous or compound heterozygous mutations were considered to be loss-of-function or truncating mutations. Only one of the 20 patients who had a single sequence variant found was probably a loss-of-function mutation. There were no discernible genotype-phenotype relationships.

NPHP4 has been found to harbor nonsense, missense, frameshift, and splice site mutations in the past; the majority of these mutations result in a shortened protein. Homogygous missense mutations, G754R, R848W, and F991S, were discovered in three kindreds without extrarenal involvement, suggesting a potential genotype–phenotype association between isolated nephronophthisis and missense mutations.

9.4.1.3.5. NPHP5

NPHP5, also known as IQCB1, is composed of 15 exons and spans 65 points 7 kb. There is no translation for the first two exons. Nephrocystin-5, a 598 amino acid protein that is widely expressed in both fetal and adult tissues, is encoded by the NPHP5 gene. It contains two IQ calmodulin-binding regions in addition to a coiled-coil domain. Nephrocystin-5 localizes to primary cilia in renal epithelial cells and their homologous structures in the retina, photoreceptor connecting cilia. Nephrocystin-5 directly interacts with calmodulin and forms a complex with retinitis pigmentosa GTPase regulator (RPGR). Senior-Løken syndrome is caused by mutations in NPHP5, resulting in nephronophthisis and early-onset retinitis pigmentosa. There were no missense mutations discovered; all eight of the initial mutations reported led to protein truncation. The majority of those afflicted possessed homozygous mutations.

9.4.1.3.6. NPHP6

NPHP6, or CEP290, is a 93.2 kb RNA polymerase with 55 exons. Nephrocystin-6, a 290 kDa protein with 2,479 amino acids, is encoded by it. It also contains three tropomyosin homology domains, an ATP/GTP-binding site motif A (P-loop), six RepA/Rep^+ protein KID motifs (KID), a bipartite nuclear localization signal (NLS_BP), and a region with homology to structural maintenance of chromosomes (SMC) chromosome segregation ATPases[14]. Nephrocystin-6 localizes to photoreceptor cilia during interphase and to renal epithelial cellular centrosomes. It engages in interactions with nephrocystin-5 and ATF4, a transcription factor implicated in the control of the cell cycle and the formation of renal cysts that are dependent on cAMP. Leber congenital amaurosis, syndromic forms of nephronophthisis like Joubert syndrome and Meckel-Graber syndrome, and exclusive cystic renal disease can all result from mutations in NPHP6. All nine of the original reported mutations were either frameshift or nonsense mutations.

9.4.1.3.7. NPHP7

GLIS2, another name for NPHP7, is a protein with six exons that span more than 7.5 kb. Nephrocystin-7, also known as "Gli-similar protein 2," is a highly expressed protein in the kidney that localizes to renal epithelial cellular primary cilia and nuclei. Given that the GLIS2 protein and the Gli transcription factor are related, there may be a connection between the sonic hedgehog signaling network and cyst formation. The first reports of NPHP7 mutations came from a consanguineous Oji-Cree kindred. A homozygous transversion (IVS5+1G>T) affecting a splice donor site was present in affected individuals. Apart from this index family, NPHP7 mutations seem to be an uncommon cause of nephronophthisis.

9.4.1.3.8. NPHP8

NPHP8, also referred to as RPGRIP1L, is a 103.2 kb gene consisting of 27 exons, the last of which is noncoding. In human embryonic and fetal tissues, the encoded protein nephrocystin-8/RPGRIP1L (retinitis pigmentosa GTPase regulator interacting protein 1-like) is widely expressed. It has two protein kinase C conserved region 2 (C2) motifs in the central region, five coiled-coil domains, and a C-terminal region homologous to the RPGR-interacting domain of RPGRIP1. Nephrocystin-8 colocalizes with renal tubular cellular basal bodies, centrosomes, and primary cilia along with nephrocystin-4 and nephrocystin-6. The type of mutation can account for a portion of the spectrum of phenotypic variability seen in people with NPHP8 mutations. A homozygous truncating mutation in NPHP8 results in Meckel-Gruber syndrome or other severe phenotypes, while a late-onset, milder disease is caused by at least one missense mutation. There have been reports of frameshift, splice site, heterozygous and homozygous missense mutations in Joubert syndrome patients. Polydactyly, liver fibrosis, pituitary agenesis, and partial growth deficiency are possible extrarenal features.

9.4.1.3.9. NPHP9

Nephronophthisis is a very uncommon cause of NPHP9 or NEK8. Only three missense mutations in NPHP9 were found in a study of 588 patients with nephronophthisis; one of these patients also had a homozygous mutation in NPHP5, indicating a potential oligogenic inheritance. Nephrocystin-9 localizes to the primary cilia of renal tubular epithelial cells, just like all other known nephrocystin proteins. Nek8 mutations increase the expression of polycystin-1 and polycystin-2 in mouse models, and it has been demonstrated to interact with polycystin-2. Nephrocystin-9/NEK8 is also believed to be involved in the control of the cell cycle.

Apart from the previously mentioned genotype-phenotype correlations, the phenotypic variation observed in nephronophthisis does not seem to be exclusively related to the type of mutation or the gene involved. There is evidence that genetic modifiers are involved. Patients with nephronophthisis and retinal degeneration had a higher frequency of the AHI1 gene's R830W allele than patients with nephronophthisis alone (1.8% vs. 25%, $P = 5.36 \times 10^{-6}$), resulting in a relative risk of 7.5. This correlation held true irrespective of the predominant mutation. Similarly, in a small cohort with nephronophthisis, the RPGRIP1L gene's Thr229 variant was linked to retinitis pigmentosa. Further elucidation of the disease mechanism may reveal additional factors.

9.4.1.4. Laboratory, Imaging, and Pathologic Findings

Severe microcytic, hypochromic, hypoproliferative anemia caused by low erythropoietin secretion is revealed by a complete blood count. Serum creatinine and BUN are elevated, but creatinine clearance is reduced. Urine osmolality after dDAVP administration or water restriction is abnormally low in comparison to serum osmolality, which indicates a decrease in the ability to concentrate urine (also referred to as nephrogenic diabetes insipidus). Pyuria and proteinuria are uncommon. Renal ultrasonography reveals diminished corticomedullary differentiation, increased echogenicity, and normal to reduced renal size. It's vital to remember that corticomedullary cysts are not required for a diagnosis, even though they may be present. Disorganized tubular basement membranes, tubular atrophy with cyst formation, interstitial lymphohistiocytic infiltration, and periglomerular and interstitial fibrosis are among the typical histopathologic findings observed in renal biopsies. If Senior-Løken syndrome is suspected, patients with nephronophthisis should also be evaluated for ocular involvement using an electroretinogram and a fundoscopic examination. Patients with Joubert syndrome may exhibit the molar tooth sign on a brain MRI.

9.4.1.5. Molecular and Prenatal Diagnosis

It might be unclear which gene to test first due to the high level of phenotypic variation and genetic heterogeneity. Furthermore, not all of the genes linked to nephronophthisis can be tested clinically using molecular genetic methods. It has been suggested that an algorithm helps with decision making. It is best to start with testing for NPHP2 mutations in children under the age of five. Since a large percentage of cases of nephronophthisis are caused by the classic homozygous deletion, testing for this gene should start with NPHP1 in individuals older than 5 years. The type of extrarenal complications will determine whether or not other genes need to be tested if no mutations are found. Recent research has demonstrated that high-throughput sequencing is a useful technique for finding uncommon mutations. 30 (25%) of the 120 patients whose 18 genes were linked to nephronophthisis and its variant forms had a molecular diagnosis. In the future, more advanced diagnostic techniques will be made available for clinical use, including this one. Notably, no mutation is found in more than two-thirds of patients, suggesting that additional genes may still be unidentified. A thorough family history should be obtained in every situation, with a focus on consanguinity, early mortality, and renal illness.

9.4.1.6. Management

The underlying disease and its neurologic and ophthalmologic manifestations are not currently treated. Erythropoietin administration results in a response from the anemia. Acidosis, electrolyte imbalances, and hypovolemia are examples of complications of renal insufficiency that require supportive care. Renal function needs to be periodically monitored to start dialysis and register for transplantation registries as soon as end-stage renal disease (ESRD) occurs. Nephronophthisis transplant recipients have excellent outcomes that are superior to those of the general pediatric transplant population, according to the analysis of the North American Pediatric Renal Trials and Collaborative Studies database.

9.4.2. Medullary Cystic Kidney Disease

The four previously mentioned criteria define a group of autosomal-dominant inherited renal disorders known as Medullary Cystic Kidney Disease (MCKD). Usually, MCKD first manifests in early adulthood. About 50 new cases have been reported in the United States, making it an uncommon condition. S. each year. MCKD1 type 1 and MCKD2 type 2 are the two varieties.

Clinically, type 2 and type 2 are identical, though type 2 may be more severe. Misdiagnosis is common because symptoms are frequently vague and subtle (with elevated serum creatinine being the most common presenting sign). Similarly, patients with MCKD are also known to experience polyuria and polydipsia, which are signs of gout, hypertension, hyperuricemia, and progressive renal insufficiency. Family history, clinical suspicion, renal biopsy (which may reveal medullary cysts with tubulointerstitial nephritis but no thickening of the tubular basement membrane), ultrasound (which may reveal shrunken kidneys with cysts), and genetic testing (available for patients with type 2 disease) can all be used to make the diagnosis. Usually, kidney failure strikes between the ages of 20 and 60. Up until a kidney transplant is necessary, the course of treatment is supportive.

9.4.2.1. Clinical Features and Natural History

It is likely that the first family with MCKD was documented in 1966. The symptoms of juvenile nephronophthisis include polyuria, polydipsia, and isosthenuria, which can be present in patients. On the other hand, MCKD develops in adulthood and is dominantly inherited, in contrast to nephronophthisis. Furthermore, the majority of patients with metastatic kidney disease (MCKD) exhibit non-nephronophthisis-related symptoms such as hypertension (40%) or microalbuminuria (5%), gout (20%), or hyperuricemia (36%). The age at which ESRD and disease onset occur exhibits a bimodal pattern, with one peak occurring in the third or fourth decade of life and another in the fifth or sixth decade. The two MCKD loci that have been found to have different phenotypes are reflected in this pattern. Although there is occasional overlap, MCKD1 typically manifests later than MCKD2, which presents earlier.

The disease advances quickly, regardless of presentation age: the average time between diagnosis and end-stage renal disease (ESRD) is five years. As renal function declines, hyperuricemia typically gets worse. In later stages of the disease, hypotension takes the place of hypertension as patients become hyponatremic and lose their ability to concentrate renal fluid. Renal failure and uremia cause death if dialysis or transplantation is not started as a form of treatment.

9.4.2.2. Gene Mapping, Structure, Function, and Genotype–Phenotype Correlations

9.4.2.2.1. MCKD1

Linkage to the NPHP1 locus was ruled out in the early studies. After a second locus was found at 1p21, linkage analysis in a Cypriot family identified a locus for MCKD, which was subsequently dubbed MCKD1. Through fine mapping, the critical region was reduced to a 3.3Mb region. When no mutations were discovered in either of the two candidate genes—the rhesus blood group B glycoprotein genes and the natriuretic peptide receptor A (NPR-A)—

they were eliminated from consideration. A 2.1 Mb interval was determined to be the final critical region. After conducting a mutational analysis on 37 genes located within the critical region, three distinct sequence variations were found in each gene, each of which segregated within a specific family. Therefore, it is still unknown which gene is the sole cause. On the other hand, several genes might be at play.

9.4.2.2.2. MCKD2

After analysis of an Italian pedigree revealed that several MCKD kindreds did not exhibit linkage to the MCKD1 critical region, 16p12 was discovered to be a second MCKD locus. One MCKD2 family did not have isosthenuria, hyperuricemia, or gout, while the Italian MCKD2 family did have an earlier disease onset, isosthenuria, and more severe hyperuricemia and gout. The critical interval was reduced to a 1.3Mb region after a family with medullary cysts and familial juvenile hyperuricemic nephropathy (FJHN) had their mapping to 16p12, indicating that both FJHN and MCKD2 were allelic.

Families with FJHN were found to have pathogenic mutations in the uromodulin gene UMOD, and sequencing of UMOD in patients with MCKD2 also revealed pathogenic mutations. The human genome's 18.6 kb is covered by the 12 exons (10 coding) of the uromodulin gene. It is translated into a 640 amino acid protein known as Tamm-Horsfall protein after being transcribed into a 2.4kb mRNA. The epithelium of the early distal convoluted tubules and the thick ascending loop (TAL) of Henle express uromodulin/Tamm-Horsfall protein (UMOD/THP). By breaking the glycosyl phosphatidylinositol linkage that anchors UMOD to the plasma membrane, the protein is released. It is composed of two zona pellucida (ZP) domains that facilitate polymerization into fibers that form a gel that is impermeable to water but allows ion flux, and two calcium-binding epidermal growth factor (cbEGF) domains. Therefore, it is believed that uromodulin gives the TAL its water impermeability, allowing the kidney to concentrate urine. It is also thought to prevent ischemia and UTIs, as well as inhibit the formation of renal stones.

Exon 4, which codes for the cbEGF domains, is the location of all known UMOD mutations, which are either missense or inframe deletions/insertions. A homozygous UMOD mutation family was found to live to adulthood, although they experienced more severe hyperuricemia and accelerated ESRD progression.

A noteworthy discovery that could potentially shed light on the pathogenesis of MCKD is the fact that most mutations impact conserved cysteine residues. Uromodulin does not contain any free sulfhydryl groups, suggesting that these mutations affect appropriate disulfide bonding and protein folding. A finding for mutated uromodulin is that misfolded endoplasmic reticulum (ER) proteins tend to aggregate within the ER rather than being secreted. The isosthenuria observed in patients with MCKD2 may be explained by decreased UMOD secretion in the TAL of the nephron, which would increase water permeability and reduce renal concentrating ability. Hyperuricemia is caused by compensatory distal convoluted tubule and collecting duct reabsorption as well as secondary urate reabsorption, which are brought on by increased excretion of salt and water. An accumulation of misfolded, non-biodegradable uromodulin causes tubular cells to undergo apoptosis. When UMOD is released into the interstitium, the body responds by becoming inflamed, which ultimately results in fibrosis.

9.4.2.2.3. Other Loci

Families that mapped neither to the MCKD1 locus nor to the MCKD2 locus were found through linkage analysis of MCKD kindreds, indicating the possibility of additional MCKD loci.

9.4.2.3. Imaging and Histopathologic Findings

Reduced cortical thickness and normal to decreased renal size are seen on renal ultrasonography. While 40% of patients may have bilateral corticomedullary or medullary cysts, these cysts are neither pathognomonic for MCKD nor required for a diagnosis. Histopathologic results of renal biopsies show the same features as those of biopsies from patients with nephronophthisis: tubular atrophy with cyst formation, interstitial lymphohistiocytic infiltration, periglomerular and interstitial fibrosis, and disorganized tubular basement membranes.

9.4.2.4. Molecular and Prenatal Diagnosis

The main methods used to make the diagnosis are imaging results, suggestive clinical features, and, if available, renal histopathologic findings. Since no particular gene has been found to cause MCKD1, testing at-risk individuals necessitates a large enough family with multiple affected members to provide adequate power for linkage analysis. For MCKD2, confirmatory molecular testing is offered on a paid basis. Testing during pregnancy or on children who show no symptoms is not advised for a disease that can be treated but does not manifest until adulthood.

9.4.2.5. Management

Treatment options are restricted to supportive care because the underlying disorder is not treatable with therapy. With allopurinol, hyperuricemia and gout are managed. When ESRD first appears, interval evaluation of renal function should be carried out to determine when dialysis and renal transplantation should be started. Family members with MCKD who want to donate their kidneys must be ruled out as donors. Renal transplantation has excellent results; cystic disease does not develop in the graft kidney.

9.5. Von Hippel–Lindau Syndrome

A rare condition known as von Hippel-Lindau (VHL) syndrome is characterized by the presence of multiple benign tumors and visceral cysts, many of which develop into malignant transformations. Hemangioblastomas of the central nervous system and retina, pheochromocytomas, and kidney, liver, and pancreatic cysts are common signs of VHL. Given the wide variation in clinical presentation among patients, a thorough investigation into the possibility of VHL is warranted upon the discovery of any of these findings or a suspicious family history.

The gene causing VHL is found on the short arm of chromosome 3, and the condition is inherited as an autosomal-dominant trait. The germ-line mutation affects about 1 in 36,000 people at birth, though the first symptoms and signs are usually not noticed until a mean of 26 years old. Similar to ADPKD, the pathophysiology of VHL most likely corresponds to the two-hit model, in which a person is born with one nonfunctioning allele. Later in life, the loss of the complementary allele causes an abnormal tumor suppressor gene, uncontrolled growth, and ultimately the VHL aftereffects.

The majority of VHL-related deaths occur from clear-cell renal carcinoma, which eventually manifests in 40% of affected individuals. Since renal cysts are thought to be premalignant, careful screening and observation are essential. To identify primary tumors, diagnostic studies use CT, MRI, and ultrasound; to verify the presence of VHL, genetic testing is used.

The mainstay of treatment is surgery, aside from routine surveillance. It has been demonstrated that renal-sparing surgical methods, such as radiofrequency ablation and partial nephrectomy, are just as successful as total nephrectomy but have fewer unfavorable side effects, such as the requirement for dialysis. With such therapeutic advancements, outcomes have improved, but VHL remains a devastating disease with an average life expectancy of 49 years.

9.6. Medullary Sponge Kidney

A diffuse or focal ectasia, cystic dilatation of the collecting ducts, and cyst formation limited to medullary pyramids are symptoms of medullary sponge kidney (MSK). It is postulated that it arises from interference with the interface between the metanephric blastema and the developing ureteral bud during embryogenesis. Though some patients may present with renal colic, hematuria, or recurrent urinary tract infections, most MSK patients are asymptomatic. Intravenous urography provides the distinctive "paint brush" appearance, contrast accumulation, and linear radiation from the calyces for the diagnosis of MSK. Because of the calcium buildup in the impacted tubules, the medullary pyramids appear uniformly hyperechoic on ultrasonography. Medullary nephrocalcinosis is frequently detected on CT examination, and stones within the dilated collecting ducts and "papillary brush" morphology are seen on CT urography. Compared to other cystic kidney diseases, MSK has a better long-term prognosis and lower morbidity; however, the consequences of recurring urinary tract obstruction and infections can lead to progressive renal failure and ESRD.

9.7. Simple Renal Cysts

The most prevalent type of acquired renal cystic lesion, simple renal cysts affect men twice as often as they do women. They are filled with fluid and can be one or more. While extremely uncommon in young children, their frequency rises with age. Although the pathogenic mechanisms underlying simple renal cysts are unknown, the diverticula of distal convoluted and collecting tubules are most likely where they begin.

Most simple cysts don't cause any symptoms. Patients may show up with flank pain, urinary tract infection, polycythemia, hematuria, or obstruction of the collecting system. While there is no enlargement of the kidneys, there may be large cysts without any smaller ones nearby. There are no cysts in the other organs. These cysts have little effect on the prognosis of the patient and do not affect renal function. It can be challenging to distinguish between a simple cyst and renal cell carcinoma because a renal mass seen on an excretory urogram by itself does not rule out cancer. To characterize the lesion, magnetic resonance imaging, computed tomography, or ultrasound are frequently needed. Differentiating between a simple renal cyst and a complex renal cyst, which is linked to a higher risk of malignancy, is the main clinical concern.

Only cysts that cause obstruction or have symptoms should be treated. Cysts of intermediate size can be percutaneously aspirated. For large cysts larger than 500 ml in volume, laparoscopic cyst unroofing might be a better option.

9.8. Acquired Cystic Kidney Disease

Patients with chronic renal failure unrelated to inherited renal cystic diseases are diagnosed with acquired cystic kidney disease (ACKD), a non-hereditary developmental disorder characterized by small cysts scattered throughout the renal cortex and medulla. Patients with ACKD present with three or more renal cysts in both kidneys. These cysts typically have a diameter of 0.5 to 2.5 cm. Even though there is clear evidence linking hemodialysis to the development of ACKD, at least 8–13% of patients experience cyst development before starting dialysis. The compensatory hypertrophy of the functioning nephrons in ESRD patients, which results in the secretion of mitogens that cause renal tubular epithelial hyperplasia and may lead to the development of renal cell carcinoma, is the first insult in the development of ACKD.

Usually asymptomatic, the disease is unintentionally found during abdominal imaging procedures. Cyst bleeding, spontaneous rupture resulting in a pericystic hematoma, cyst infection, ureteric stone development, and renal cell carcinoma are among the complications linked to ACKD. The absence of a family history of ADPKD and small or normal-sized kidneys with a smooth contour help to distinguish ACKD from ADPKD. After a successful kidney transplant, the cysts might stabilize or shrink.

9.9. Multicystic Dysplastic Kidney Disease (MKD)

Congenital MDK is identified by ultrasonography as cysts of varying sizes with lost lobar organization. Subtle ductules and cartilage are present, along with a loss of normal structure under the microscope that suggests abnormalities in renal differentiation. Cysts resulting from dysplasia can be large or small, solid or cystic. The function is not fixed.

Typically, MDK manifests as an abdominal mass during the neonatal stage. Uncommon additional notable symptoms include flank pain, dysuria, frequent urination, failure to thrive, and urinary tract infections. The majority of MKD cases are intermittent. MKD, however, can present as a renal symptom in several syndromes. These include certain chromosomal trisomies, brachio-oto-renal syndrome, Williams syndrome, Beckwith-Wiedemann syndrome, Meckel-Gruber syndrome, Jeune asphyxiating thoracic dystrophy, Zellweger syndrome, VACTERL association, and others.

9.10. Genetic Syndromes With Cystic Renal Disease as a Major Component

9.10.1. Tuberous Sclerosis Complex

A neurocutaneous condition known as tuberous sclerosis complex affects one in 5,000 to 10,000 live births. It is characterized by the involvement of numerous organ systems, including the skin, liver, kidney, heart, brain, eye, and lung in addition to benign hamartomas.

The most prevalent renal manifestations are angiomyolipomas, which are followed by renal cysts and lymphangiomas. Bleeding is more likely in angiomyolipomas, especially if the enlargement progresses. In 1–2% of cases, renal cell carcinoma develops. For patients with TSC, the Consensus Conference recommended the following surveillance imaging studies. When a patient is diagnosed, renal ultrasonography should be done to determine whether they have angiomyolipomas or the polycystic variant of TSC. Renal ultrasonography screening should be performed on all children with TSC every 1–3 years (or every 3 years if no previous lesions are visible on imaging). Abdominal CT or MRI should be done to assess any abnormalities if malignant transformation or the emergence of large angiomyolipomas (larger than 3–5 cm) are found. To stop bleeding, interventional radiology can be consulted for treatment of lesions larger than 3–5 cm.

The expression of tuberous sclerosis complex varies and it is inherited autosomally dominantly. The disorder is known to be caused by two genes: TSC1, which is found on chromosome 9q34, and TSC2, which is found on chromosome 16p13.3, which is near the PKD1 gene. The combined phenotype of ADPKD and tuberous sclerosis is caused by a contiguous gene deletion syndrome involving TSC2 and PKD1. Whereas TSC2 encodes tuberin, TSC1 encodes hamartin. By interacting, the two proteins create a complex. 70 to 80% of affected individuals who meet specific clinical criteria have a detectable mutation in one of these two genes, with TSC2 being more commonly implicated. Most mutations are due to sequence variants, although both genes have also been reported to have significant deletions and rearrangements. People with a TSC1 mutation seem to have a milder disease than those with a TSC2 mutation, according to genotype-phenotype correlations. In one study, patients with TSC1 mutations had lower rates of mental retardation and seizures, fewer cortical tubers and subependymal nodules, milder kidney involvement, no retinal hamartomas, and less severe facial angiofibroma. Furthermore, compared to de novo TSC2 mutations, mutations in familial TSC2 cases seem to be linked to less severe clinical manifestations.

9.10.2. Bardet–Biedl Syndrome

With 14 gene loci found so far, Bardet-Biedl syndrome (BBS) is a genetically heterogeneous disorder. Although most forms have a distinct triallelic inheritance pattern requiring recessive mutations at one locus and an additional mutation at a second locus, it is usually inherited in an autosomal recessive manner. Due to significant phenotypic variability, a classification scheme with a minimum of four major diagnostic criteria has been proposed. Learning disability (62–187%), rod-cone dystrophy (92–100%), postaxial polydactyly (58–74%), truncal obesity (72–196%), hypogonadism in males (74–66%), and renal anomalies (46–45) are the main diagnostic criteria. Additional common characteristics include speech impairment (54%), motor and speech delay (50%), hypertension (50%), ataxia (40%), "difficult," immature, volatile behavior with no inhibition and easy frustration (33%), dental crowding (27%), and asthma (25%). Commercial molecular diagnostic testing is available.

Certain characteristics of nephronophthisis are also present in BBS patients, including polyuria, polydipsia, nyctalopia that progresses to total blindness in the second decade of life, hepatic fibrosis, and chronic renal failure. Sometimes renal pathology can be confused with MCKD and nephronophthisis. However, progression to ESRD is uncommon. Cortical cysts, calyceal blunting, hydronephrosis, vesicoureteral reflux with recurrent UTI, renal dysplasia, and fetal lobulation are examples of structural renal anomalies.

The BBS8 protein's ability to localize to centrosomes and co-localize with tubulin provided evidence for a potential connection to inversin (NPHP2), cilia, and cell cycle regulation. Additionally, it was discovered that patients with homozygous BBS8 mutations had randomization of body situs. BBS proteins typically localize to basal bodies, centrosomes, or cilia.

9.10.3. Jeune Asphyxiating Thoracic Dysplasia and the Short-Rib Polydactyly Syndromes

Because of their shortened, horizontal ribs, patients with asphyxiating thoracic dysplasia (ATD) have extremely constricted and narrow thoracic cages. Because of the small chest cavity, severe pulmonary hypoplasia frequently results in death in infancy. Recurrent pneumonia and the risk of respiratory failure due to restrictive lung disease are challenges faced by survivors. Postaxial polydactyly of the hands and/or feet is present in certain patients, and long bones and phalanges are shortened. Radiographs reveal transient irregularity of epiphyses and metaphyses, hypoplastic iliac wings with trident-shaped acetabulae, short ribs with irregular costochondral junctions, and cone-shaped phalangeal epiphyses. Along with hepatic fibrosis, pancreatic cysts and fibrosis, polycystic kidneys, and biliary ductal plate malformations, children also experience improvements with age in short stature and relative thoracic cage size. Cystic renal tubular dysplasia, tubular atrophy, possibly disordered tubular basement membranes, interstitial infiltration, and fibrosis observed in nephronophthisis are all observed in renal histopathology. It's interesting to note that some ATD patients experience situs inversus and tapetoretinal degeneration, conditions that are also common in nephronophthisis patients. ATD is currently linked to two causative genes: DYNC2H1 and IFT80. Like BBS and nephronophthisis, IFT80 and DYNC2H1 are involved in microtubular and/or ciliary function.

ATD is a member of the short-rib dysplasia family of skeletal dysplasias, which also includes Barnes thoracolaryngopelvic dysplasia, Ellis-van Creveld dysplasia, and the four neonatal lethal short-rib polydactyly (SRP) syndromes. SRP syndrome-affected infants are hydropic and pass away from respiratory insufficiency during the perinatal stage. There is cystic renal disease in each of the four forms of SRP. They are all affected by gastrointestinal malformations (esophageal, intestinal, or anal atresia in SRP I, II, and III, malrotation in IV), micromelia, postaxial polydactyly, and CNS malformations (Dandy–Walker malformation, pachygyria, holoprosencephaly, and anencephaly). SRP types II and IV have a median cleft lip and palate along with a bifid epiglottis. Similar to ATD and ARPKD, hepatic and pancreatic cysts with fibrosis are also observed in SRP IV infants.

9.10.4. Hajdu–Cheney Syndrome

The middle and distal phalanges of the hands and feet gradually and slowly resorb due to this autosomal dominant skeletal dysplasia, which is an acroosteolytic disorder that starts in adolescence. In affected infants, sagittal and/or lambdoid suture widening is the first abnormality seen. Persistently open sutures, Wormian bones, elongation of the Sella turcica, coarse hair and facies, broad forehead, hypertelorism with down-slanting palpebral fissures, broad nasal bridge, and early tooth loss are additional craniofacial abnormalities that develop with age. Osteoporosis, joint laxity, and short stature are also noted. About 10–14% of affected children had polycystic kidneys, which are similar to ADPKD. These kidneys frequently had concurrent hypertension and CRI. There have been reports of additional renal abnormalities, including glomerulonephritis, vesicoureteral reflux, and unilateral multicystic dysplastic kidney.

9.10.5. Campomelia, Cumming Type

Premature stillbirth, cervical hygromas with hydrops fetalis, narrow chest, shortened limbs with bowing of all long bones, especially the tibiae and ulnae, and a cloverleaf skull are the hallmarks of this autosomal recessive skeletal dysplasia. Hepatic fibrosis, pancreatic fibrosis, renal cortical and medullary cysts, and biliary ductal plate malformation are observed. There have been reports of multiple fetuses with situs anomalies, including dextrocardia, left-sided superior vena cava, right-sided aortic arch, total anomalous pulmonary venous return, and polysplenia.

9.10.6. Glutaric Acidemia Type II

Mutations in the ETFA, ETFB, or ETFDH genes, which encode the electron transport flavoprotein (ETF) and ETF ubiquinone oxidoreductase (ETF:QO), result in glutaric acidemia type II, also known as multiple acyl-CoA dehydrogenase deficiency, an autosomal recessive disorder. In the metabolism of branched-chain amino acids, long-chain fatty acids, and choline, ETF is the most important electron acceptor. Electrons are moved from ETF to the electron transport chain via ETF:QO. A combination of fatty acid oxidation disorders, isovaleric acidemia, metabolic acidosis, hypoketotic hypoglycemia, hepatomegaly, hypotonia, and a "sweaty foot" odor characterize the phenotype caused by an enzyme deficiency. There may be deformities like telecanthus, high forehead, flat nasal bridge, enlarged anterior fontanel, and ear abnormalities. Particularly in patients with more advanced disease, bilaterally enlarged, polycystic kidneys with medullary dysplasia can be observed. Urine organic acid analysis and plasma acylcarnitine can be used to make a preliminary diagnosis. The diagnosis is confirmed by the fibroblast assay of ETF and ETF:QO activity and the molecular genetic testing of ETFA, ETFB, and ETFDH.

9.10.7. Carnitine Palmitoyltransferase II Deficiency, Neonatal Lethal Form

After translocation into the mitochondrion, the enzyme carnitine palmitoyltransferase II (CPT II) catalyzes the reconjugation of long and very-long-chain acylcarnitines to coenzyme A. As a result, individuals with CPT II deficiency cannot metabolize long-chain fatty acids and experience energy deficits when fasting. Although severely affected infants with lethargy, poor feeding, tachypnea, metabolic acidosis, hepatomegaly, hypothermia, and hypoglycemia in the first few days of life may have enlarged, polycystic kidneys with parenchymal dysplasia, CPT II deficiency can manifest at any time. Urine organic acid analysis, plasma acylcarnitine profile, and free and total carnitine levels can all be used to make an assumption diagnosis. By assessing CPT II activity in fibroblasts or performing molecular testing on the CPT2 gene, the diagnosis is verified.

9.10.8. Zellweger Syndrome

Zellweger syndrome, also called cerebrohepatorenal syndrome, is a peroxisome biogenesis disorder at the severe end of a clinical spectrum that also includes infantile Refsum disease and neonatal adrenoleukodystrophy. There is genetic diversity in this group of disorders. 12 distinct genes encoding proteins required for regular peroxisome assembly have been found to be mutated. The most frequently implicated gene is PEX1, and autosomal recessive inheritance governs all forms. Early infancy: Patients exhibit poor feeding, severe hypotonia, and hyporeflexia. Many people are first thought to have a particular kind of myopathy. A dysmorphologic examination reveals hepatomegaly, hypertelorism with upslanting palpebral fissures, flat facies, high forehead, and macrocephaly with an exceptionally large anterior fontanelle. Stippling of the patellae and long bone epiphyses are visible on plain-film X-rays. The majority of patients experience myoclonic or generalized tonic-clonic seizures in addition to brain abnormalities. The survivors are profoundly mentally retarded, and the great majority pass away before turning one year old. Most patients have kidneys with polycystic kidneys. Measurements of plasma very-long-chain fatty acids, which are elevated in Zellweger syndrome, can be used to screen for the condition. Measurements of phytanic acid and pristanic acids in plasma, bile acid intermediates, and analysis of plasmalogens in erythrocytes are possible additional tests. Fibroblasts can be used in complementation studies to determine which peroxisomal gene is lacking. For many of the PEX genes, molecular diagnostic testing is offered in the commercial domain (Wilson, 2004).

A Closer Look

Mechanisms of Cystogenesis

How do mutations in the polycystins, fibrocystin, and nephrocystins result in cyst formation? While all the mechanisms are not clear, increasing knowledge of the primary cilia of renal tubular epithelial cells has shed light on some of the mechanisms.

Each epithelial cell of the distal convoluted tubule and collecting duct contains a single primary cilium that is nonmotile, with microtubules arranged in a $9_{+}0$ pattern. Once thought to be a vestigial organelle, the primary cilium is now known to be necessary for sensing extracellular shear stress from perpendicular fluid flow and transducing an increase in intracellular calcium ion concentration. Studies have also shown that primary cilia are necessary for the maintenance of planar cell polarity through various cellular signaling pathways (e.g., Wnt signaling), and loss of cilia results in abnormal orientation of cell division and cystogenesis.

Polycystin-1, polycystin-2, fibrocystin, and the nephrocystins all localize to the primary cilia of renal epithelial cells, and some at basal bodies, centrosomes, focal adhesions or adherens junctions. Likewise, the genes associated with syndromic forms of cystic kidney disease (i.e., Joubert syndrome, BBS, Meckel–Gruber syndrome, etc.) demonstrate similar localization.

Polycystin-1 and polycystin-2 directly interact with one another through their C-terminal coiled-coil domains to form a complex. This complex mediates calcium influx in response to shear stress by sensing the bending of the primary cilium. The large extracellular domain of polycystin-1 functions as a mechanosensor of urine flow, which triggers calcium influx through polycystin-2 channels. The initial calcium current has been shown to "feed forward" and trigger the release of intraorganellar calcium stores via the ryanodine receptor. The polycystin complex is also believed to play a role in the regulation of the cell cycle. Expression of mutant PKD1, blockade with polycystin-1- and polycystin-2- specific antibodies or other disruptions of this system results in impaired calcium influx, leading to increased cAMP levels, and ultimately, abnormal cell proliferation and cell dedifferentiation. The flow-sensor function of the polycystins in the primary cilium may be a contributing pathway in the pathogenesis of cyst formation in kidneys with obstructed flow, such as ureteropelvic or ureterovesicular junction obstruction.

Nephrocystin-1 and fibrocystin have also been found at the primary cilium in association with the polycystin protein complex and are also thought to participate in the same mechanotransduction pathway.

The Wnt signaling pathway is an integral part of the pathogenic process of renal cyst formation. Under normal circumstances, cilia respond to fluid flow, and the calcium signaling cascade is initiated. As a result, several proteins, including nephrocystin-2/inversin and the BBS proteins, are activated and shift the Wnt pathway from its canonical to noncanonical mode. As a result of this shift, β-catenin, which normally acts as a transcriptional activator, is degraded by proteasomes, and normal planar cell polarity is maintained. When calcium signaling or ciliary proteins are defective, the canonical Wnt pathway predominates, and β-catenin can translocate into the nucleus where it forms an active transcription factor complex with the T-cell-specific transcription factor/lymphoid enhancer binding factor (TCF/LEF) and promotes the expression of fetal genes to induce cell proliferation and differentiation, ultimately resulting in cyst formation.

Polycystin-1, polycystin-2, and nephrocystin-1 also aggregate into a complex that co-localizes in vivo with α2β1 integrin and co-immunoprecipitate with multiple focal adhesion adaptor proteins, most notably focal adhesion kinase, c-src, and p130cas. In response to ligand binding, the polycystin complex activates c-Jun kinase and mitogen-associated protein kinase via focal adhesion adaptor proteins, leading to phosphorylation and activation of the c-Jun protein, a member of the AP-1 transcription factor family. Phosphorylated c-Jun dimerizes with ATF, another member of the AP-1 family, to create an active transcription factor that drives the expression of genes responsible for differentiation and reduction of proliferation in developing renal tubular epithelium. Inactivation of AP-1 transcription factor-mediated gene expression by abrogation of polycystin-1 and/or 2 signaling results in inability to downregulate proliferation and fetal gene expression, leading to conditions that foster cyst formation. The exact role of nephrocystin-1 at the focal adhesion complex is not well defined, although its SH3 domain may be responsible for recruiting c-src and p130cas to the polycystin protein complex.

The function of the other nephronophthisis genes, especially in relation to cerebral and ocular development, is less well defined. While nephrocystin-3 and nephrocystin-4 have been found to associate with nephrocystin-1, it is not yet known which signaling pathways they participate in and how. Inversin interacts with the anaphase-promoting complex via its two "destruction-box" domains, possibly linking environmental stimuli sensed by primary cilia to the centrosome and regulation of cell division. Finally, inversin is involved in early embryogenesis as one of the determinants of left–right axis patterning, perhaps through its interaction with mechanosensory cilia.

Much progress has been made in our understanding of renal cystogenesis. Although questions remain to be answered, our increasing knowledge of the genetic and molecular basis of cystic kidney diseases will enhance insight into the pathogenesis, clinical consequences, and ultimately, the treatment of these disorders.

Summary

- Cystic diseases of the kidney include a broad range of disorders, presenting in infants, children and adults with numerous phenotypic expressions. These account for around 10% of patients with end-stage renal disease (ESRD) and are prevalent worldwide irrespective of gender, race or ethnicity. Usually, their clinical diagnosis is aided by the age of presentation, clinical features, and renal imaging studies including cyst location and distribution and extra-renal manifestations.
- In simple terms, a cyst is described as a cavity lined by epithelium and filled with liquid or semisolid material. There may be single or multiple cysts in one or both kidneys. They may be small, non-enlarging, and clinically insignificant, or large, enlarging and harmful.
- ADPKD is one of the most common genetic disorders in humans affecting all ethnic groups worldwide with an incidence of 1 in 400 to 1,000 births. It accounts for more than 5% of cases of ESRD in Europe and North America. There are two genetic mutations that have been linked with ADPKD. Mutation of the PKD1 gene which is located on chromosome 16 and encodes polycystin-1 and the PKD2 gene located on chromosome 4 which encodes polycystin-2 can lead to ADPKD.
- Autosomal recessive polycystic kidney disease (ARPKD) is a cystic kidney disorder usually affecting children. This is a recessively inherited disorder, therefore, it may occur in siblings but not in parents.
- The term NPH refers to a group of autosomal-recessive inherited renal disorders that are characterized by the four previously listed criteria. NPH typically presents during childhood, and it is often associated with extrarenal involvement. It is the most common genetic cause of kidney failure in European children and adolescents (>15%), although it is seen less frequently among the U.S. population.
- Medullary Cystic Kidney Disease (MCKD) is a group of autosomal-dominant inherited renal disorders that are characterized by the four criteria listed previously. MCKD typically presents during early adulthood. It is a rare condition, with approximately 50 new cases reported in the U.S. every year. There are two types: MCKD1 type 1 and MCKD2 type 2.
- von Hippel–Lindau (VHL) syndrome is an uncommon disorder that is characterized by the presence of various visceral cysts and benign tumors, many of which undergo malignant transformation. Common manifestations of VHL include hemangioblastomas of the central nervous system and retina, pheochromocytomas, and cysts of the kidney, liver, and pancreas. Because the clinical presentation varies widely from patient to patient, the discovery of any of these findings or a suspicious family history warrants a thorough investigation into the possibility of VHL.
- Medullary sponge kidney (MSK) is a diffuse or focal ectasia and cystic dilatation of the collecting ducts and cyst formation confined strictly to medullary pyramids. It is hypothesized to result from disruption of the interface between the developing ureteral bud and metanephric blastema during embryogenesis. A majority of patients with MSK are asymptomatic; however, some patients may present with renal colic, hematuria, or recurrent urinary tract infections.

- Simple renal cysts are the most commonly acquired renal cystic lesions, and occur twice as frequently in men as in women. They may be solitary or multiple and are filled with fluid. They are very rare in children, but the frequency increases with age. For simple renal cysts the pathogenic mechanisms are unknown but most likely they originate from the diverticula of distal convoluted and collecting tubules.
- Acquired cystic kidney disease (ACKD) is a non-hereditary developmental disorder presenting with three or more renal cysts in both kidneys and is characterized by small cysts distributed throughout the renal cortex and medulla of patients with chronic renal failure unrelated to inherited renal cystic diseases. These cysts are usually small, 0.5 to 2.5 cm in diameter.
- Tuberous sclerosis complex is a neurocutaneous disorder with an incidence of 1 in 5.000 to 10,000 live births and is characterized by the involvement of many organ systems including benign hamartomas of the brain, eye, heart, lung, liver, kidney, and skin. Bardet–Biedl syndrome (BBS) is a genetically heterogeneous disorder with 14 gene loci identified to date. It is usually inherited in an autosomal recessive manner, but some forms have a unique triallelic inheritance pattern requiring recessive mutations at one locus and an additional mutation at a second locus.

References

1. Auranen, M., et al. (2001). Further evidence for linkage of autosomal-dominant medullary cystic kidney disease on chromosome 1q21. *Kidney International, 60*(4), 1225–1232.
2. Butler, W. E., Barker, F. G., 2nd, & Crowell, R. M. (1996). Patients with polycystic kidney disease would benefit from routine magnetic resonance angiographic screening for intracerebral aneurysms: A decision analysis. *Neurosurgery, 38*(3), 506–515, discussion 515–516.
3. Caridi, G., et al. (2000). Clinical and molecular heterogeneity of juvenile nephronophthisis in Italy: Insights from molecular screening. *American Journal of Kidney Diseases, 35*(1), 44–51.
4. Errasti, P., et al. (2003). Autosomal-dominant polycystic kidney disease: High prevalence of graft loss for death-related malignancies and cardiovascular risk factors. *Transplantation Proceedings, 35*(5), 1717–1719.
5. Everson, G. T., Taylor, M. R., & Doctor, R. B. (2004). Polycystic disease of the liver. *Hepatology, 40*(4), 774–782.
6. Hildebrandt, F. (2004). Nephronophthisis–Medullary cystic kidney disease. In E. D. Avner & W. E. Harmon (Eds.), *Pediatric Nephrology* (5th ed., p. 665). Lippincott Williams & Wilkins.
7. Maschio, G., et al. (1996). Effect of the angiotensin-converting enzyme inhibitor benazepril on the progression of chronic renal insufficiency. The Angiotensin-Converting-Enzyme Inhibition in Progressive Renal Insufficiency Study Group. *New England Journal of Medicine, 334*(15), 939–945.
8. Maschio, G., et al. (1999). Angiotensin-converting enzyme inhibitors and kidney protection: The AIPRI trial. The ACE Inhibition in Progressive Renal Insufficiency (AIPRI) Study Group. *Journal of Cardiovascular Pharmacology, 33*(Suppl. 1), S16–S20, discussion S41–S43.

9. Parisi, M. A., et al. (2006). AHI1 mutations cause both retinal dystrophy and renal cystic disease in Joubert syndrome. *Journal of Medical Genetics, 43*(4), 334–339.
10. Schrier, R. W., et al. (2003). The role of parental hypertension in the frequency and age of diagnosis of hypertension in offspring with autosomal-dominant polycystic kidney disease. *Kidney International, 64*(5), 1792–1799.
11. Torres, V. E., & Harris, P. C. (2009). Autosomal dominant polycystic kidney disease: The last 3 years. *Kidney International, 76*(2), 149–168.
12. Wilson, P. D. (2004). Polycystic kidney disease. *New England Journal of Medicine, 350*, 151–164.
13. Wolf, M. T., & Hildebrandt, F. (2011). Nephronophthisis. *Pediatric Nephrology, 26*(2), 181–194.
14. Yendt, E. R. (1993). Medullary sponge kidney. In R. W. Schrier & C. W. Gottschalk (Eds.), *Diseases of the Kidney* (5th ed., pp. 525–532). Little, Brown.

Chapter 10

POLYCYSTIC KIDNEY DISEASE (PKD)

Contents

Introduction

A genetic condition known as polycystic kidney disease (PKD) is typified by the development of multiple kidney cysts. The two organs that make up the kidneys are roughly the size of a fist each and are situated toward the back of the upper abdomen. Urine is produced by the kidneys filtering wastes and surplus fluid from the blood. They also control the body's levels of a few essential chemicals. Kidney cysts are fluid-filled when they develop. Kidney failure can arise from PKD cysts that cause the kidneys to enlarge significantly and replace a large portion of their natural structure.

Dialysis and kidney transplantation are necessary for patients with Parkinson's disease (PD) when their kidneys fail, usually after many years of the disease. Kidney failure, also known as end-stage renal disease (ESRD), is experienced by about half of those with the most common type of Parkinson's disease (PKD). In addition to causing issues with other organs like the brain and heart's blood vessels, PKD can also result in liver cysts. Doctors can differentiate between "simple" cysts in the kidneys, which are usually benign, and PKD based on the quantity of cysts and the complications they cause. About 600,000 people in the US have PKD, and the fourth most common cause of kidney failure is cystic disease. Two major inherited forms of PKD exist:

- Autosomal dominant PKD is the most common inherited form. Symptoms usually develop between the ages of 30 and 40, but they can begin earlier, even in childhood. About 90% of all PKD cases are autosomal dominant PKD.
- Autosomal recessive PKD is a rare inherited form. Symptoms of autosomal recessive PKD begin in the earliest months of life, even in the womb.

Orientation and Directional Terms

Term	Definition	Illustration
Polycystic Kidney Disease (PKD)	Polycystic kidney disease (PKD) is a genetic disorder that causes many fluid-filled cysts to grow in your kidneys. Unlike the usually harmless simple kidney cysts that can form in the kidneys later in life, PKD cysts can change the shape of your kidneys, including making them much larger.	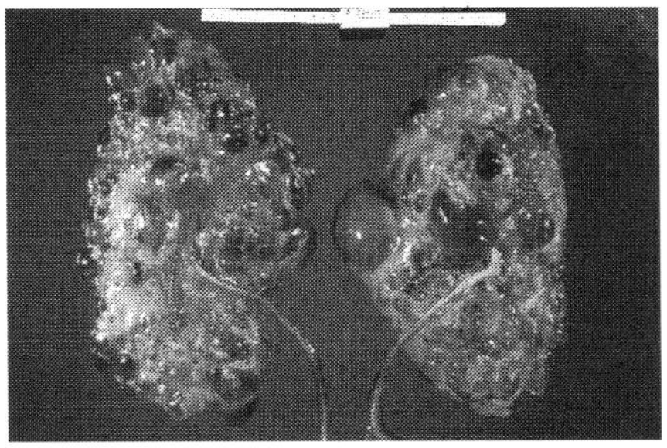
Autosomal Recessive Polycystic Kidney Disease (ARPKD)	Autosomal recessive polycystic kidney disease (ARPKD) is a rare genetic disorder that affects 1 in 20,000 children. A fetus or baby with ARPKD has fluid-filled kidney cysts that may make the kidneys too big, or enlarged. ARPKD can cause a child to have poor kidney function, even in the womb.	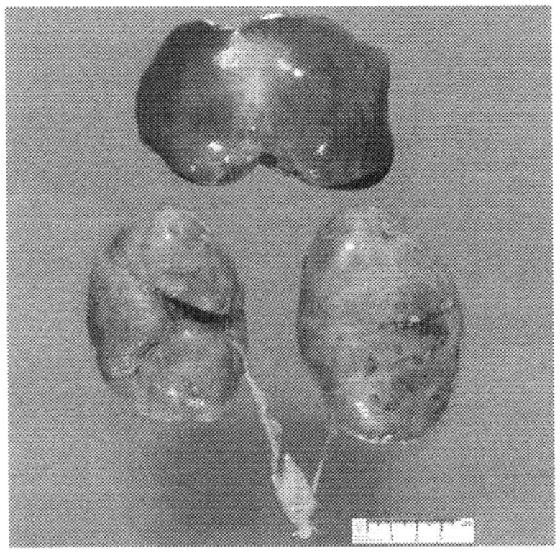
Angiotensin Receptor Blockers (ARBs)	Angiotensin receptor blockers (ARBs), also known as angiotensin II receptor antagonists, are used to treat high blood pressure and heart failure. They are also used for chronic kidney disease and prescribed following a heart attack. They include irbesartan, valsartan, losartan and candesartan.	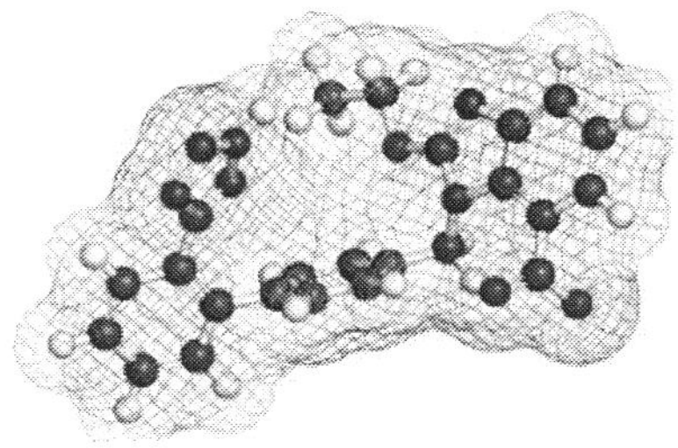
Angiotensin Converting Enzyme Inhibitors (ACEIs)	Angiotensin-converting-enzyme inhibitors are a class of medication used primarily for the treatment of high blood pressure and heart failure.	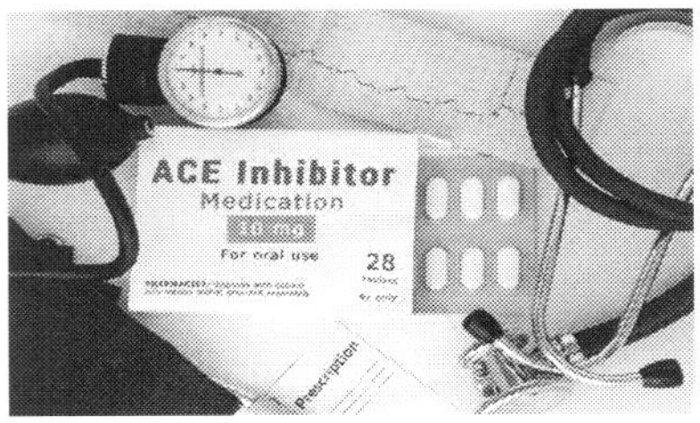

Estimated Glomerular Filtration Rate (eGFR)	The rate naturally declines as you age and lose muscle mass. The average eGFR for someone in their 20s is about 116 mL/min/1.73m2. It drops to 85 mL/min/1.73m2 for people in their 60s. An eGFR higher than 60 means you have at least 60% kidney function.	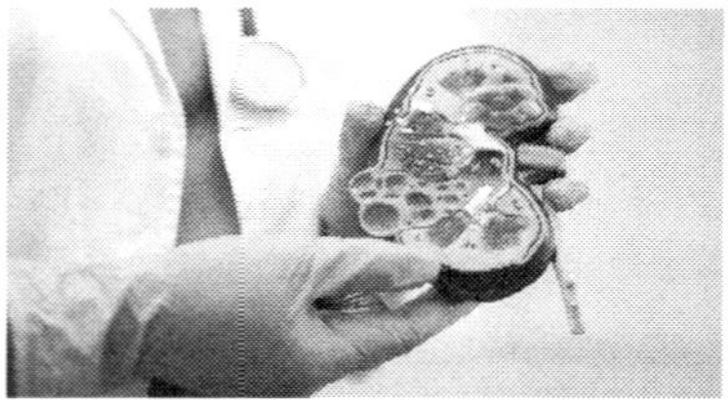
Kidney Infection	A kidney infection is a type of urinary tract infection (UTI). A kidney infection may begin in the tube that carries urine from the body (urethra) or in the bladder. The infection can travel to one or both kidneys. A kidney infection is also called pyelonephritis.	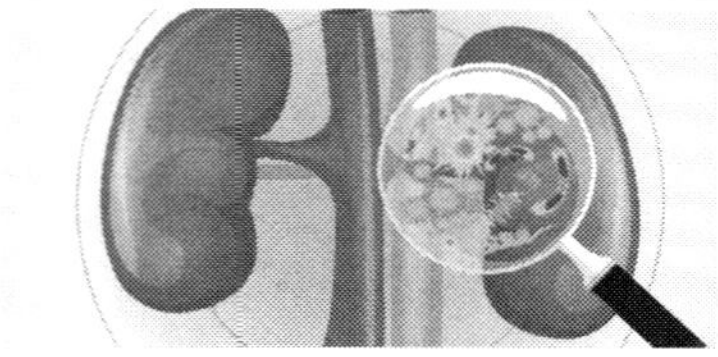

10.1. Overview of Polycystic Kidney Disease

Polycystic kidney disease (PKD or PCKD, also known as polycystic kidney syndrome) is a genetic disorder that causes the development of multiple cysts within the kidney due to abnormal renal tubules. These cysts can appear in utero, infancy, childhood, or adulthood and vary in size from microscopic to large, impacting nearby normal tubules. The condition is caused by abnormal genes producing a specific protein that disrupts tubule development. PKD encompasses two types, autosomal dominant polycystic kidney disease (ADPKD) and autosomal recessive polycystic kidney disease (ARPKD), each with their own genetic causes. The abnormal gene can also lead to cysts forming in other organs like the liver, seminal vesicles, and pancreas, as well as cause aortic root aneurysms and cerebral artery aneurysms, potentially leading to serious complications like subarachnoid hemorrhage.

A positive family history, palpation of enlarged kidneys on physical examination, an incidental finding on abdominal sonography, new-onset flank pain or red urine, or an incidental finding of abnormal kidney function on routine lab work (BUN, serum creatinine, or eGFR) can all raise suspicions about the diagnosis. An abdominal CT scan is used to make the final diagnosis. Renal decline, recurrent cyst infections, bleeding in the urine, and hypertension brought on by the renin-angiotensin-aldosterone system (RAAS) activation are among the complications. Angiotensin receptor blockers (ARBs) or angiotensin converting enzyme inhibitors (ACEIs) are used to treat hypertension. Antibiotics are used to treat infections. Renal replacement therapy (RRT), which includes dialysis and/or transplantation, is used to treat declining renal function. From the moment of the suspected or confirmed diagnosis, care is provided by a medical professional with the necessary training (Figure 10.1).

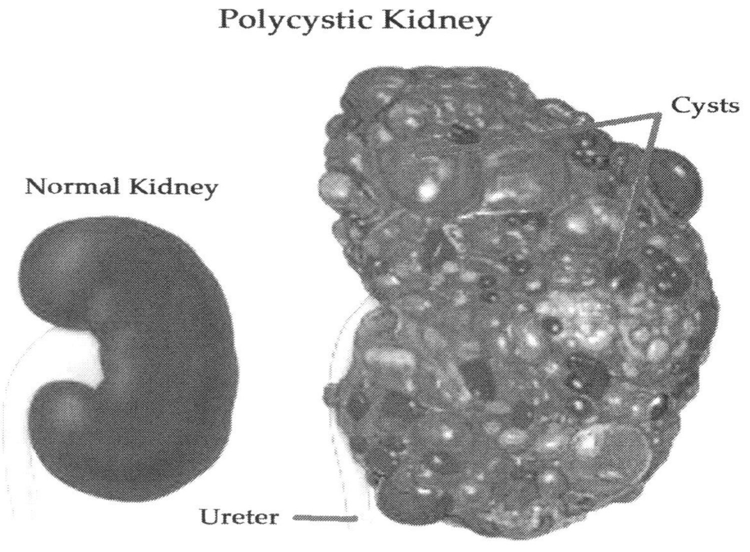

Figure 10.1. *Polycystic kidney disease is a genetic disorder that causes many fluid-filled cysts to grow in your kidneys.*

Source: *https://www.niddk.nih.gov/health-information/kidney-disease/polycystic-kidney-disease/what-is-pkd#:~:text=Polycystic%20kidney%20disease%20(PKD)%20is,including%20making%20them%20much%20larger.*

10.2. Genetic Variability in Autosomal Dominant Polycystic Kidney Disease

ADPKD is an autosomal dominant disease with a genetically heterogeneous inheritance pattern. The majority of cases are caused by mutations in either the PKD1 gene on chromosome 16 that codes for polycystin (PC)-1 or the PKD2 gene on chromosome 4 that codes for PC-2, with the former accounting for 78% of the cases and the latter for roughly 15%. The disease is characterized by a wide range of phenotypic variability. In comparison to PKD2 mutations, PKD1 mutations show more severe disease manifestations, such as more cysts, larger height-adjusted total kidney volume (TKV), lower estimated glomerular filtration rate (eGFR), and earlier development of ESKD. Apart from the genotype, multiple other factors also play a role in the phenotypic variability seen in ADPKD. These variables include the rate of cystic growth, mosaicism, and environmental factors like diet, water intake, hormones, obesity, and smoking. Additionally, kidney cysts can be a presenting symptom of other diseases that may mimic ADPKD. Because the prognosis and treatment plan will be impacted by an accurate diagnosis, it is imperative to comprehend these subtleties. Renal cysts and an ADPKD-like phenotype can be caused by mutations in PRKCSH, SEC63, LPR5, ALG8, and SEC61B, which are linked to autosomal dominant polycystic liver disease (ADPLD), but there is no increased risk of the condition progressing to end-stage liver disease (ESKD).

Recently, it was discovered that mutations in GANAB, which encodes the glucosidase II subunit α protein required for PC-1 protein maturation, cause mild to severe polycystic liver disease, mild renal cystic disease (average total of 10 cysts), and a mild decline in kidney function. Out of ADPKD patients, 0.3% have GANAB-associated disease. ADPKD can be mimicked by mutations in PKHD1, which are linked to autosomal recessive polycystic kidney disease (ARPKD) and manifest as congenital hepatic fibrosis. Moreover, renal cysts and impaired kidney function that mimic ADPKD can be present in individuals with mutations in UMOD, REN, MUC1, and HNF1B, which are linked to autosomal dominant tubulointerstitial kidney disease (ADTKD). Patients with ADTKD typically have a smaller cystic burden than those with ADPKD. comparatively few kidney cysts, normal to slightly enlarged kidneys). Interstitial fibrosis, the main characteristic of ADTKD, causes a progressive loss of kidney function. DNAJB11 mutations were linked to an ADPKD-like phenotype in a recent study by Cornec-Le Gall et al., which included liver cysts and an overlap of ADTKD clinical features. ALG9 mutations are among the other mutations that result in kidney and liver cysts without kidney enlargement.

Mutations linked to ciliopathies and impaired ciliary apparatus function, like those in OFD1 and NPHP1, can cause corticomedullary cysts in the kidneys that resemble ADPKD but have different extrarenal symptoms and early onset of ESKD. Kidney cysts that resemble ADPKD can also be a presenting feature of other systemic syndromes, such as Von Hippel Lindau disease and tuberous sclerosis complex, which are caused by mutations in the TSC and VHL genes, respectively. Because of this, there is a significant phenotypic overlap between ADPKD and other hereditary cystic kidney diseases. This underscores the significance of accurately diagnosing ADPKD since it influences the prognosis for the kidneys and the course of treatment aimed at slowing down the disease's progression.

10.2.1. Cyst Formation

Cysts on the kidneys appear to be caused by increased cell growth in autosomal dominant polycystic kidney disease (ADPKD). Nephrons are the fundamental building blocks of the kidney, and each kidney has about a million of them. Every nephron is made up of a glomerulus, which is a group of tiny arteries mixed in with many tubules. Together, the glomeruli and tubules remove waste from the bloodstream and excrete it in the urine. In a tiny percentage (5%) of nephrons with ADPKD, cyst formation starts as an expansion, or ballooning, most frequently of a tubule. After that, the cyst typically grows larger as a result of fluid secretion inside it. Cysts enlarge due to the proliferation of the cells that comprise them. Other organs such as the liver, pancreas, thyroid gland, and/or spleen can also develop cysts.

10.2.2. Effects on the Kidney

Chronic cyst enlargement and replacement of normal kidney tissue are the main causes of ADPKD, which frequently results in progressive kidney failure. Other kidney-related issues that can arise include hypertension, kidney infections, hematuria (blood in the urine), and kidney stones. Pain in the abdomen and flanks is also typical.

- **Kidney Failure**: End-stage kidney disease is defined as renal failure severe enough to require dialysis or kidney transplantation. In early childhood, ADPKD rarely results in end-stage kidney disease; instead, it usually manifests itself in middle age or later in life. Individuals with ADPKD are estimated to have a less than 2% chance of needing dialysis if they are under 40 years old, and a 50 to 75% chance if they are 70 to 75 years old. Kidney failure does not always occur in patients with ADPKD, especially in those with PKD2.
- **Risk Factors**: In ADPKD, there are several factors that influence the risk of developing kidney failure. For instance, the most accurate indicator of kidney failure in patients with ADPKD is having enlarged kidneys. Maleness, PKD1 illness (especially a mutation that shortens the protein), episodes of visible blood or detectable protein in the urine, and high blood pressure (especially before the age of 35) are additional factors that raise the risk of developing kidney failure. The most significant risk factor for the development of kidney failure is enlarged kidneys or increased total kidney volume as a result of a high cyst burden. These complications are linked to each other.
- **High Blood Pressure**: High blood pressure is a common feature of ADPKD, occurring in 60 to 70% of patients with normal kidney function by the age of 29 years. Over 90% of patients will have high blood pressure by the time they reach end-stage kidney disease. Men have higher blood pressure than women and high blood pressure is associated with bigger kidneys and faster rates of kidney growth.
- **Kidney Infection**: People with ADPKD will experience at least one cyst infection in their lifetime in between 30 and 50% of cases. For those with ADPKD, fever and flank pain are the main signs of a kidney infection. Either a kidney or a cyst could be infected. Certain antibiotics are less effective when the infection is inside the cyst. Since the exact location of the infection is often unknown, most doctors will prescribe an oral antibiotic that can enter the cyst cavity. Intravenous antibiotics are necessary

for certain individuals who have high fevers or severe symptoms. When treating a cyst or kidney infection, the course of treatment is usually longer than when treating a simple kidney infection in a person without ADPKD.

- **Blood in the Urine**: About 35 to 50% of individuals with ADPKD experience hematuria, or blood in the urine, which may be the initial indication of the illness. Urine may appear pink or red when hematuria is present. Frequent episodes of hematuria are typical. Hematuria is linked to larger kidneys and a quicker rate of kidney growth. Bleeding into a cyst that connects to the bladder and urinary tract typically results in hematuria. This can happen after hard exercise, and bleeding can result in flank pain, which is low back pain on the side. In addition to flank pain and hematuria, kidney stones can occur in patients with ADPKD. In most cases, bleeding cyst-related hematuria goes away in two to seven days. Bed rest and increasing fluids are the standard treatments until the bleeding stops. If bed rest and more fluids don't stop the bleeding, a procedure to stop the bleeding might be necessary. In this scenario, patients usually experience localized flank pain and, in rare instances, a low-grade fever. Bleeding into a cyst that is not in communication with the urinary system may not result in visible blood.
- **Kidney Stones**: Up to 25% of patients with ADPKD develop kidney stones. Kidney stones can sometimes obstruct the urine's flow without causing any pain. For patients with ADPKD, treating kidney stones that obstruct urine flow is crucial. That kidney's function could be lost if the obstruction is not cleared. Urologists may be needed to assist in clearing the obstruction. Because of the cysts, it is more difficult to break up the stone with shock waves (extracorporeal shock-wave lithotripsy, or ESWL).
- **Flank and Abdominal Pain**: The most prevalent symptom of ADPKD is pain, which is usually underreported by patients. At least 30% of patients experience persistent discomfort in their abdomen or flanks. Abdominal and flank pain unrelated to kidney stones, infections, or bleeding into cysts is common in people with ADPKD. It is believed that the pain, which is frequently dull and persistent, is brought on by a cyst's wall stretching or by pressure from large kidneys or livers pressing on other organs. The most typical symptom among ADPKD patients is this one. On the other hand, sudden onset pain is more likely to be the result of kidney stone, kidney twisting, or bleeding into or infection of a cyst.

For most people with dull or persistent flank and abdominal pain, no special treatment is needed, though acetaminophen or other painkillers are frequently advised. Nonsteroidal anti-inflammatory drug (NSAID) users, such as those with ADPKD, may occasionally benefit from taking these drugs; however, before using

NSAIDs, patients should discuss the advantages and disadvantages with their healthcare provider. When renal function is compromised or long-term use of NSAIDs is required to treat chronic pain, patients with ADPKD are not advised to take them. Some people experience chronic pain that interferes with their everyday activities to a considerable extent. Kidney imaging is typically used to assess severe pain to determine whether a large cyst is present in the painful area. If so, the cyst can be drained by inserting a needle through the skin. This requires the use of suitable imaging and the expertise of a radiologist skilled in this kind of procedure. Most people experience noticeable pain relief following drainage. But pain can return, and in certain cases, surgery is necessary to treat chronic pain that lowers quality of life.

10.2.3. Associated Conditions Outside of the Kidney

In patients with ADPKD, many conditions other than kidney disease can arise. Numerous systems, including the connective tissue, vascular system, and liver, may be impacted by these conditions.

- **Intracranial Aneurysm**: A cerebral or brain aneurysm, which is a bulging blood vessel caused by the weakening of the blood vessel wall, is the most serious potential PKD complication. Subarachnoid hemorrhage, or bleeding into the brain, can occur when aneurysms burst. This can result in irreversible brain damage or even death if treatment is not received before the aneurysm rupturing. People with larger aneurysms (>10 mm) are more likely to experience aneurysm rupture. The most typical sign of a subarachnoid hemorrhage is a strong headache that starts out of nowhere, usually with a pop, and is frequently accompanied by nausea and vomiting. Brain aneurysms are estimated to affect 3 to 7% of adults with ADPKD; if another member of the patient's family has experienced an intracranial aneurysm, this frequency rises to 12 to 15%. When it comes to ADPKD, the risk of aneurysm development is roughly five times higher than in the general population. The greatest risk factor for developing an aneurysm is having a first-degree relative with a history of subarachnoid hemorrhage or intracranial aneurysm.
  Patients with ADPKD may also be more susceptible to aneurysm development if they smoke or have high blood pressure.

For those who are at high risk, early detection of intracranial aneurysms is advised—that is, before symptoms appear. When screening is necessary to find an aneurysm before it bursts, magnetic resonance angiography (MRA) or, if MRA is not available, a computed tomography (CT) scan is typically used. Only high-risk patients, such as those who have experienced a prior rupture, have a positive family history of brain hemorrhage or stroke, exhibit warning signs (such as unusual headaches), or work in a high-risk profession (such as aviation), where losing consciousness would put them or others in grave danger, are advised to undergo routine screening.

- **Liver Cysts**: People with ADPKD are frequently affected by liver cysts. At 30 years of age, over 85% of patients will have liver cysts. As patients age, liver cysts grow bigger and more prevalent. Women also tend to have larger liver cysts than men, especially after multiple pregnancies, long-term use of oral contraceptives, or hormone replacement therapy. Most liver cyst sufferers don't have any symptoms and their liver function is normal or almost normal. But occasionally, people experience symptoms like breathing difficulties, early satiety, fullness in the abdomen, or, less frequently, pain that may need to be relieved by draining the cyst if it is severe and persistent, or infection that may require antibiotic treatment and, in certain situations, drainage. In the worst situations, a liver transplant may not always be necessary to replace the damaged liver.

- **Heart Valve Disease**: Heart valve abnormalities have been found in as many as 25% of ADPKD patients. The majority of heart valve disease patients don't need treatment and don't exhibit any symptoms. Rarely, though, is the possibility that the valve disease will worsen over time and necessitate valve replacement. Certain patients with mitral valve prolapse may exhibit palpitations and require specific medication, such as beta-blockers.
- **Abdominal Wall Hernias**: A muscle weak spot is called a hernia. When a person increases the pressure in their abdomen, such as when coughing or carrying a heavy package, the area may protrude if the organs behind the muscle press against the weak spot. About 45% of patients with ADPKD have abdominal wall hernias, which are a relatively common condition. Typically, abdominal wall hernias are found in the groin (inguinal), at the level of the belly button (umbilical), or on the midline directly above the belly button (ventral). For painful abdominal wall hernias, surgery is the best course of action; however, not all hernias need to be surgically repaired. Over time, small hernias may be observed.

10.3. Differential Diagnosis of Autosomal Dominant Polycystic Kidney Disease

Finding one or more kidney cysts is a fairly common occurrence, particularly as people age, and it is not particularly significant. Conversely, there exist individuals with multiple cysts who may fall under the category of patients with polycystic kidney diseases based on many factors, such as age, the number of cysts, and how they are distributed across multiple organs. These illnesses primarily affect the liver or kidneys and are typically genetically based (Figure 10.2). The significance of their differential diagnosis, which is predominantly determined by imaging criteria, lies in the fact that polycystic kidney diseases comprise multiple clinical entities, each with distinct symptoms, course, and outlook. Early diagnosis enables careful monitoring and management of renal function as well as the treatment of related issues like nephrolithiasis or hypertension, which can halt the development of renal failure.

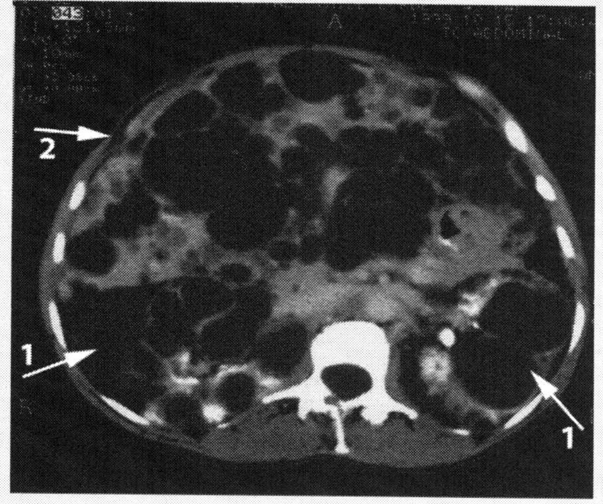

Figure 10.2. *Polycystic kidney and liver disease. 1, Enlarged kidneys due to multiple cysts; 2, Enlarged liver with multiple cysts.*

Source: *Alves M, Fonseca T, de Almeida EAF. Differential Diagnosis of Autosomal Dominant Polycystic Kidney Disease. In: Li X, editor. Polycystic Kidney Disease [Internet]. Brisbane (AU): Codon Publications; 2015 Nov. Chapter 1. Available from: https://www.ncbi.nlm.nih.gov/books/NBK373390/ doi: 10.15586/codon.pkd.2015.ch1.*

10.3.1. Autosomal Dominant Polycystic Kidney Disease

The most prevalent type of monogenic, inherited kidney disease in the world, autosomal dominant polycystic kidney disease (ADPKD) affects one in 500–1,000 people. Two genes are known to be involved in ADPKD: PKD1 (discovered in 1994), which is found on chromosome 16's short arm and produces polycystin 1 (PC1), a transmembrane protein with an extracellular tail that is long and can act as a mechanosensor; and PKD2 (discovered in 1996), which is found on chromosome 4's long arm and produces polycystin 2 (PC2), a smaller glycoprotein that is involved in calcium transport. It is possible that there is a third unknown gene because a small subset of all ADPKD families is unrelated to either of the two identified genes. Some families that had previously fit into this group were reevaluated and found to have a linkage to PKD1 or PKD2 mutations. A small number of reports describe patients with ADPKD phenotype who do not have mutations in the two genes described. Therefore, it seems doubtful that a third gene for ADPKD exists at this time.

In clinically identified populations, 85% of ADPKD cases are caused by the PKD1 mutation, with PKD2 being responsible for the remaining 15%. High degrees of variability are seen in the phenotypes linked to ADPKD with regard to the age at which end-stage kidney disease (ESKD) first manifests, associated liver disease, or other extrarenal symptoms. Environmental factors as well as genetic and allelic heterogeneity can be blamed for this. In terms of genetic heterogeneity, PKD1 mutations are known to be linked to more severe disease than PKD2 mutations (median age: 54 vs 74 years old). This includes earlier age at diagnosis, a higher prevalence of hypertension, and an earlier onset of ESKD. From an allelic perspective, patients with truncating mutations have a more severe disease than those with non-truncating mutations. Certain mutations are linked to a more severe disease phenotype than others. It is reported that truncating mutations affect the majority of ADPKD patients. According to a study, mutations in the PKD1 gene near the 5' end are linked to an earlier onset of ESKD and a higher risk of intracranial aneurysm rupture.

Research has indicated a dose-dependent effect of genes on the severity of ADPKD. Humans with homozygous complete penetrance mutations in PKD1 or PKD2 are expected to be embryonically lethal. While heterozygous inheritance of the same alleles was linked to mild cystic disease, homozygous inheritance of incompletely penetrant PKD1 or PKD2 alleles can be linked to a more severe phenotype. Since studies have shown intrafamilial phenotypic variability in families where patients share the same mutation but show significant differences in disease severity and presentation, the involvement of modifier genes (e.g., endothelial nitric oxide synthesis/ENOS and angiotensin-converting enzyme/ACE) and epigenetic regulators (e.g., histone deacetylases/HDACs) may add to the complexity of phenotypic variability in ADPKD.

10.3.2. Diagnosis of ADPKD

Even though our understanding of the genetic characteristics of this illness is always growing, imaging criteria based on an individual's age, family history, and number of cysts are used for screening and diagnosis. Although ultrasound is a low-cost, safe way to diagnose and screen individuals who have a high risk of ADPKD, the cost of this screening will keep it from being available to the general public. Consequently, the McGovern et al. system to determine clinical characteristics that may be applied in the early detection of ADPKD patients who are at high risk. Diastolic blood pressure (BP) greater than 90 mmHg, proteinuria, hematuria, chronic kidney disease stage 3A or worse, and being on multiple antihypertensive medications were the clinical features that best-distinguished people with polycystic kidney disease.

In the past, patients with a family history of PKD1 were the basis for the diagnostic criteria. The criteria were changed in 2009 to include at-risk adults of unknown gene type and patients with a family history of PKD2 who started cyst development later in life and had fewer cysts overall (Table 10.1). In older subjects, where the finding of simple cysts is common, four or more cysts in both kidneys are required for the definite diagnosis of ADPKD. In younger subjects (15–29 years old), who are at-risk due to an affected first-degree relative, three cysts in both kidneys are sufficient for the diagnosis. It is significant to remember that these unified criteria only apply to patients who have a positive family history of ADPKD, which eliminates roughly 10–15% of potential cases of ADPKD that do not have a history of the disease in their family. It is possible for a positive family history to be absent because of non-truncating PKD1 mutations, mosaicism, mild disease from PKD2, new mutations, or missing parental medical records. Given the patient's multiple cysts and bilaterally enlarged kidneys, along with the lack of additional findings that would point to a different cystic disease (Table 10.2), ADPKD is most likely the diagnosis in this case.

Table 10.1. Unified Criteria for Ultrasound Diagnosis of ADPKD

Age	Number of Cysts	Sensitivity	Positive Predictive Value
15 – 29 years	A total of 3 cysts in both kidneys	81.7%	100%
30 – 39 years	A total of 3 cysts in both kidneys	95.5%	100%
40 – 59 years	2 or more cysts in each kidney	90%	100%

Source: *Alves M, Fonseca T, de Almeida EAF. Differential Diagnosis of Autosomal Dominant Polycystic Kidney Disease. In: Li X, editor. Polycystic Kidney Disease [Internet]. Brisbane (AU): Codon Publications; 2015 Nov. Chapter 1. Available from: https://www.ncbi.nlm.nih.gov/books/NBK373390/ doi: 10.15586/codon.pkd.2015.ch1.*

Table 10.2. Differential Diagnosis of ADPKD

Condition	Gene	Inheritance	Prevalence	Differentiating Signs/Symptoms
Simple renal cysts	–	Acquired	Common	Normal renal function; normal-sized kidneys with smooth contour
Acquired renal cystic disease	-	Acquired	Common	Associated with CKD or ESKD; multiple renal cysts associated with small- to normal-sized kidneys
Medullary cystic kidney disease	MCKD1–2	AD	Unknown	Interstitial fibrosis on renal biopsy. Rarely cysts in the corticomedullary junction; slowly progressive renal failure; small- to normal-sized kidneys; Hyperuricemia, gout
Polycystic liver disease	PRKCSH / SEC63	AD	Unknown	Small number of renal cysts; predominantly liver cystic disease
Autosomal Recessive Polycystic kidney disease	PKHD1	AR	1: 20.000	Early in life kidneys cystic, enlarged and echogenic. With increasing age, kidneys are smaller with macroscopic cysts, nephrocalcinosis and/or small medullary calcifications common; Oligohydramnios (Potter's phenotype) and pulmonary hypoplasia in utero, congenital hepatic fibrosis, Caroli's disease
Tuberous Sclerosis	TSC 1–2	AD	1: 10.000	Angiomyolipoma. Contiguous deletion of PKD1/TSC2 results in severe early onset PKD with ESKD typically occurring in the first 2 decades of life. Skin lesions (facial angiofibromas, periungal fibroma, hypomelanotic macules and Shagreen patch); retinal hamartomas; seizures; mental retardation; cortical tuber; subependymal giant cell astrocytoma; cardiac rhabdomyoma; lymphangioleiomyomatosis

Von Hippel-Lindau	VHL	AD	1:50.000	High risk of renal cell carcinomas. CNS and retinal hemangioblastomas, pancreatic cysts, pancreatic endocrine tumors, pheochromocytoma
Orofaciodigital syndrome I	OFD1	X-linked, dominant	Very rare (1:250.000)	Embryonic male lethal, cleft palate, bifid tongue, hyperplastic frenula, hypertelorism, broadened nasal ridge, digital abnormalities including syndactyly, CNS malformations
Nephronophtisis	NPHP1–6	AR	1:10.000	Normal-sized kidneys with corticomedullary junction cysts; Interstitial fibrosis; Retinitis pigmentosa; Cerebellar vermis aplasia, polydactyly, occipital encephalocele (NPHP 1 / 6); ocular motor apraxia (NPHP 1–2); liver fibrosis (NPHP2–3), situs inversus (NPHP 2)
Bardet-Biedl syndrome	BBS 1–12	AR	1:140.000	retinal degeneration, childhood obesity, mental retardation, malformations of the urogenital tract, polydactyly
Medullary sponge kidney	Unknown	Unknown	1:5000	Malformation of the distal collecting tubules with nephrolithiasis (hematuria), renal function impairment, tubular acidosis, recurrent urinary tract infections
Localised cystic disease	--	Unknown	Unknown (very rare)	Benign disease, unilateral cysts, no progression to chronic renal failure, no extrarenal involvement
Meckel-Gruber syndrome	MGS 1–6	AR	1:13.250 to 1:140,000	Occipital encephalocele, and postaxial polydactyly
Renal cysts and diabetes syndrome	HNF1B	AD	Unknown	Renal malformation, diabetes mellitus, hypomagnesemia, genital tract abnormalities, hyperuricemia and elevated liver enzymes

AD, autosomal dominant; AR, autosomal recessive; CKD, chronic kidney disease; ESKD, end-stage kidney disease; CNS, cerebral nervous system.

Source: Alves M, Fonseca T, de Almeida EAF. Differential Diagnosis of Autosomal Dominant Polycystic Kidney Disease. In: Li X, editor. Polycystic Kidney Disease [Internet]. Brisbane (AU): Codon Publications; 2015 Nov. Chapter 1. Available from: https://www.ncbi.nlm.nih.gov/books/NBK373390/ doi: 10.15586/codon.pkd.2015.ch1.

Regardless of the gene type, ADPKD diagnosis in older subjects requires the presence of at least four kidney cysts. However, a small percentage of patients who fulfilled the ADPKD diagnostic criteria do not exhibit the typical clinical characteristics, such as a degree of renal impairment or known gene mutations. Van Gulick et al. went beyond the most typical renal phenotype. highlighted a subset of patients who suffer more from their polycystic liver (> 20 cysts) and whose hepatic cysts are more noticeable than their renal cysts. On rare occasions, patients with ADPKD may exhibit normal renal function, extensive hepatic disease, and both liver and renal cysts. Cnossen and associates. found that the third locus linked to isolated polycystic liver disease was the LRP5 gene. It was postulated that LRP5 variants may contribute to the heterogeneity of hepatic and renal disease in ADPKD since polycystic liver disease is the most prevalent extrarenal feature in patients with ADPKD. It was hypothesized that LRP5 variants may make ADPKD patients more prone to the development of polycystic liver, though further research is required. Physicians should be aware of other renal cyst diseases that should be taken into consideration as a differential diagnosis of ADPKD in light of these few cases where the diagnosis is not linear. A significant proportion of patients with ADPKD go on to develop ESKD, which accounts for 6–10% of patients receiving renal replacement therapy. Early diagnosis is crucial because treating related issues like nephrolithiasis or hypertension can halt the development of ESKD. Furthermore, many medications that target particular pathways that are altered in ADPKD have recently been tested in randomized controlled studies and should soon be made available for human use.

10.3.3. Direct Molecular Genetic Tests for Diagnosis

The majority of the time, clinical criteria—including history, especially family history, physical examination, and renal ultrasonography—are used to diagnose ADPKD. Follow-up studies will confirm the diagnosis if there is an increase in the size and number of renal cysts, as well as if hepatic cysts appear, hypertension, urologic symptoms, and cardiovascular disease. Due to their high cost and lack of benefit for clinical follow-up, genetic studies are currently not widely accessible for clinical diagnosis; however, we anticipate that this will change as more evidence emerges suggesting a relationship between the type of mutation and the prognosis of the illness. Furthermore, the high degree of allelic heterogeneity and the duplication of the PKD1 gene's 1–32 exons as pseudogenes in chromosome 16 may complicate this analysis. About 8% of the families that took part in the HALT-PKD trial had no mutation found in them overall. Genetic studies are therefore only performed in a restricted number of circumstances, such as living-related kidney transplant donors, to rule out ADPKD in the donor, for prenatal counseling, especially in the context of pre-implantation in vitro fertilization, and to treat complex renal cystic disease, if clinically significant.

10.3.4. Which Diagnosis Should Doctors Consider When the Patient has Multiple Renal Cysts?

Making an ADPKD diagnosis is generally not too difficult. The typical patient has a positive family history and enlarged cystic kidneys when they first arrive. In cases where there is no family history of ADPKD, cystic kidney disease necessitates a thorough examination of the medical history to identify any unusual clinical or radiologic features. A summary of the ADPKD differential diagnosis can be found in Table 10.2. In adults, renal cysts are common. When renal cysts are discovered on ultrasonography in a patient who is asymptomatic, there are multiple possibilities for diagnosis, including simple cysts, ADPKD, or acquired renal cysts. A thorough history and physical examination, along with additional clinical findings like liver cysts, hypertension, or renal failure, help to differentiate between these common conditions. However, in certain circumstances, particularly with atypical clinical presentations the following entities should be excluded:

- **Multiple Benign Simple Cysts:** Simple renal cysts are more common as people age, and sensitive imaging techniques like computed tomography (CT) or magnetic resonance imaging (MRI) are frequently used to find them. 93% of subjects aged 45–59 have at least one renal cyst found by an MRI-based series. Out of 617 patients, simple renal cysts were found in 41% of them using spiral CT. About half of men (mean age 66 years) and three-quarters of women (mean age 63 years) have renal cysts.
- **Localized Renal Cystic Disease:** A rare and benign condition is localized renal cystic disease. Patients may exhibit flank mass, hematuria, hypertension, or flank pain. Due to its unilateral location, lack of a family history, lack of progression to chronic renal failure, and lack of extrarenal involvement, the clinical features of this disease differ from those of ADPKD.
- **Acquired Renal Cystic Disease:** Acquired renal cystic disease is typically detected in individuals with longstanding renal failure and can be found in up to 20% of patients with ESKD. The main distinction is the presence of cysts in a normal or small kidney with signs of chronic kidney disease.
- **Medullary Sponge Kidney:** Medullary sponge kidney is a cystic renal disease with unknown inheritance characterized by malformation of the distal collecting tubules with nephrolithiasis, impairment of renal function, tubular acidosis and recurrent urinary tract infections—but rarely evolves to ESKD.
- **Bilateral Parapelvic Cysts:** Parapelvic cysts are a subset of simple cysts that arise within the renal parenchyma adjacent to the renal sinus and account for 5% of all renal cysts in adults. Clinically they may manifest through obstruction of the ureter or renal pelvis.
- **Autosomal Recessive Polycystic Kidney Disease:** In 30% of cases, ARPKD results in neonatal deaths and affects 1 in every 20,000 births. Due to a mutation in the PKHD1 gene on chromosome 6, patients typically exhibit enlarged, echogenic kidneys and sporadic cortical cysts when they first appear in the neonatal period. In addition, pulmonary hypoplasia, portal fibrosis, and Potter's phenotype are perinatal symptoms. Though adult forms have been reported, ARPKD is typically diagnosed

in childhood. The presence of congenital hepatic fibrosis and/or Caroli's disease in addition to the absence of liver cystic disease and poor differentiation in both of the large echogenic kidneys—which, in contrast to ADPKD, have few macrocysts—are identifiable characteristics.

- **Tuberous Sclerosis Complex:** Mutations in the TSC1 or TSC2 gene cause the autosomal dominant disease known as tuberous sclerosis complex, which has an incidence of 1:5,000 to 10,000. In two thirds of families, there is no family history of the illness. Particularly in the so-called contiguous gene syndrome, mutations of TSC2, which is paired with the PKD1 gene in the short arm of chromosome 16, may cause polycystic renal abnormalities that mimic ADPKD. Kidney angiomyolipomas, facial angiofibromas, retinal hamartomas, subependymal giant cell astrocytomas, cerebral pathology, and benign neurocutaneous tumors permit differentiation.
- **Von Hippel-Lindau Syndrome:** The features of autosomal dominant-inherited von Hippel-Lindau (VHL) syndrome include a combination of renal cell cancers, pheochromocytoma, endocrine tumors (retina and cerebellum), and, less commonly, pancreatic hemangioblastomas. Precancerous renal cysts, which cause kidney enlargement and may be misdiagnosed as ADPKD, can develop in the early stages. Kidney failure, however, is not a significant characteristic of VHL syndrome.
- **Autosomal Dominant Medullary Cystic Disease:** Autosomal dominant medullary cystic disease may be present in adulthood (30–60 years) with renal dysfunction and, occasionally, renal cysts. The gene involved is uromodulin (encoding Tamm-Horsfall protein) on chromosome 16. Distinguished features are tubular interstitial fibrosis with normal- to small-sized kidneys usually accompanied by early hyperuricemia and gout.
- **Autosomal Dominant Polycystic Liver Disease:** The primary distinction between mild ADPKD and autosomal dominant polycystic liver disease is the lack of cystic kidney disease. These patients typically have polycystic liver disease and do not develop ESKD, but in some cases, they may have few renal cysts, prompting the physician to consider an ADPKD diagnosis (Figure 10.3). Few patients with ADPKD exhibit a predominant liver cyst phenotype. It might not be possible to differentiate between ADPKD and polycystic liver disease if there is no family history of the condition, the kidneys also have cysts, and there are few liver cysts. Clinical follow-up and genetic studies could be useful in these situations.
- **Orofaciodigital Syndrome Type I:** This is an X-linked disease due to mutation of the OFD1 gene, and craniofacial and digital defects are associated with polycystic kidney disease.

- **Bardet-Biedl Syndrome:** With a frequency of 1:140,000, Bardet-Biedl syndrome is an extremely rare disease caused by a variety of gene mutations coding for proteins involved in primary cilium functions. This condition is referred to as a ciliopathy. Numerous extrarenal abnormalities, including childhood obesity, mental retardation, urogenital tract malformation, polydactyly, and vision loss from retinal degeneration, coexist with polycystic kidney disease.

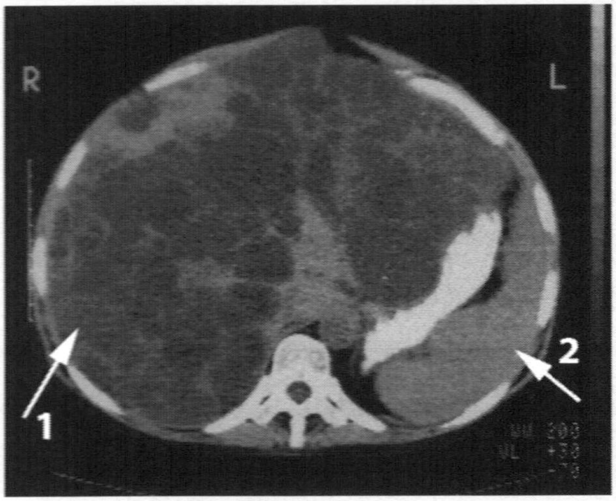

Figure 10.3. *Polycystic liver disease. 1, Enlarged liver due to uncountable cysts; 2, Spleen.*

Source: Alves M, Fonseca T, de Almeida EAF. Differential Diagnosis of Autosomal Dominant Polycystic Kidney Disease. In: Li X, editor. Polycystic Kidney Disease [Internet]. Brisbane (AU): Codon Publications; 2015 Nov. Chapter 1. Available from: https://www.ncbi.nlm.nih.gov/books/NBK373390/ doi: 10.15586/codon.pkd.2015.ch1.

- **Renal Cysts and Diabetes Syndrome:** Renal cysts and mutations in hepatocyte nuclear factor 1β (HNF-1β) cause the rare monogenic disease known as Type 5 MODY (Maturity Onset Diabetes of the Young). De novo mutations cause about half of this autosomal-dominant disease, which manifests as renal cysts or malformations in 90% of cases. Additionally, genital tract abnormalities and hyperuricemia account for 20% of cases, hypomagnesemia for 40%, elevated liver enzymes for 15%, and diabetes mellitus for 45% of patients.

In children with the finding of renal cysts in absence of a family history of ADPKD, the differential diagnosis should consider the following entities:

- **Contiguous PKD1-TSC2 Syndrome:** This syndrome is caused by deletions in the TSC2 and PKD1 genes located on the short arm of chromosome 16. These patients typically have characteristics of polycystic kidneys and tuberous sclerosis when they first appear in infancy, and their ESKD progresses quickly. Since the parents are somatic mosaics or the result of de novo mutations, there is frequently no family history.
- **Meckel-Gruber Syndrome**: This is a rare autosomal recessive lethal malformation, characterized by the triad occipital encephalocele, bilateral polycystic kidneys and post axial polydactyly.
- **Nephronophtisis:** This condition typically results in ESKD before the second decade of life and is characterized by the formation of cysts at the corticomedullary junction without kidney

enlargement. There are several extrarenal manifestations observed, including hepatomegaly, cerebellar ataxia, oculomotor apraxia, and Retinitis Pigmentosa. This autosomal recessive disease (NPHP1 to NPHP6) is primarily caused by six different gene mutations and is a leading cause of renal failure in children.

10.4. Autosomal Recessive Polycystic Kidney Disease (ARPKD)

The rare hepatorenal fibrocystic disease known as ARPKD (OMIM 263200) is caused by a malformation of the biliary ductal plate and is characterized by non-obstructive, fusiform, cystic distension of the renal collecting ducts with variable degrees of congenital hepatic fibrosis (CHF). A cystic widening of the intrahepatic bile ducts, known as Caroli disease, and the common bile duct are two conditions that can result from progressive biliary disease. It also causes periportal fibrosis, or CHF. Despite a great deal of variation in phenotype, mutations in a single gene, the PKHD1 gene, cause ARPKD, which has an incidence rate of 1/20,000 and is frequently diagnosed in utero or at birth. Despite a great deal of variation in phenotype, mutations in a single gene, the PKHD1 gene, cause ARPKD, which has an incidence rate of 1/20,000 and is frequently diagnosed in utero or at birth. Even though ARPKD typically manifests in a neonatal form, there is a considerable variation in the age at which the condition first manifests as well as in the degree of renal and biliary abnormalities. Although it is widely acknowledged, the degree of organ involvement in ARPKD varies. This is not well understood. Other disease-modifying genes, the combination of the two distinct parental PKHD1 mutations, epigenetic factors, hormonal effects, and environmental factors all play a role in regulating this phenotypic variability.

10.4.1. Epidemiology and Genetics

The PKHD1 gene, which encodes the FPC, is mutated in ARPKD. Two different research teams successfully cloned PKHD1 in 2002. PKHD1 is an incredibly large gene, spanning about 470 kb of genomic DNA. It is composed of 86 exons, of which the longest open-reading frame transcript includes 67 exons. The precise purpose and therapeutic importance of these isoforms remain unknown despite the identification of several alternatively spliced transcripts. To date, approximately 750 mutations in PKHD1 have been found. Attempts have been made to define genotype-phenotype correlations since PKHD1 was identified as the causative gene in ARPKD through cloning; however, thus far, only general correlations have been possible. The latest findings on transcriptional complexities have further complicated even the most tenuous correlations, and these must be taken into account for appropriate genetic counseling.

Several documented ARPKD families show that mutations in PKHD1 are spread out throughout the gene, rather than concentrated in specific hotspots, and the majority of families have unique mutations. Furthermore, almost all patients have two different mutations on their alleles, known as compound heterozygotes. Various types of mutations, including missense, nonsense, frame shift, and truncating mutations, have been identified in these families.

Individuals who had truncating mutations on both alleles usually had a severe phenotype and a high death rate during the perinatal or neonatal stages. Individuals who have at least one missense mutation—a substitution of an amino acid—have a higher chance of surviving into the neonatal stage and beyond. Boddu and associates. discovered 22 new renal transcripts produced by various alternative splicing techniques. These include exon skipping, the use of alternative acceptor/donor splice sites, and the inclusion of novel exons in a particular animal model of Pkhd1. According to these studies, PKHD1 splicing events that are not typical may be another pathogenic mechanism that results in ARPKD. Although the functional role of these transcripts is unknown, these findings raise the bar for genetic counseling.

Autosomal recessive inheritance means that parents are carriers without any clinical manifestation. There is a 25% chance of having an affected offspring in any pregnancy, and a 50% chance that unaffected offspring will carry a mutation in PKHD1. ARPKD does not show a gender preference and affects all ethnic and racial groups equally.

10.4.2. Diagnosis

As modern obstetrical ultrasonography (US) becomes more widely available, an increasing number of patients with ARPKD are being diagnosed during the prenatal period. The identification of ARPKD is typically made based on clinical observations and our current knowledge of the disease's progression. The diagnostic criteria proposed by Zerres et al (1996). with modifications, are generally used and include:

1. US features typical of ARPKD, including enlarged, echogenic kidneys, with poor corticomedullary differentiation; and
2. One or more of the following:
    i. Absence of renal cysts in both parents, particularly if they are at least 30 years old,
    ii. Clinical, laboratory or radiographic evidence of hepatic fibrosis,
    iii. Hepatic pathology demonstrating characteristic ductal plate abnormalities,
    iv. Previous affected sibling with pathologically or genetically confirmed disease,
    v. Parental consanguinity suggestive of autosomal recessive inheritance.

ARPKD is often identified before birth or shortly after, presenting with worsening kidney function and portal hypertension (PH). In severe cases, affected fetuses may exhibit the classic "Potter" phenotype, characterized by enlarged, echogenic kidneys with poor corticomedullary differentiation caused by dilated collecting ducts. Additional symptoms can include respiratory issues, cranial abnormalities, and clubbed feet. Although oligohydramnios can be seen in prenatal screenings, it may not appear in ARPKD cases until the later stages of pregnancy.

About one-third of neonates with large, echogenic kidneys present with pulmonary insufficiency, a serious complication that usually results from oligohydramnios and causes respiratory failure and neonatal death. The survival rate for patients who make it through the neonatal period is 82% after one year and 85% after ten. An ever-smaller but increasingly recognized subgroup of ARPKD patients is identified as older children or adults with hepatosplenomegaly or enlarged kidneys causing abdominal enlargement. These patients usually exhibit PH and esophageal hemorrhage as well as other symptoms associated with congenital hepatic fibrosis. Additional related comorbidities include progressive renal insufficiency, systemic hypertension, and, less frequently, chronic lung disease in older children, particularly in those who were born with respiratory insufficiency. Neonatal survival rates have increased as a result of advancements in critical care for the newborn, and as more ARPKD patients live to adulthood, complications related to the liver and other organs are expected to rise in frequency. Pre-implantation genetic diagnosis through linkage analysis or mutational analysis is possible in families with at least one pathologically or genetically confirmed affected child when the mutation on both the maternal and paternal allele can be identified. Linkage analysis can also be used to identify the carrier status of an unaffected child. In "genetically informative" families, the accuracy of prenatal diagnosis using linkage analysis is >95% (Alves, Fonseca, & de Almeida, 2015).

10.4.3. Pathology

Fusiform dilatation of the collecting ducts results in loss of corticomedullary differentiation, and enlarged echogenic kidneys are characteristic of the kidney phenotype. When newborns and early children undergo renal ultrasonography, both kidneys are bilaterally enlarged and show poor corticomedullary differentiation (Figure 10.4a). Figure 10.4b shows the kidneys' reniform contour, while Figure 10.4c shows several small cysts that are limited to collecting ducts. The spindle-shaped collecting duct cysts that extend into the renal cortex can be seen macroscopically on the cut surface in a radial pattern (Figure 10.4c). Microscopically, the cysts (Figure 10.4d) are typically less than 2 mm in diameter. Studies involving immunohistology and microdissection have shown that these so-called "microcysts" are actually dilated collecting ducts.

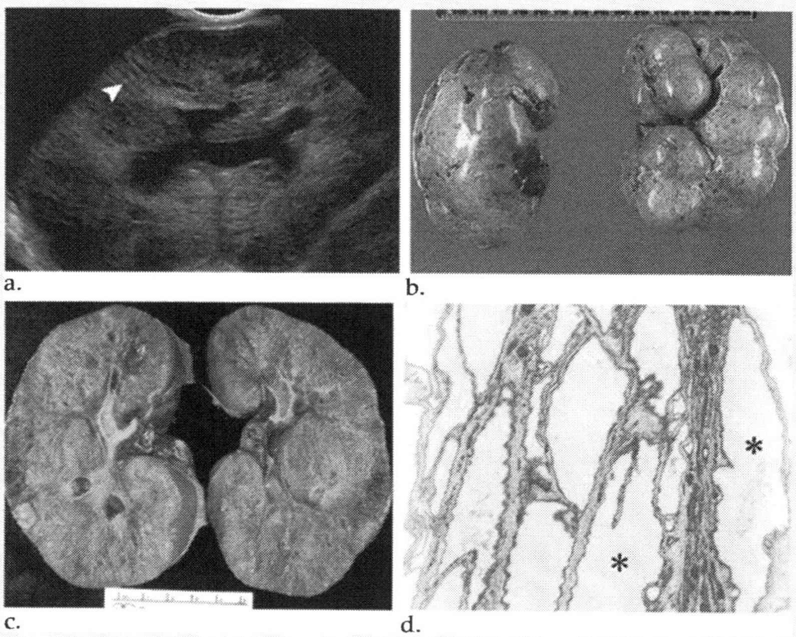

Figure 10.4. *ARPKD in a 2-month-old boy. (a) Longitudinal high-spatial-resolution (8-MHz) ultrasonographic (US) image of the right kidney shows diffuse tubular ectasia involving the medulla and extending to the cortical surface (arrowhead).*

Source: *Patil A, Sweeney WE Jr., Avner ED, et al. (2015). Childhood polycystic kidney disease. In: Li X, editor. Polycystic Kidney Disease [Internet]. Brisbane (AU): Codon Publications. Chapter 2. Available from: https://www.ncbi.nlm.nih.gov/books/NBK373381/ doi: 10.15586/codon.pkd.2015.ch2.*

Squeezing and atrophying the renal parenchyma, collecting duct ectasia, and interstitial changes appear to be the cause of the decreased number of glomeruli and other tubular segments. Although they have been found in the kidneys of fetuses, proximal tubular cysts are typically undetectable after birth. The renal pelvis, renal vessels, and calyces all seem normal.

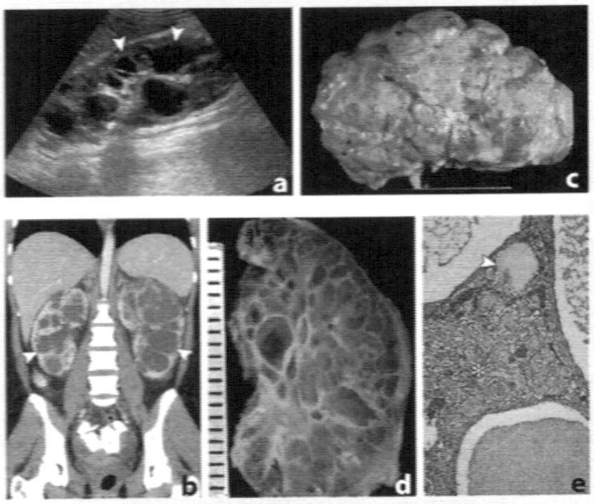

Figure 10.5. *Renal cysts in ADPKD.*

Note: (a) Longitudinal ultrasound (US) image of the right kidney in a 14-year-old girl reveals multiple round renal cysts (arrowheads). (b) Coronal computed tomography (CT) image in the same patient after administration of intravenous.

Source: *Patil A, Sweeney WE Jr., Avner ED, et al. (2015). Childhood Polycystic Kidney Disease. In: Li X, editor. Polycystic Kidney Disease [Internet]. Brisbane (AU): Codon Publications. Chapter 2. Available from: https://www.ncbi.nlm.nih.gov/books/NBK373381/ doi: 10.15586/codon.pkd.2015.ch2.*

The fusiform cystic tubules in ARPKD stay in contact with the urinary stream, in contrast to renal cysts in ADPKD, where the tubular cysts separate from the tubule of origin. There are two significant implications from this: 1) obstruction does not play a role in the formation of cysts in ARPKD patients, and 2) the urine is more likely to reflect changes that arise from cystic formation and growth because the afferent and efferent openings of an ARPKD collecting duct cyst remain continuous with the urinary stream. Urine changes in the cystic lesion are unlikely to correspond with changes in the tubular segment of origin in ADPKD, where cysts pinch off. Hyperplasia leads to larger renal cysts and interstitial fibrosis develops, producing a pattern more akin to ADPKD as the disease progresses and patient survival increases (see Figure 10.5).

The clinical manifestations of PH include splenomegaly, thrombocytopenia, low platelet counts, hypersplenism, enlarged hemorrhoids, and gastric and esophageal varices. PH is defined as an increase in blood pressure within the portal venous system. In the context of CHF (Caroli's syndrome), intrahepatic dilatation of the large and small peripheral bile ducts as well as the central bile ducts can occasionally progress to macrocysts and dilatation of the extrahepatic bile duct in ARPKD. ARPKD is the only condition that has both renal collecting duct and biliary ectasia along with periportal fibrosis.

10.4.4. Clinical

Amniotic fluid is necessary for lung development to expand the growing fetal lung, and sufficient physical room is needed for diaphragmatic movement. Pulmonary hypoplasia in ARPKD is caused by oligohydramnios and diaphragmatic movement restriction as a result of large cystic kidneys. In neonates with ARPKD, pulmonary insufficiency is the primary cause of morbidity and mortality. Despite neonatal interventions, infants with true pulmonary hypoplasia remain hypoxemic and seldom survive. Patients typically have palpably large flank masses at birth, which could make delivery more difficult. The majority of newborns with ARPKD (70–80%)

have some degree of impaired renal function; however, as respiratory problems resolve and renal development proceeds, there is frequently a brief improvement. If hyponatremia occurs, it usually goes away fast unless the patient is experiencing acute renal failure. The majority of patients have polyuria and polydipsia symptoms in addition to a urinary concentrating defect. While some newborns have noticeably larger kidneys, most eventually exhibit stable to reduced renal size.

Even though all ARPKD patients have microscopic evidence of CHF from birth, the implications of these findings are uncertain. Between infancy and adulthood, CHF complications can manifest at any point, or they can go unnoticed until later in life. For unknown reasons, the renal and hepatobiliary disease components of ARPKD progress at different rates. However, hepatobiliary disease can cause the development of PH, which can be quite serious, so the progressive biliary ductal ectasia and CHF need to be closely watched.

Chronic heart failure (CHF) commonly leads to pulmonary hypertension (PH), which is the predominant complication associated with CHF. Symptoms of PH can include enlargement of the liver and spleen, decreased platelet counts, bleeding from varicose veins and hemorrhoids, and most significantly, an elevated vulnerability to acquiring bacterial infections from cholangitis. Recent research on PH in autosomal recessive polycystic kidney disease (ARPKD) indicates that this condition may begin at an early age, characterized by liver enlargement that initially occurs in the left lobe.

As ARPKD survival rates rise, the clinical significance of severe hepatobiliary disease has taken on greater significance. According to recent research on the hepatobiliary aspect of ARPKD, 40% of patients who survive the condition will likely have severe renal and hepatobiliary disease. Depending on the severity of dual-organ disease, the remaining 60% of ARPKD survivors will either have mild/severe hepatobiliary disease, severe kidney/mild hepatobiliary disease, or mild kidney/mild hepatobiliary disease. Platelet count has been found to be a reliable indicator of PH severity in patients with ARPKD and has a strong positive correlation with spleen size. A common presenting feature in both infants and children, hypertension is frequently severe, challenging to treat, and necessitates multiple drug regimens. Patients with normal renal function frequently have hypertension, which eventually affects almost all children with ARPKD. The intrarenal renin-angiotensin system is believed to play a significant role in the multifactorial pathophysiology of hypertension in ARPKD.

10.4.5. Treatment and Complications

Neonatals with ARPKD are now more likely to survive thanks to developments in neonatal critical care. It is currently impossible to predict which neonates with ARPKD who need artificial ventilation right away will have pulmonary hypoplasia to the point of life-threatening severity. This is because there are three possible causes of severe pulmonary distress: true neonatal pulmonary hypoplasia, a potentially reversible fluid overload, or restricted diaphragm motion from greatly enlarged kidneys. In certain instances, peritoneal dialysis in conjunction with continuous venovenous hemofiltration or unilateral or bilateral nephrectomy to permit diaphragmatic movement can yield a more accurate assessment of the patient's long-term pulmonary prognosis.

Young people with ARPKD need to be closely watched, even if they don't have severe renal insufficiency. These patients have a significant risk of dehydration with coexisting illnesses due to their loss of concentration. In ARPKD, hyponatremia resulting from decreased urine dilution—as opposed to sodium wasting—is frequently observed. When it is, fluid consumption should be reduced without sacrificing nutritional value. Thiazide diuretics may be used to reduce distal nephron solute and water delivery in patients with severe polyuria. Patients who suffer from metabolic acidosis will need to take additional bicarbonate medication.

In patients with ARPKD, rates of urinary tract infections (UTIs) have been reported to reach 50%, with girls experiencing UTIs more frequently than boys. Clinical features and properly obtained urine cultures should guide antibody therapy for any child with an abnormal urinalysis. When a UTI is identified, it is advised to have an assessment to rule out bladder dysfunction, obstruction, and vesico-ureteral reflux. The consequences of progressive CKD, such as growth failure, anemia, renal osteodystrophy, and cognitive deficits, are a risk for infants and children with ARPKD, and this risk increases as renal function declines. The preferred treatment for patients with symptomatic end-stage kidney disease (ESKD) is peritoneal dialysis, which has been demonstrated to be effective even in the presence of intra-abdominal organomegalies, such as those involving the liver, spleen, and kidneys. A renal transplant should be properly thought out. In patients with large kidneys, a nephrectomy might be required to make room for the transplant and might be recommended to manage hypertension if transplantation is required. A combined liver and kidney transplant should be considered for patients with severe renal and severe biliary diseases. Telega et al. (2013) provide a decision tree that facilitates the making of suitable decisions.

Even in patients without renal insufficiency, feeding difficulties and stunted growth are frequently reported. In these situations, routine nutritional assessment can help determine the best course of treatment, and feeding specialists ought to be a member of the multidisciplinary care team. Normal growth curves can be attained with the right support measures, according to data from the NIH-sponsored Natural History Study of ARPKD. Hepatic complications are now the main clinical concern for many ARPKD patients due to advancements in renal replacement therapy and improvements in neonatal critical care, which have improved patient survival. 37–65% of neonatal survivors of ARPKD experience PH, an increase in portal venous pressure. Hepatocellular function usually stays normal even when PH develops.

Bleeding varices and bacterial cholangitis are the most dangerous side effects of PH. Patients suffering from ARPKD who have significant dilations in both the intrahepatic and extrahepatic bile ducts are more likely to experience ascending bacterial cholangitis. Fever or, in rare cases, an abrupt elevation in liver function tests at any point should raise the possibility of cholangitis, prompting an appropriate assessment and the start of antibiotic therapy.

All patients with ARPKD should be evaluated by a gastroenterologist at the time of initial diagnosis and should have routine evaluations for complications related to the liver and biliary system. Periodic imaging by magnetic resonance cholangiopancreatography (MRCP), magnetic resonance imaging (MRI), or ultrasound on an annual basis for elevated liver echogenicity, hepatobiliary abnormalities, and splenomegaly should be part of recommended evaluations. It is recommended to check platelet counts right away because they have been reported to be a surrogate marker of the severity of PH. To detect varices early and treat them with endoscopic bind ligation (EBL), which can stop potentially fatal bleeding, endoscopy is frequently necessary. Hemoglobin/hematocrit and platelet count, which serve as proxy markers for the degree of PH, are regularly checked for signs of hypersplenism, splenic sequestration, and gastrointestinal hemorrhage with varices. In situations where variceal sclerotherapy is either inappropriate or has not worked, porto-systemic shunting may be necessary; however, Telega et al. advise that this be carried out after consulting a transplant surgeon. Individuals who have moderate to severe renal disease along with severe PH should be considered for a dual kidney and liver transplant.

Despite the lack of evidence to support clinical practice, patients with ARPKD may be at risk for neurocognitive and behavioral dysfunction as a result of their early onset severe hypertension and chronic kidney disease. The psychosocial effects of ARPKD on the patient and family can be quite severe in addition to the serious medical issues, and this should be kept in mind. When a person experiences exhaustion from the demands of a new role, depleted finances, or other aspects of a changed lifestyle, social support measures may be necessary. To provide the best possible comprehensive care for patients with ARPKD, a multidisciplinary team comprising pediatric gastroenterologists, pediatric nephrologists, dietitians, social workers, and, if necessary, psychiatrists and other support staff may be required (Patil et al, 2015).

10.5. Autosomal Dominant Polycystic Kidney Disease (ADPKD)

More common than ARPKD, ADPKD affects 13 million people globally, with an incidence rate of 1:400–1:1,000. It accounts for 7–10% of adult cases of ESKD. Historically, ADPKD was referred to as "adult" polycystic kidney disease because of the typical late-life onset of clinical symptoms. An early-onset hypertensive disease, ADPKD is characterized by extrarenal manifestations such as cystic lesions in the pancreas, liver, and spleen as well as vascular abnormalities such as mitral valve prolapse and, less frequently, intracranial aneurysms (ICAs). Although ADPKD is commonly an adult disease, there are significant clinical manifestations of the disease in children and in some cases, even in utero. When pediatric patients do present as children, their renal findings are comparable to adult patients with the same condition. In contrast, pediatric patients seldom or never experience the extrarenal manifestations of ADPKD that are frequently seen in adults (such as ICAs and cysts in the pancreas and liver). The notion that pediatric ADPKD patients who present with early disease manifestations are most likely to benefit from early therapeutic interventions is becoming more widely accepted. Thus, when providing care for children who have ADPKD or are at risk of developing it, it is critical for clinicians to be aware of these manifestations.

In ADPKD, renal cysts develop in the womb, and newborns, kids, and teenagers may experience bilateral enlarged cystic kidneys, left ventricular hypertrophy with or without systemic hypertension, proteinuria, gross hematuria, nephrolithiasis, flank pain, and impaired renal function. Rarely occurring in children, ICAs represent the most clinically significant and potentially fatal extrarenal manifestation of ADPKD. The clinical course of ADPKD is influenced by factors other than the primary mutation, as evidenced by the significant degree of phenotypic variability in the rate of progression even among family members in patients with the disease. These consist of altering genes, diet, environment, and epigenetics.

10.5.1. Diagnosis

The clinical range of pediatric or early-onset ADPKD is particularly wide, and it can occasionally be challenging to differentiate ADPKD from ARPKD, particularly in infants.

On the other hand, unilateral or bilateral renal cysts in normal or slightly enlarged kidneys are the typical presentation of ADPKD in early childhood. Regretfully, with this presentation, it remains difficult to predict how ADPKD will progress in children. The illness may either progress to more severe clinical symptoms or continue to be asymptomatic well into adulthood.

10.5.2. Pathology

According to research, children with ADPKD typically have one or more renal cysts inside enlarged kidneys (see Figure 10.5a). Kidney cysts develop in all tubular segments and glomeruli in children with ADPKD (refer to Figures 10.5b, 10.5c, 10.5d, and 10.5e). The cyst formation is usually asymmetrical, though unilateral presentation is possible on occasion. Simple renal cysts are exceedingly uncommon in children, so the discovery of even one solitary renal cyst in an at-risk pediatric or adolescent patient should generally prompt additional evaluation. Glomerular cysts can arise as a distinct autosomal dominant disease entity or as a part of ADPKD. Enlarging cysts in ADPKD "pinch off," or separate from the tubule, and do not stay connected to the urinary stream, in contrast to ARPKD, where the cystic lesions are ectatic and stay in continuity with the nephron of origin.

10.5.3. Clinical Features

Pediatric or early-onset ADPKD has a very wide range of clinical manifestations, and there is currently insufficient data to reliably identify patients who will advance quickly. Rarely, it might manifest as the above-mentioned severe disease that is indistinguishable from ARPKD. Pediatric ADPKD most often manifests as renal cysts, either unilateral or bilateral, in near-normal or mildly enlarged kidneys. Children who present in this way may show symptoms as adults or they may not show any symptoms at all. In addition to micro- and gross hematuria, hypertension, proteinuria, and infrequently back, flank, or abdomen pain, childhood ADPKD also causes renal manifestations. Although there is rarely overt proteinuria in children with ADPKD, overt proteinuria is typically a sign of more severe structural kidney disease. However, there is little to no evidence linking microalbuminuria to kidney function or volume in ADPKD children.

Similar to ARPKD, ADPKD in children can manifest as hypertension as early as the newborn stage. Hypertension is a crucial screening tool for kids who are at risk because it frequently occurs before the biochemical and clinical signs of ADPKD. Larger kidneys and hypertension have been found to be strongly correlated in several cohorts of children with ADPKD. In offspring with ADPKD, hypertension is more likely to develop more frequently and at a younger age if the affected parent has the condition.

Blood pressure (BP) abnormalities in ADPKD patients have been made visible and greater precision in BP assessments has been made possible by the use of ambulatory blood pressure monitoring (ABPM). In children with ADPKD, only nocturnal hypertension is seen in about 33% of cases. An important fraction of young adults with ADPKD who are normotensive also have "prehypertension" according to ABPM. It has also been reported that endothelial dysfunction in this population is linked to blunted "nocturnal dipping" on ABPM.

Cardiovascular disease is a major feature of ADPKD, and children with ADPKD demonstrate a substantial correlation between left ventricular mass index (LVMI) and systolic blood pressure. Hypertensive and pre-hypertensive (blood pressure in the upper range of normal (75–95th percentile for age, sex, and height) children with ADPKD have a statistically significantly higher LVMI than normotensive ADPKD children.

Heart valvular abnormalities, such as mitral valve prolapse, are more common in adult ADPKD patients; these abnormalities have also been observed in pediatric ADPKD patients. Other presenting symptoms, in addition to hypertension, may include inguinal or abdominal hernias, gross or microscopic hematuria, abdominal pain, and palpable abdominal masses. In children who are at risk, the development of gross hematuria following mild trauma to the side or back should be taken more seriously. Although it is usually uncommon, renal insufficiency in children with ADPKD has been documented. Within a cohort of children with ADPKD, 58% of them had a renal concentrating defect. By using ABPM, it was demonstrated that the presence of hypertension was correlated with the discovery of a renal concentrating defect. These results imply that in children with ADPKD, reduced renal concentrating ability may serve as a crude indicator of the severity of the disease. An infant or child with ADPKD may present with renal infections. Children with ADPKD may also have pain from ruptured cysts or renal stones. Rarely do pediatric patients with ADPKD develop the extrarenal cysts that are observed in adult patients. If discovered in a child with ADPKD, they could, nevertheless, offer clinical criteria for a differential diagnosis. Previously believed to be an uncommon finding in children with ADPKD, liver cysts were discovered in 55% of adolescents and young adults with ADPKD, according to a MRI study. When they do occur, pediatric liver cysts are typically not linked to hepatomegaly, pain, or infection.

10.5.4. Treatment and Complications

The management of renal and extrarenal complications is the only available course of treatment for patients with ADPKD at this time. Children who are asymptomatic but at risk for ADPKD should be closely watched, particularly if hematuria, polyuria, proteinuria, hypertension, or palpable abdominal masses develop. Any of these conclusions ought to encourage more research. In ADPKD, identifying and treating childhood hypertension is essential to delaying the onset of ESKD. More stringent blood pressure control (<120/80) was found to have a higher effect on LVH reduction in adults with ADPKD than standard control (<140/90). Angiotensin receptor blocker (ARB) telmisartan combined with angiotensin-converting enzyme inhibitor (ACEi) lisinopril did not appear to be beneficial for the progression of ADPKD in adult patients with early or moderately advanced kidney disease, according to a recent report from the HALT/PKD study. In contrast, a second arm of the HALT/PKD study found that using an ACEi to lower blood pressure to a target level improved total kidney volume (TKV), decreased urinary albumin excretion, and reduced left ventricular hypertrophy (LVH) in younger patients with moderately preserved renal function. These findings might be especially relevant to children, especially in the early stages of the illness. Pravastatin was found to be effective in slowing the progression of structural kidney disease in older children and young adults with ADPKD in a phase III clinical trial that was randomized, double-blind, placebo-controlled and measured height-corrected total kidney volume (HtTKV) and LVMI by MRI.

Despite these factors, it is important to adhere to recognized international guidelines for the staged treatment of hypertension in pediatric patients. Although there is little information on the precise characteristics of UTIs or renal cyst infections in children with ADPKD, the clinical course and most likely the course of treatment would be comparable to those of ADPKD patients in adulthood. Pediatric ADPKD patients rarely experience flank pain, most likely because they have fewer cysts. But as the illness worsens, especially in teenagers, flank pain might need medical attention. The multifactorial pathophysiology and treatment of chronic pain in ADPKD are summed up in a recent review.

Roughly 10% of patients with ADPKD experience cerebral aneurysms and bleeding, and this characteristic appears to run in families. However, since this rarely happens before the age of 20, it is not advised to screen pediatric ADPKD patients on a routine basis until they turn 20. After turning 20, patients with symptoms or a positive family history may be referred for magnetic resonance angiography (MRA) screening.

10.5.5. Prognosis

A low prognosis was previously believed to be associated with early-onset ADPKD that manifests in pregnancy or in the newborn. Though the prognosis is not as bad as is commonly believed, new research on "very early onset" ADPKD indicates otherwise. Screening at-risk patients to identify those at risk for rapid progression has become increasingly important, given the findings that aggressive treatment of hypertension reduces LVH and the use of pravastatin slows the progression of structural kidney disease as well as reduces LVH. When new treatments are initiated early in the course of the disease, they are likely to have the greatest impact on reducing the number and/or size of renal cysts while remaining safe (Patil et al, 2015).

10.6. Pathophysiology of Cyst Formation in Childhood PKD

The pathophysiology of cyst formation in Parkinson's disease is becoming increasingly clear as we work to define its molecular drivers. However, the disease burden is ultimately caused by aberrant cell-signaling networks. Since this complicated aberrant cellular signaling defines the cystic cellular phenotype mentioned below, therapeutic interventions are therefore primarily focused on addressing it.

10.6.1. Molecular Pathogenesis

It is evident that neither the severity of extrarenal manifestations in childhood PKD nor the rate of progression of the renal disease can be predicted using standard Mendelian genetics. In childhood PKD, complex transcriptional events are undoubtedly important disease modifiers. The severity and progression of ADPKD and ARPKD are influenced by complex inheritance patterns, as evidenced by recent discoveries of hypomorphic or incompletely penetrant alleles, homozygosity involving either PKD1 or PKD2, compound heterozygosity, digenic inheritance or trans-heterozygosity, somatic and germline mosaicism, genetic modifiers, and epigenetic regulators co-inheritance of mutations in either PKD1 or PKD2 with other PKD-causing genes like HNF1B or the tuberous sclerosis 2 (TSC2) gene.

10.6.2. Cellular Pathophysiology of Cyst Formation in PKD

The process of cyst development and growth is intricate and involves multiple factors working together, rather than acting independently. The exact mechanisms that result in the PKD phenotype are still not fully understood, but various cellular defects have been identified. Molecular factors that are known to impact the extent or seriousness of cyst formation include the timing of PKD1 inactivation during development, the decrease in functional PC1 levels, variations in sensitivity to PC1 levels among cells and nephrons, and the potential snowball effect of one cyst affecting neighboring nephrons and leading to cyst development in adjacent tubules.

A PKD cystic epithelial cell is identified by its altered rates of proliferation and apoptosis, as well as its transition from a fully differentiated, nonproliferative, absorptive cell to a partially dedifferentiated secretory cell with particular polarization defects. Since mathematical modeling of renal cystic epithelia establishes proliferation and secretion as necessary and sufficient to account for cyst growth in PKD, these changes leading to a proliferating secretory cell are fundamental and critical.

10.6.3. Cyst Formation in PKD

The phenotypic abnormalities of ADPKD and ARPKD cells are similar, regardless of when they manifest clinically. The distinct phenotype of the cystic epithelial cell is caused by aberrant multiprotein complexes whose aberrant function results in aberrant signaling events caused by mutated PKD genes. Although the exact mechanisms by which these aberrant complexes interfere with normal signaling and result in the formation of renal cysts remain unclear, considerable progress has been made in comprehending the cellular processes that lead to cyst formation. Important pathogenic characteristics of the distinct cystic phenotype have been determined. These phenotypic abnormalities provide therapeutic targets for the development of PKD therapies and include:

- abnormalities of in expression of one or more members of the epidermal growth factor (EGF) family of receptors and/or ligands, the (EGFR –axis), leading to an autocrine-paracrine cycle of proliferation through activation of the Ras-Raf-MEK-ERK pathway
- increased cAMP in concert with decreased intracellular calcium levels leads to aberrant intracellular cAMP signaling resulting in the activation of the β-Raf /MEK-ERK pathway and stimulates both proliferation and tubular fluid secretion.
- abnormal activity of C-terminal Src kinase or cellular Src (c-Src). A critical molecule that mediates cross-talk between the EGFR axis and G-protein-cAMP pathways
- abnormal function of the primary cilia;
- changes in cell-cell, and cell-matrix interactions, and
- alternative activation of renal interstitial macrophages that contribute to the development of progressive fibrosis.

The aforementioned pathogenic processes—tubular epithelial proliferation, abnormal tubular secretion, changes in the extracellular matrix, structure, and/or function, and the recruitment of macrophages and inflammatory mediators—all most likely play a role in the development of renal cysts and their progressive enlargement. Both orthologous and non-orthologous models of ADPKD and ARPKD have provided important new insights into the cellular processes that result in renal cyst formation in PKD. A comprehensive listing of these models would not be possible due to the rapid advancements in molecular techniques that have made it possible to create genetically manipulated or conditionally targeted models of disease. The following provides an overview of the most important models created thus far for the interested reader (Patil et al, 2015).

10.6.4. The Cystic Phenotype and Targeted Future Therapy

A distinct "cystic phenotype" has been identified by studies intended to clarify the molecular and cellular biology of ADPKD and ARPKD. This phenotype offers several possible targets for pharmacological therapy, both now and in the future (see Figure 10.6).

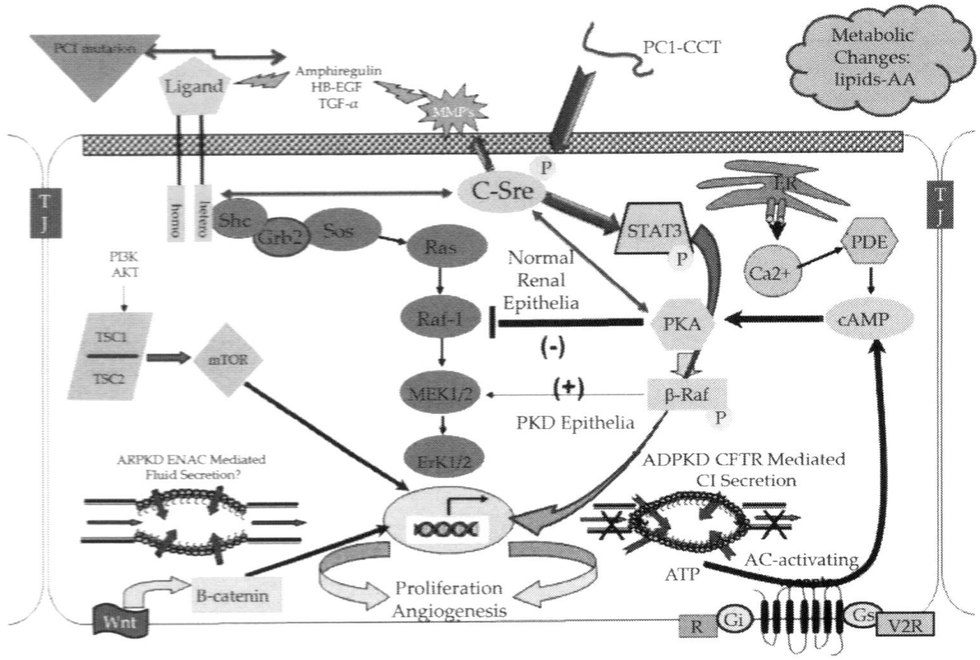

Figure 10.6. *An abridged composite of the abnormally active signal transduction pathways in PKD.*

Source: *Patil A, Sweeney WE Jr., Avner ED, et al. (2015). Childhood Polycystic Kidney Disease. In: Li X, editor. Polycystic Kidney Disease [Internet]. Brisbane (AU): Codon Publications. Chapter 2. Available from: https://www.ncbi.nlm.nih.gov/books/NBK373381/ doi: 10.15586/codon.pkd.2015.ch2.*

Based on our understanding of the pathophysiology of cyst formation in Parkinson's disease (PKD) and the abnormal integration of signaling pathways that have been found thus far, targeted therapeutic approaches can be categorized into three groups. These include treatments aimed at lowering levels of cAMP, reducing fluid secretion, and reducing cell proliferation. For any therapy to be effective, proliferation is a necessary process that needs to be targeted and controlled. The EGFR family of receptors and ligands and a G-protein-regulated axis that results in elevated cAMP and a phenotypic change in renal epithelia's response to cAMP are the two main signaling pathways that cause unchecked proliferation. A crucial intermediary that links the two pathways and contributes to their continued activity is c-Src. The following hypothetical chain of events could replace this detailed explanation: a mutation in PKD1 causes an increase in amphiregulin production, which in turn activates the EGFR axis. This leads to reciprocal phosphorylation (activation) of Src, which interacts with the cAMP pathways by changing the renal epithelia's response to cAMP levels from an anti-mitotic to a pro-proliferative response. Finally, in the presence of PC1's terminal tail, Src-dependent activation of STAT3 results in the proliferative signal persists. Potentially, the most effective treatments will probably focus on key signaling intermediates that integrate multiple pathways, like Src, and/or combination therapies, which use different compounds to target different pathways at the same time, or a single compound that targets different pathways, like multi-kinase inhibitors (MKI) like tesevatinib.

10.7. Treatment and Management of Autosomal Dominant Polycystic Kidney Disease

The most prevalent single-gene disease that poses a serious risk to life and is linked to a high rate of morbidity and death is autosomal dominant polycystic kidney disease or ADPKD. It is the fourth most common cause of end-stage kidney disease (ESKD) worldwide, affecting up to 15 million people. A multi-systemic, progressive illness, ADPKD is typified by kidney and other organ enlargement and cyst formation. Progressive increases in renal volume and decreases in glomerular filtration rate (GFR) were features of ADPKD's natural history. By the time they are 60 years old, up to 50% of ADPKD patients need renal replacement therapy. In contrast to the treatment of other kidney diseases, this disease's management and treatment have not advanced significantly over a long period of time.

10.7.1. Management of Kidney Disease Progression in ADPKD

ADPKD progression varies greatly between families and between members of the same family, and the population as a whole has a significantly different relative risk of renal decline. Because ADPKD is such a highly variable illness, it can be difficult to predict how a particular patient will progress. When long-term cohort data sets and trustworthy biomarkers are unavailable, disease modeling can help define the broader clinical assessment of patients who are at-risk and support useful decision-making. The most accurate indicator of CKD progression is total renal volume.

Vasopressin and related cAMP-related signaling pathways have been shown to play a significant role in the growth of cysts in ADPKD, which justifies the study of the effects of vasopressin (V2) receptor antagonism on the development and growth of cysts. ADPKD patients showed a slower rate of decline in kidney function and a decreased rate of growth in total renal volume in a 5-year prospective study comparing Tolvaptan to placebo. Many factors must be taken into account to ensure the safe and effective use of Tolvaptan, including the cautious selection of treatment-eligible patients based on progression risk. The patient will require assistance during the start of treatment and ongoing care. Tolvaptan has been approved by the European Medicines Agency and Japan for the treatment of adult-onset stage 1 to 3 chronic kidney disease (ADPKD) in adults who also exhibit rapidly progressing disease. To better assess the effectiveness and safety of this medication, the FDA in the USA has asked for more information. To determine which scores to use for ADPKD patients who exhibit signs of a rapidly progressing disease, a consensus must be reached. Furthermore, the results of randomized studies conducted in later stages of ADPKD are not promising, indicating that Tolvaptan use is not advised in the absence of additional data from sizable clinical trials (Patil et al, 2015).

10.7.2. Hypertension Management in ADPKD

A common and dangerous side effect of ADPKD is hypertension, which affects 50–70% of patients early in the disease before renal dysfunction manifests. In ADPKD, the median age at hypertension diagnosis is 32 years for men and 34 years for women. This is an earlier age than in the general population. Moreover, 30% of kids with ADPKD experience hypertension. It is critical to treat hypertension early and effectively to reduce ADPKD patients' morbidity and mortality. The etiology of hypertension in ADPKD is intricate and contingent upon numerous interrelated factors. The development of hypertension in ADPKD has been linked to many factors, including activation of the renin-angiotensin-aldosterone system (RAAS), vascular dysfunction associated with ciliopathy, activation of efferent sympathetic nerves, renal handling of sodium, and others. In patients with ADPKD, activation of the RAAS appears to play a major role in the pathophysiology of hypertension.

A blood pressure of less than 130/80 mm Hg is the target for patients with renal disease. We must use this blood pressure target when treating patients with ADPKD. Since better blood pressure control can slow the progression of kidney disease, hypertension is the most significant modifiable risk factor in ADPKD. The best course of treatment for ADPKD patients with hypertension is to combine ACE inhibitors or angiotensin II receptor blockers (ARBs) with RAAS inhibitors, according to pathogenic data. Even though research on the RAAS hasn't been able to provide solid evidence that it contributes significantly to the pathophysiology of ADPKD, these medications are still the most often prescribed ones for treating hypertension in ADPKD patients. Studies that have looked at how controlling hypertension affects the development of kidney disease and the incidence of cardiovascular events are currently insufficient in number. The rate of total kidney volume growth was not considerably slowed down in the early stages of ADPKD by the dual inhibition of RAAS caused by the combination of ACE inhibitor and ARB. Severe blood pressure control was linked to a higher decline in the left ventricular mass index, a greater reduction in urinary albumin excretion, and a slower rate of total kidney volume growth than standard blood pressure control. On kidney function, however, no effect was noted. Monotherapy blockade of RAAS with an ACE inhibitor was linked to blood pressure control in ADPKD patients with stage 3 chronic kidney disease later on in the disease. The progression of kidney function remained unchanged with the addition of an ARB.

The prognosis for ADPKD patients in the US, Denmark, and the UK is improving, according to recently released data. Early diagnosis, improved blood pressure management, increased use of RAAS inhibitors, improved renal function preservation, delayed onset of ESKD, and improved survival have all occurred. For this reason, it's critical for patients with ADPKD to have early control of their hypertension to delay the course of their kidney disease and avoid cardiovascular events. More research is necessary on this topic because there is no doubt that factors other than better blood pressure management and renal function preservation contribute to the improved survival.

10.7.3. Extrarenal Complications Management

Adult patients are primarily the only ones who experience co-morbidity from extrarenal manifestations. Rarely seen in children, hepatic cysts develop later than renal cysts. After 60 years of age, their prevalence rises to 80%. The majority of patients continue to have liver function and are asymptomatic. Women typically have larger and more frequent cysts due to their higher estrogen usage and higher rates of multiple pregnancies. Cyst decompression may be necessary in cases of severe and ongoing pain. Hepatic cyst infection is uncommon and is treated with antibiotics and occasionally drainage. With continued use, medical management with somatostatin analogs has resulted in a significant reduction in liver volume. It is rare to find epithelial cysts in other organs. These comprise the thyroid, endometrium, seminal vesicle, pancreas, ovaries, spleen, and epididymis. Many vascular abnormalities are also more common in patients with ADPKD, in addition to the kidney and other organs developing cysts over time. Compared to 1.2% of the general population, intracranial aneurysms have been detected in 8% of patients and seem to be grouped in families. The most dangerous side effect of ADPKD is aneurysm rupture, which can cause 7–13% of fatalities. An expert center's multidisciplinary team should be consulted regarding the management of unruptured aneurysms. There have also been reports of cardiac valve abnormalities and aortic aneurysms. It's unclear if the hypertension and renal failure in these patients cause the vascular complications, or if the genetic defect causes them directly. Extrarenal manifestations in young children are extremely uncommon.

Urinary tract infections are thought to be risk factors in the progression of renal disease because they can result in sepsis, renal abscesses, and cyst infections. Treatment for these infections might be challenging. It's essential to receive adequate treatment with antibiotics that can pass through cyst walls. Both microscopic and macroscopic hematuria are typically self-limiting and can be caused by a ruptured cyst. Rarely, it may be advised to reduce physical activity when there is prolonged bleeding. Analgesics can be used to treat ADPKD pain, which is occasionally linked to perinephric hemorrhage. One needs to rule out renal infection, stones, or tumors when the pain lasts longer than a few days. Additionally, pain may be linked to cyst enlargement. Percutaneous aspiration or surgical cyst reduction may provide some relief in these cases. Cyst decortications may be carried out in conjunction with renal denervation, which has been utilized with success. About 50% of patients with ADPKD progress to ESKD by the time they are 60 years old. Those with the PKD1 genotype seem to progress more quickly than those with the PKD2 genotype. The two most significant modifiable risk factors for the onset of renal failure are hypertension and kidney infections, both of which need to be appropriately managed. Although it hasn't been proven, it may be hypothesized that treating normotensive patients with ACE inhibitors at an early age can slow the progression to ESKD. Reduction in dietary protein intake has shown disappointing results in slowing the progression of renal disease.

A younger age at diagnosis, larger kidneys, episodes of hematuria, proteinuria, and multiple pregnancies have all been linked to an earlier onset of chronic kidney disease. Comprehending the factors that contribute to the swift advancement of this illness has grown in significance due to the possibility of novel therapeutic approaches. In the modern era, several risk factors influencing the progression of kidney disease in ADPKD have been discovered. Urinary molecular markers, glomerular hyperfiltration, renal blood flow, uric acid, and total kidney volume have all been linked to early emergent markers of the progression of ADPKD renal disease. Dialysis and renal transplantation are equally possible for ADPKD patients with EKRD as they are for patients with the majority of other renal disorders. Individuals who have a positive family history of cerebral aneurysm development should also be screened with cerebral computed tomography and/or magnetic resonance imaging. Children in ADPKD families who are at-risk but do not exhibit symptoms are typically monitored annually for the emergence of hypertension, hematuria, and UTIs. Prompt and sufficient treatment is required for hypertension and urinary tract infections, as these conditions may accelerate the development of renal lesions.

10.7.4. Lifestyle Modifications, Consultations and Long-Term Monitoring in ADPKD

ADPKD patients ought to stay away from violent sports. Counselling regarding the possibility of exogenous estrogen or progesterone exposure exacerbating polycystic liver disease should be provided to all female ADPKD patients who are capable of becoming pregnant. Patients with non-hypertensive ADPKD and normal kidney function should have annual renal ultrasounds as well as blood and urine tests. Depending on the degree of hypertension and stage of chronic kidney disease, ADPKD patients with high blood pressure, cardiovascular problems, or both need more frequent monitoring. The most prevalent genetic renal disease in adults is ADPKD. Every patient with ADPKD should have a unique treatment and management plan. The most recent methods and state of knowledge regarding the assessment, handling, and therapy of ADPKD (Table 10.3). New guidelines for ADPKD have been released to aid in bettering the diagnosis, management, and course of therapy (Patil et al., 2015).

Table 10.3. Management of ADPKD Patients

Manifestation	Recommendation
Assess for the Presence of Risk Factors for Rapidly Progressing Disease	• PKD-1 gene mutation; • Male gender; • Young age at diagnosis; • Presence of hypertension, • Hematuria • Proteinuria; • Young age at onset of hypertension • Increased total kidney volume
Reduce Hypertension Risk	• Lifestyle changes -- Smoking cessation -- Dietary salt restriction -- Moderate alcohol consumption -- Maintain BMI between 18.5 and 24.9 kg/m2 through diet and exercise -- Avoid caffeinated drinks • BP: assess and maintain BP <130 / 80 mmHg with RAAS inhibitors

Slow Kidney Disease Progression	• Lifestyle changes, • Tolvaptan approved for ADPKD adults patients with CKD stage 1 to 3 and evidence of rapidly progressing disease
Assess and Manage Other Renal Complications • Chronic kidney disease • Renal pain • Kidney stones • Hematuria • Urinary tract and cyst infection • Large symptomatic cyst	• Monitor eGFR and refer to nephrologist • Symptom review • Maintain adequate fluid intake (3 liters per day) for primary prevention • Reduced physical activity • Antibiotics, fluoroquinolones • Consider avoiding oral contraceptive pill and hormone replacement therapy in women with severe polycystic liver disease • Aspiration and sclerotherapy, • Cyst fenestration, resection
Assess and Manage Other Systemic Complications • Intracranial aneurysms	• Consider screening for intracranial cerebral aneurysm in ADPKD patients with high risk • Clipping or endovascular procedure

Source: Patil A, Sweeney WE Jr., Avner ED, et al. Childhood Polycystic Kidney Disease. In: Li X, editor. Polycystic Kidney Disease [Internet]. Brisbane (AU): Codon Publications; 2015 Nov. Chapter 2. Available from: https://www.ncbi.nlm.nih.gov/books/NBK373381/ doi: 10.15586/codon.pkd.2015.ch2.

A Closer Look

End-Stage Renal Disease (ESRD)

End-stage renal disease (ESRD) represents the final stage of chronic kidney disease (CKD) where the kidneys are no longer able to function adequately to meet the body's needs. This stage is characterized by a glomerular filtration rate (GFR) of less than 15 mL/min/1.73 m^2, signifying that kidney function is at a critical low. The primary causes of ESRD include diabetes and hypertension, which are responsible for about two-thirds of all cases. Other contributing factors can be glomerulonephritis, polycystic kidney disease, and prolonged obstruction of the urinary tract. Symptoms of ESRD are severe and varied, encompassing fatigue, swelling (edema), shortness of breath, and changes in urination patterns, among others. As kidney function deteriorates, the accumulation of waste products and excess fluids can lead to life-threatening complications such as heart disease, bone disease, anemia, and nerve damage.

The management of ESRD typically involves renal replacement therapies, either through dialysis or kidney transplantation. Dialysis, which can be either hemodialysis or peritoneal dialysis, performs the crucial functions of waste removal and fluid balance maintenance that failing kidneys can no longer accomplish. Hemodialysis involves the use of a machine and a dialyzer to filter the blood, whereas peritoneal dialysis utilizes the lining of the abdomen as a natural filter. While dialysis can significantly prolong life and improve symptoms, it does not cure kidney failure and often involves a significant lifestyle adjustment, including strict dietary and fluid restrictions, regular sessions, and potential complications such as infections or cardiovascular issues.

Kidney transplantation, on the other hand, offers a more definitive solution by replacing the failed kidneys with a healthy one from a donor, which can restore more natural kidney function and improve the quality of life. However, this option is limited by the availability of suitable donor organs and the need for lifelong immunosuppressive medications to prevent rejection. Transplant patients must also adhere to regular medical follow-ups to monitor for complications.

Preventive measures and early detection are critical in managing CKD and preventing its progression to ESRD. This includes controlling blood pressure and blood sugar levels, following a healthy diet, avoiding smoking, and regular check-ups, especially for those with risk factors like diabetes, hypertension, or a family history of kidney disease. Public health initiatives aimed at raising awareness about CKD and its risk factors, along with better access to medical care and early interventions, are essential strategies in reducing the burden of ESRD.

Living with ESRD poses substantial physical, emotional, and financial challenges. Patients often experience a significant impact on their daily lives, requiring adjustments to work, family responsibilities, and social activities. The high cost of treatment, particularly for those undergoing dialysis or seeking transplantation, adds another layer of difficulty, often necessitating support from government programs or private insurance. The mental health implications, including depression and anxiety, are also notable, necessitating comprehensive care that includes psychological support and counseling. Overall, ESRD is a complex, multifaceted condition that necessitates a holistic approach to care. Advancements in medical treatment, improved access to healthcare, and robust support systems are crucial for enhancing the quality of life for those affected by this severe stage of kidney disease. Continued research into better treatment options and preventive strategies holds the promise of more effective management and eventual reduction in the incidence of ESRD.

Summary

- Polycystic kidney disease (PKD) is a genetic disorder characterized by the growth of numerous cysts in the kidneys. The kidneys are two organs, each about the size of a fist, located in the upper part of a person's abdomen, toward the back.
- Polycystic kidney disease (PKD or PCKD, also known as polycystic kidney syndrome) is a genetic disorder in which the renal tubules become structurally abnormal, resulting in the development and growth of multiple cysts within the kidney.
- Mutations associated with impaired ciliary apparatus function and ciliopathies such as those found in OFD1 and NPHP1 can present with corticomedullary cysts in the kidneys that might mimic ADPKD but with distinct extrarenal manifestations and ESKD onset at a younger age.
- Autosomal dominant polycystic kidney disease (ADPKD) appears to cause increased cell growth that leads to cysts on the kidneys. The basic unit of the kidney is the nephron, with each kidney containing approximately 1 million nephrons.
- Autosomal dominant polycystic kidney disease (ADPKD) often leads to progressive kidney failure due primarily to continued enlargement of the cysts and replacement of normal kidney tissue.
- Kidney failure severe enough to require dialysis or kidney transplantation is called end-stage kidney disease. ADPKD rarely leads to end-stage kidney disease in early childhood; it most commonly occurs in middle age or later in life.
- A hernia is an area of weakness in a muscle. The area may protrude if the organs behind the muscle press against the area of weakness, especially as a person increases the pressure in their abdomen (such as during a cough or while carrying a heavy package).
- Parapelvic cysts are a subset of simple cysts that arise within the renal parenchyma adjacent to the renal sinus and account for 5% of all renal cysts in adults. Clinically they may manifest through obstruction of the ureter or renal pelvis.
- Tuberous sclerosis complex is an autosomal dominant disease, with incidence 1:5000 to 10 000 and is caused by mutations of the TSC1 or TSC2 gene. Family history of the disease is absent in two-thirds of families.
- ARPKD (OMIM 263200) is a rare, hepatorenal fibrocystic disease, characterized by non-obstructive, fusiform, cystic distension of renal collecting ducts with unpredictable degrees of congenital hepatic fibrosis (CHF), as a result of biliary ductal plate malformation.
- Lung development requires amniotic fluid to distend the developing fetal lung and adequate physical space for diaphragmatic movement is required. In ARPKD, oligohydramnios and restriction of diaphragmatic movement due to large cystic kidneys results in pulmonary hypoplasia.
- The clinical spectrum of pediatric or early-onset ADPKD is particularly broad and there is still little evidence to allow accurate prediction of those patients that will rapidly progress. It may present infrequently as severe disease as noted above may be indistinguishable from ARPKD.

- Cardiovascular disease is a major feature of ADPKD, and children with ADPKD demonstrate a substantial correlation between left ventricular mass index (LVMI) and systolic blood pressure.
- ADPKD and ARPKD cells share phenotypic abnormalities regardless of when they become clinically evident. Mutated PKD genes result in abnormal multiprotein complexes whose abnormal function leads to aberrant signaling events resulting in the unique phenotype of the cystic epithelial cell.
- Autosomal dominant polycystic kidney disease (ADPKD) is the most common life-threatening single-gene disease associated with significant morbidity and mortality. It affects up to 15 million people and represents the 4th most common cause of end-stage kidney disease worldwide (ESKD).
- ADPKD progression is highly variable among families and among individuals within families, with a relative risk of renal decline varying significantly across the population. ADPKD is a significantly heterogeneous disease, predicting progression for a given individual a challenging process.
- Hypertension is a common and serious complication of ADPKD, often occurring in 50% – 70% of ADPKD patients early in the disease, before the appearance of renal dysfunction.

References

1. Ali, H., Hussain, N., Naim, M., Zayed, M., Al-Mulla, F., Kehinde, E. O., Seaburg, L. M., Sundsbak, J. L., & Harris, P. C. (2015). A novel PKD1 variant demonstrates a disease-modifying role in trans with a truncating PKD1 mutation in patients with autosomal dominant polycystic disease. *BMC Nephrology, 16*, 26.
2. Alves, M., Fonseca, T., & de Almeida, E. A. F. (2015). Differential diagnosis of autosomal dominant polycystic kidney disease. In X. Li (Ed.), *Polycystic Kidney Disease* [Internet]. Codon Publications. Available from: https://www.ncbi.nlm.nih.gov/books/NBK373390/ (accessed on 31 July 2024).
3. Ariza, M., Alvarez, V., Marín, R., Aguado, S., López-Larrea, C., Alvarez, J., Menéndez, M. J., & Coto, E. (1997). A family with a milder form of adult dominant polycystic kidney disease not linked to the PKD1 (16p) or PKD2 (4q) genes. *Journal of Medical Genetics, 34*(7), 587–589.
4. Bennett, W. M. (2009). Autosomal dominant polycystic kidney disease: 2009 update for internists. *Korean Journal of Internal Medicine, 24*(3), 165–168.
5. Binu, P. A., et al. (2014). Evidence of a third ADPKD locus is not supported by re-analysis of designated PKD3 families. *Kidney International, 85*, 383–392.
6. Boddu, R., Yang, C., O'Connor, A. K., Hendrickson, R. C., Boone, B., Cui, X., et al. (2014). Intragenic motifs regulate the transcriptional complexity of Pkhd1/PKHD1. *Journal of Molecular Medicine (Berlin, Germany), 92*(10), 1045–1056.
7. Bogdanova, N., Dworniczak, B., Dragova, D., Todorov, V., Dimitrakov, D., Kalinov, K., Hallmayer, J., Horst, J., & Kalaydjieva, L. (1995). Genetic heterogeneity of polycystic kidney disease in Bulgaria. *Human Genetics, 95*, 645–650.

8. Braun, W. E. (2014). Advances in autosomal dominant polycystic kidney disease–2014 and beyond. *Cleveland Clinic Journal of Medicine, 81*(9), 545–556.
9. Chapman, A. B. (2007). Autosomal dominant polycystic kidney disease: Time for a change? *Journal of the American Society of Nephrology, 18*, 1399–1407.
10. Chapman, A. B. (2015). Autosomal-dominant polycystic kidney disease: Executive summary from a kidney disease improving global outcomes (KDIGO) controversies conference. *Kidney International.*
11. Cnossen, W. R., et al. (2015). LRP5 variants may contribute to ADPKD. *European Journal of Human Genetics, 24*, 237–242.
12. Daoust, M. C., Reynolds, D. M., Bichet, D. G., & Somlo, S. (1995). Evidence for a third genetic locus for autosomal dominant polycystic kidney disease. *Genomics, 25*, 733–736.
13. De Almeida, E., Lopes, J. A., Prata, M. M., & da Costa, A. G. (2009). Progression of autosomal dominant polycystic kidney disease: A follow-up study of a large cohort in a single center. In E. Kruger & K. Hahn (Eds.), *Nephrology, Dialysis Transplantation* (pp. 109–123). Nova Science Publishers.
14. De Almeida, E., Martins Prata, M., de Almeida, S., & Lavinha, J. (1999). Long-term follow-up of a family with autosomal dominant polycystic kidney disease type 3. *Nephrology Dialysis Transplantation, 14*(3), 631.
15. Igarashi, P., & Somlo, S. (2007). Polycystic kidney disease. *Journal of the American Society of Nephrology, 18*, 1371–1373.
16. McConnell, R. S., Rubinsztein, D. C., Fannin, T. F., McKinstry, C. S., Kelly, B., Bailey, I. C., & Hughes, A. E. (2001). Autosomal dominant polycystic kidney disease unlinked to the PKD1 and PKD2 loci presenting as familial cerebral aneurysm. *Journal of Medical Genetics, 38*, 238–239.
17. McGovern, A. P., Jones, S., van Vlymen, J., Saggar, A. K., Sandford, R., & Lusignan, S. (2014). Identification of people with autosomal dominant polycystic kidney disease using routine data: A cross-sectional study. *BMC Nephrology, 15*, 182.
18. Patil, A., Sweeney, W. E., Jr., Avner, E. D., et al. (2015). Childhood polycystic kidney disease. In X. Li (Ed.), *Polycystic Kidney Disease* [Internet]. Codon Publications. Available from: https://www.ncbi.nlm.nih.gov/books/NBK373381/ (accessed on 31 July 2024).
19. Paul, B. M., & Vanden Heuvel, G. B. (2014). Kidney: Polycystic kidney disease. *Wiley Interdisciplinary Reviews: Developmental Biology, 3*(6), 465–487.
20. Pei, Y., & Watnick, T. (2010). Diagnosis and screening of autosomal dominant polycystic kidney disease. *Advances in Chronic Kidney Disease, 17*(2), 140–152.
21. Pei, Y., et al. (2009). Unified criteria for ultrasonographic diagnosis of ADPKD. *Journal of the American Society of Nephrology, 20*(1), 205–212.
22. Rossetti, S., Consugar, M. B., & Chapman, A. B. (2007). Comprehensive molecular diagnostics in autosomal dominant polycystic kidney disease. *Journal of the American Society of Nephrology, 18*(7), 2143–2160.
23. Saigusa, T., & Bell, P. D. (2015). Molecular pathways and therapies in autosomal-dominant polycystic kidney disease. *Physiology (Bethesda), 30*(3), 195–207.

24. Telega, G., Cronin, D., & Avner, E. D. (2013). New approaches to the autosomal recessive polycystic kidney disease patient with dual kidney-liver complications. *Pediatric Transplantation, 17*, 328–335.

25. Temmerman, F., Missiaen, L., Bammens, B., Laleman, W., Cassiman, D., Verslype, C., van Pelt, J., & Nevens, F. (2011). Systematic review: The pathophysiology and management of polycystic liver disease. *Alimentary Pharmacology & Therapeutics, 34*(7), 702–713.

26. Turco, A. E., Clementi, M., Rossetti, S., Tenconi, R., & Pignatti, P. F. (1996). An Italian family with autosomal dominant polycystic kidney disease unlinked to either the PKD1 or PKD2 gene. *American Journal of Kidney Diseases, 28*, 759–761.

27. Van Gulick, J., Gevers, T., Van Keimpema, L., & Drenth, J. (2011). Hepatic and renal manifestations in autosomal dominant polycystic kidney disease: A dichotomy of two ends of a spectrum. *Netherlands Journal of Medicine, 69*(9), 367–371.

28. Wołyniec, W., Jankowska, M. M., Król, E., Czarniak, P., & Rutkowski, B. (2008). Current diagnostic evaluation of autosomal dominant polycystic kidney disease. *Polski Archiwum Medycyny Wewnętrznej, 118*(12), 767–773.

29. Zerres, K., Rudnik-Schöneborn, S., Deget, F., Holtkamp, U., Brodehl, J., & Geisert, J., et al. (1996). Autosomal recessive polycystic kidney disease in 115 children: Clinical presentation, course, and influence of gender. *Acta Paediatrica, 85*(4), 437–445.

INDEX

B

C

D

E

J

K

L

M

N

O

P

R

S

T

Kolibri 360 GmbH
Ferdinand-Jühlke-Straße 7
99095 Erfurt, Deutschland
produktsicherheit@kolibri360.de